RISK, CULTURE, AND HEALTH INEQUALITY

Shifting Perceptions of Danger and Blame

Edited by
Barbara Herr Harthorn
and
Laury Oaks

Foreword by
Dorothy Nelkin

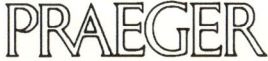

Westport, Connecticut
London

Library of Congress Cataloging-in-Publication Data

Risk, culture, and health inequality : shifting perceptions of danger and blame / edited by
Barbara Herr Harthorn and Laury Oaks; foreword by Dorothy Nelkin
    p. cm.
  Includes bibliographical references and index.
  ISBN 0–275–97869–9 (alk. paper)
  1. Health risk assessment. 2. Equality—Health aspects. 3. Public health—Social
aspects. 4. Applied anthropology. I. Harthorn, Barbara Herr, 1951– II. Oaks, Laury,
1967–
RA427 .R52 2003
362.1′042—dc21   2002029878

British Library Cataloguing in Publication Data is available.

Library of Congress Catalog Card Number: 2002029878
ISBN: 0–275–97869–9

First published in 2003

Praeger Publishers, 88 Post Road West, Westport, CT 06881
An imprint of Greenwood Publishing Group, Inc.
www.praeger.com

Printed in the United States of America

The paper used in this book complies with the
Permanent Paper Standard issued by the National
Information Standards Organization (Z39.48–1984).

10 9 8 7 6 5 4 3 2 1

Copyright Acknowledgment

The editors and publisher gratefully acknowledge permission to reprint "Risk, Remediation, and the Stigma of a Technological Accident in an African American Community" by Theresa A. Satterfield from *Human Ecology Review* vol. 7 (1):1–11, Summer
2000. Copyright 2000 by the Society for Human Ecology.

Contents

Foreword: The Social Meanings of Risk

Dorothy Nelkin

During the summer of 2000, a group of actors in New York City performed a street theater play called "Biotech" in public parks throughout the city. The play was about the risks of a new crop called "dicktater"—a genetically modified crossbreed of penis and potato. The tuber had infiltrated a community garden, causing an epic battle. The issues were less about health risks than about an array of social and political issues: lack of consumer choice, abuse of corporate power, mistrust of science, appropriate use of public space, and police brutality when corporate interests fought off local activists.

Risk disputes are ubiquitous—controversies occur over the risk of genetically modified food and other products of biotechnology, the spread of infectious agents, workplace and environmental hazards, the siting of large technological facilities, global warming and ozone depletion, and the risks imposed by diagnostic and reproductive technologies (Nelkin 1992). "Risk" has become one of the defining cultural characteristics of Western society (Beck 1992; Robertson 2001). And some would argue that we have become a risk-averse society.

For years, risk assessments were based on technical assumptions. Risks were technically manageable: identification and measurement of risk were sufficient as a basis for effective public decisions. Social psychologists then examined the character of different risks to find what was influencing public perceptions. They concluded that risks that were involuntary, uncertain, unfamiliar, and potentially catastrophic were most difficult for people to accept (Fischhoff, Lichtenstein, and Slovic 1991). Most recently, attention has focused on inherent risks—often called predispositions. The anticipation of illness, of future risks, has become a preoccupation of our time (Lock 2001). This anticipatory notion of risk, writes Robert Castel (1991), calls for systematic pre-detection of future risks in asymptomatic people—the interpretations of the expert become more important than the perceptions of the person. It has also depoliticized risk, diverting attention toward individual predisposition and away from the social and institutional factors that contribute to risk (Tesh 1988).

At the same time, there is growing awareness that risk is a social and cultural concept and that risk perceptions depend less on the nature of a hazard than on political, social, and cultural contexts. Narratives of risk are pervaded by concepts of accountability, responsibility, liability, and blame. Community groups, as in the Biotech skit, are calling attention to abuses of corporate power and inequities in the distribution of costs and benefits. And they demand greater choice and participation in decisions. Risks, writes anthropologist Mary Douglas, are embedded in a complex system of beliefs, values, and ideals (Douglas 1992). This is the approach that guides the chapters in this book.

Following similar assumptions, I suggest that risk disputes express the points of tension and the value conflicts in a society; that, in many ways, risk is a surrogate issue, a proxy for many other concerns. Although risk disputes often dwell on scientific questions—after all, public policy has privileged scientific expertise—risk perceptions are shaped by social issues that are troubling to the participants in disputes. The way people interpret risks and benefits may be influenced less by the details of scientific evidence than by social, political, and ethical concerns and especially by questions of participation and control. In this context, the globalization of science and technology and their attendant risks has further complicated risk disputes and amplified the critical question of "who controls."

In this introductory essay, I briefly lay out some features of risk disputes, suggesting ways in which risk perceptions are changing in the contemporary social context. This context has several features: growing corporate control of the scientific and regulatory environment, concerns about declining consumer choice and public participation in highly technical decisions, and the globalization of science, with the uncertainty and unpredictability associated with its application. These features are expressed in the language of risk and in the debates over the role of technical evidence in the resolution of disputes.

SOCIAL CONTEXTS

People perceive risks through different "frames" that reflect their values, world views, and concepts of social order. These frames can influence definitions of risk, allocations of responsibility and blame, evaluations of scientific evidence, and ideas about appropriate decision-making authority. Is risk to be defined as a technical matter to be resolved by measuring the extent of harm? A bureaucratic issue of appropriate regulatory mechanisms and jurisdictions? An economic question of allocating costs and benefits? A political issue involving consumer choice and control? A moral issue involving questions of social responsibility, religious values, equity, and rights?

Definitions of risk are frequently tied to contested social and political issues. Fears about the spread of infectious disease are exploited by those opposed to immigration. The risk from new medical procedures is tied to resentment toward the growing power of corporate management of medical care. Worries about the safety of genetically modified foods and crops are linked to concerns about the dominance of large pharmaceutical companies and also to opinions about Third World politics and the problems of exploitation. Cancer fears reflect a broader fear of industry out of control. Risks may be perceived differently in different cultures. The risk of genetically modified food has been more of a concern in France and England than in the United States, reflecting recent experience with food-borne disease, the politics of regulation, and the power of affected interest groups.

The narratives of the companies advocating particular technologies focus on technically manageable risks, emphasizing the benefits of technology, and communicating scientific evidence indicating minimal risk (Silverman 2001). But a shared feature of most risk disputes is mistrust of corporate policies and promises. This is most apparent in the case of environmental and workplace risks, but the disputes over genetically modified food also reflect public mistrust. Is economic concentration in the production of food for the world appropriate? Is corporate accountability really possible? Will not the desire for corporate profit trump the demand for consumer safety?

Following the discovery that StarLink, a genetically engineered corn, was polluting the Mexican corn supply, this product has come to represent the difficulty of containing genetically modified crops and, symbolically, of controlling the policies and practices of transnational corporations. Incidents and accidents in many disputed areas have assumed iconic importance. Ultimately, critics argue, questions of human health cannot depend on the good will of multinational corporations. They fear that policy decisions about food or environmental risks will be based on market rather than moral considerations and that public interests will be sacrificed to the imperatives of private gain.

Mistrust is compounded by an erosion of trust in regulatory authorities. One critic writes about the "testosterone" in the State Department, comparing American environmental policies to "the old colonial game" (Burrows 1999). Regulatory bodies such as the Food and Drug Administration (FDA), critics claim, are hostage to corporate interests, slaves to industry. Policies of self-policing in the United States allow companies to tailor their tests to get the results they need to avoid regulation—a form of "regulatory relief." This voluntary system of regulation has helped erode public confidence, though trust remains higher in the United States than in Western Europe where the outbreak of "mad cow disease" (BSE) and other food disasters created a crisis of public confidence in the effectiveness of regulation and the efficacy of scientific expertise.

A related political concern is the lack of consumer choice and the absence of public participation in policy decisions about risk. French farmers want a say in the introduction of new food products, patient rights are at issue in medical disputes, and community participation is demanded in the siting of toxic-waste dumps or other noxious facilities. Labeling—of modified foods, chemicals, and pharmaceuticals—has become a critical issue as individuals seek greater consumer choice and feel themselves increasingly excluded from the decision-making process (Kinderlerer 2000). Some demands for consumer choice arise from moral and religious interests. Controversies over risk can be a proxy for concerns that science is violating ethical and religious values—tampering with nature or threatening the sanctity of life. These concerns reflect the strongly embedded fundamentalist tradition in American society, where religious interests have had a powerful influence on policy decisions.

Globalization is dramatically changing the social context of many risk disputes. The risks of science and its applications are no longer contained within national boundaries, and this has greatly amplified and complicated questions of cultural acceptability, choice, and control. Should a few pharmaceutical companies be able to monopolize the food supply for the entire world? Should farmers throughout the world be dependent on American and European firms? Will farmers and food safety be hostage to multinational enterprises? The issues of risk are increasingly tied to broader issues of Third World politics and the past and current role of Western powers in developing countries. These themes of corporate mistrust, concerns about choice, and globalization appear in the language of risk disputes, providing rhetorical resources for activists.

THE LANGUAGE OF RISK

This is a time of technology "hype" (Nelkin 1994). In corporate public relations and media reports we hear that the biotechnology "revolution" will radically alter agricultural practices so that food production will be independent of the vagaries of soil, sun, and rain. Advances in biotechnology will be used to create plants that are resistant to disease and drought and vegetables able to survive salinity and frost. There will be fields of higher yields and foods with higher nutritional value. Biotech, we are told, is an economic engine for agricultural growth—enhancing the world's food supply. It will solve the world's problems of hunger.

For those of us who study risk, this language is eerily familiar. In 1907, physicist Frederick Soddy predicted that the energy of radium would transform deserts and make the whole world one Garden of Eden. In the 1950s, promoters of nuclear power promised that the technology would solve the problem of world hunger, turning deserts into flourishing agricultural regions and ending inequality throughout the world. Gene therapy, stem cells, and other medical procedures are promoted with futuristic promises that encourage inflated expectations. They also contribute to cynicism when promises fail or involve unanticipated risks.

New words have entered our risk vocabulary: chemophobia, cancerphobia, chemical sensitivity, toxic terrorism, frankenfoods. Critics employ the language of rights and concepts of justice. They accuse industry of bio-colonialism and use metaphors of pollution and contamination (Levidow 2000). The words used to describe risks and prescribe solutions are judgmental. Some words imply disorder or chaos; others suggest certainty and scientific precision. Selected metaphorical images can trivialize an event or render it important, marginalize some groups and empower others, define a controversial technology as a problem or reduce it to a routine. Language is a rhetorical resource. Interest groups filter facts about risk, select information, and compress and package it for public scrutiny (Hilgartner 1985).

Rhetorical strategies are intended to win public support for technologies and to dismiss opposing positions. The parties to risk disputes dismiss each other as irrational and immoral. Critics of new technologies claim that market interests ("callous capitalists") are overriding moral imperatives. Proponents dismiss critics as emotional and unrealistic, marginal, uninformed, risk adverse, or Luddites afraid of technological change. No technology, they argue, is free of risk. Both sides in risk disputes employ a moral and religious rhetoric to dramatize their views. The rhetoric of risk is full of exaggerated dichotomies (chemicals versus starvation, nuclear power or freeze in the dark, profits versus health). The media perpetuate these language wars and amplify the issues. They play a critical role in helping convince the public to accept or reject certain risks (Nelkin 1989).

Media language can point the finger of blame and imply responsibility. If health risks are a technical problem, regulation is properly the province of technical expertise. And risk assessment, with its connotation of neutrality and scientific objectivity, is appropriate. But if the problems are embedded in the moral context of responsibility and social justice, this calls for a more political approach to public policy that considers social, ethical, and political concerns. Interestingly, moral critics in risk disputes rely on technical evidence as a political resource and a tool of persuasion in their efforts to find resolutions.

DISPUTE RESOLUTION

Technical studies about health and safety, however, often fail to stop opposition; in a context of uncertainty, there are deep disagreements about what constitutes adequate evidence. What is the relevance of animal data to judgments about human health effects? What is the relative importance of specific incidents of harm as opposed to statistical or epidemiological data? What level of statistical uncertainty constitutes significant risk?

The preoccupation with risk reflects concerns that have developed over many years. People have been deluged with dire warnings about invisible hazards: PCBs, radiation, chemicals in the workplace, food additives, mad cow disease,

toxic wastes, and infectious organisms. The cumulative nature of these warnings of risk has fostered mistrust of science, industry, and regulation. Science—
once an arbiter of truth, a trusted source of neutral knowledge—is now
perceived as embedded in corporate agendas and imbued with conflicts of interest. The Euro-Barometer surveys of public opinion in 12 countries found that
some people trust environmental and consumer groups to tell the truth more
than they trust public authorities, industry, or scientists (Durant, Bauer, and
Gaskell 1998). Surveys in the United States found that Americans believe
environmental groups over federal agencies by a margin of 63 percent to 26
percent. Some scientists seek to resolve disputes through improved public communication of technical information. Their efforts assume that people's concerns reflect lack of knowledge and that better information will enhance
confidence. But information may have little impact on perceptions. Indeed, efforts to convince the public about the safety and benefits of a controversial
technology may only amplify mistrust, because consumer information is often
viewed as public relations and resented as a way to dismiss social concerns
(Wynne 1991).

The evolution of risk disputes, their media visibility, and their influence on
corporate and regulatory policies depend less on the actual nature of risk than
on the existence of powerful groups—community organizations, farm lobbies,
and mobilized activists organized to respond to new developments and skilled
at attracting financial resources and media attention. These mobilized critics
have had a striking influence in framing broader public responses. Using concepts such as fairness and justice as well as technical arguments, they create a
moral imperative to protect nature. "They have succeeded in claiming issues
from the scientific realm of true and false and … moving them to the ethical
realm of right and wrong" (Tesh 2000:125).

To focus on the proxy issues raised by risk disputes is not to dismiss concerns
about health. Clearly these are an important part of the story. But the social,
ethical, and political issues associated with risk—such as those raised by the
New York City street theater performance—are also a critical aspect of disputes. Ignoring these issues will preclude long-term dispute resolution.

Over the coming years, several factors will shape the public's construction of
risk. The economic and political autonomy of large corporations, and especially
their role in the process of economic globalization, are bound to influence future
controversies. Third World issues will become increasingly important. The debates over genetically modified (GM) foods are calling public attention to—and
compounding resentment of—resource disparities and exploitation, the growing
power of transnational corporations of unprecedented size and wealth, and the
limits of consumer choice and participation in decisions that affect their health
and their lives. To dismiss concerns about risk is to underestimate the popular
perception that science and technology are out of control, that scientific hubris
and corporate greed are generating dangerous products, and that many governments have neither the ability nor the will to impose adequate regulations.

REFERENCES

Beck, Ulrich. 1992. *Risk Society: Towards a New Modernity.* London: Sage.

Burrows, Beth. 1999. "Resurrecting the Ugly American." *Rachel's Environmental and Health News,* June 17, #655.

Castel, Robert. 1991. "From Dangerousness to Risk." In *The Foucault Effect,* eds. Graham Burchell, Colin Gordon, and Peter Miller, 281–298. Chicago: University of Chicago Press.

Douglas, Mary. 1992. *Risk and Blame.* New York: Routledge.

Durant, John, Martin Bauer, and George Gaskell. 1998. *Biotechnology in the Public Sphere.* London: British Science Museum.

Fischhoff, Baruch, S. Lichtenstein, and Paul Slovic. 1991. *Acceptable Risk.* New York: Cambridge University Press.

Hilgartner, Stephen. 1985. "The Political Language of Risk." In *The Language of Risk,* ed. Dorothy Nelkin, 25–66. Beverly Hills: Sage.

Kinderlerer, Julian. 2000. "Genetically Modified Organisms: A European Scientist's View." *New York University Environmental Law Journal* 8(3): 556–565.

Levidow, Les. 2000. "Pollution Metaphors in the UK Biotechnology Controversy." *Science as Culture* 9(3): 325–351.

Lock, Margaret. 2001. "Introduction to Special Issue on Medical Innovation and Public Knowledge." *Health* 5(3): 285–901.

Nelkin, Dorothy. 1989. "Communicating Technological Risk." *Annual Reviews of Public Health* 1: 95–113.

———. 1992. *Controversy: The Politics of Technical Decisions.* 3rd ed. Newbury Park: Sage.

———. 1994. *Selling Science: How the Press Covers Science and Technology.* New York: W. H. Freeman.

Robertson, Ann. 2001. "Biotechnology, Political Rationality and Discourses on Health Risk." *Health* 5(3): 293–309.

Silverman, Chloe. 2001. "Molecular Stories." *Science As Culture* 10(2): 255–263.

Tesh, Sylvia Noble. 1988. *Hidden Arguments.* New Brunswick, NJ: Rutgers University Press.

———. 2000. *Uncertain Hazards: Environmental Activists and Scientific Proof.* Ithaca, NY: Cornell University Press.

Wynne, Brian. 1991. "Public Understanding and the Management of Science." In *The Management of Science,* ed. Douglas Hague, 143–169. London: Macmillan.

Acknowledgments

Early discussions of the issues raised in this book were part of a faculty reading group at UC Santa Barbara whose participants were Francesca Bray, Sabine Frühstück, Barbara Herr Harthorn, Jessica Jerome, and Laury Oaks. Several of the chapters (Bray, Harthorn, Hunt and de Voogd, Murphy-Lawless, and Oaks) were presented originally at the 2000 American Anthropological Association meetings as part of a panel organized by Barbara Herr Harthorn and Laury Oaks, "Revising Risk: Shifting Perceptions of the Public's Health and the Social Contract." We solicited additional contributions from a range of anthropologists and sociologists whose work has analyzed the social and cultural dimensions of risk in relation to health. Sarah Rodriguez has provided invaluable editorial and bibliographic assistance.

Part I

Introduction and Overview

Introduction: Health and the Social and Cultural Construction of Risk

Laury Oaks and Barbara Herr Harthorn

Risks to health and safety perhaps were never more prominently at the center of public discourse and private anxieties in the United States than in the weeks following the events of September 11, 2001. This tragic circumstance provides ample evidence for the main arguments in this book: risk meanings are primarily socially, culturally, and politically constructed; judgments about relative safety or appropriate risks are almost entirely social/cultural, particularly when attached to categories of ethnicity, class, gender, immigration experience, sexuality, religion, and numerous other identifiers; and shifting assessments of risk provide fertile ground for the dynamic analysis of social/cultural systems of meaning.

The purpose of this book is to examine what one scholar has deemed "the epistemology of risk" (Hayes 1992), which we take to mean a critical analysis of the way risk is discussed, deployed, and disentangled by multiple actors and across varied cultural and social divides. Building on the pivotal analyses of the social and cultural construction of risk by anthropologists and sociologists (Douglas 1970, 1992; Nelkin 1985, 1989, [1979, 1984] 1992; Lupton 1999a, 1999b), our contributors' case studies expand understandings of the perception of health-risk categories and the social, political, and cultural uses of risk assessment and risk warnings. The main contributions of this book are its dual focus on health risks and health inequality and the breadth of its analysis of risk in distinct cultural contexts and in relation to pressing health issues.

An important argument of this book is to show the strong connection between health-risk perceptions and both risk-taking and risk-reducing behavior. The study of risk perception emerged in the early 1980s and was primarily designed to explore divergent views of laypersons from those of "experts." That is, experts' views were taken to have scientific truth value, while laypersons' views represent a (mis-) perception, meriting exploration due to the political difficulties encountered when "the public" sees things differently from "the experts." Risk in these studies is defined as a statistical probability of an event's occurring within a population. In contrast, our use of risk redirects attention to the culturally contingent nature of this category and signals how the related concepts of hazard, harm, and danger are measured in multiple discourses— everyday, popular, and political—in ways that are largely disengaged from population-based probability statistics. Health-risk perceptions and reactions to health-risk warnings are based on cultural knowledge and practical experience, not simply on expert risk probability calculations. We draw attention to risk as a fluctuating, socially seismic field in which definitions of danger, harm, safety, and blame are constantly shifting. Social difference and health inequality figure largely in the cultural landscape of risk precisely because risk is used in the production of health inequality.

Recent events have forced into public view contesting versions of what constitutes risk, who is responsible for risk prevention, which risk-taking actions are socially acceptable, and who is to blame when risk warnings are not heeded. Yet rapid and contradictory shifts in the valences of risk perception and risk messages are not limited to times of national or international crisis. As Dorothy Nelkin's foreword so precisely points out, social, political, and cultural forces are reflected in the ever-present controversies over defining what constitutes danger and how individuals should respond to threats and hazards. The studies in this book point to how various actors—scientists, medical professionals, government officials, corporate leaders, social movement activists, and lay individuals—employ discourses and practices that mobilize fear, blame, trust, and control in ongoing controversies over health risk and uncertainty.

RISK AS SOCIALLY CONSTRUCTED AND CULTURALLY EMBEDDED

Questions of risk and danger have been at the center of anthropological and sociological inquiry at least since Douglas's classic analysis in *Purity and Danger* (1970), in which she showed how societies socially construct categories of safe behavior and persistently displace danger and blame onto external sources. Social theorists Giddens (1990) and Beck (1992, 1999) have detailed the erosion of public trust in governments and science as conditions of late modernity and argue that diminished trust and increased perception of risk are directly connected. Others, taking a Foucauldian approach, have illuminated how social control is effected through various disciplinary regimes, including public health (see Lupton 1994, 1999a, 1999b). Social, economic, and political position all have profound effects on perceptions of what is dangerous and the level of perceived danger attached to specific experiences (Slovic 1987, 1992, 2000; Slovic, Fischhoff, and Lichtenstein 1982). Moreover, perception of risk is best argued to be socially and culturally constructed through a complex process that depends on a range of social and cultural factors and may be contributed to through processes of risk communication (Freudenburg 1988; Nelkin 1989; Douglas 1992; Balshem 1993; Lupton 1994, 1995; Petersen and Lupton 1996; Lock 1998; Rapp 1999; Caplan 2000; Oaks 2001). In short, this body of literature argues that, at its essence, risk is socially constructed.

Crucial to the aims of this book, Douglas (1992) has also pointed out how the "forensic needs" of global culture are well served by judgments of risk acceptability, which she argues are necessarily social, rather than scientific. Although Douglas views risk perception as "a culturally standardized response," others argue persuasively that risk perception is better conceptualized as a multiplicity of views that vary according to a wide range of factors (Sobo 1995). Some scholars have also provided an even more pointed critique of the concept of acceptable risk, including attention to its intrinsic idea that there are expendable people (Sobo 1995; Farmer 1999; Satterfield, this volume). Thus, the chapters in this book demonstrate that the politics of risk perception is an imperative site for analyzing processes of discrimination by gender, race, ethnicity, class, sexual identity, political views, and other social categories.

Another foundational thinker about the social construction of risk is sociologist Nelkin. Her important early work on this (Nelkin and Brown 1984; Nelkin 1985) showed how the language of risk reflects key aspects of social position and political aims, for example, among workers and employers. In a key article, Nelkin (1989) laid essential foundation to the work in this book, and more recently her work has argued across a number of cases to show how science and its pronouncements are always underwritten by social and political agendas (Nelkin 1992, [1987] 1995, 2000).

The work of sociologist Lupton offers another signal contribution to the study of the social construction of risk. A cultural critic of the politics of public health (Lupton 1995; Petersen and Lupton 1996), she has recently provided an elegant summary and analysis of social risk theory in her book, *Risk* (1999a). In it, she argues there are three main theoretical approaches to the social aspects of risk. Lupton terms these the "cultural/symbolic" perspectives, typified by Douglas; "risk-society" perspectives at a macro level, of which the key proponents are Giddens and Beck; and "governmentality" perspectives, which expand on Foucault's scholarship. Lupton's significant contribution is to show the startling lack of interaction among these lines of inquiry, and she highlights new studies that work across these boundaries in her companion edited volume, *Risk and Sociocultural Theory: New Directions and Perspectives* (1999b). Although her scholarship has not focused exclusively on health risk, it provides an excellent base from which to extend discussions of the concept of risk in relation to health and health inequality.

HEALTH INEQUALITY AND RISK

A crucial argument that runs throughout this book is that risk and judgments about risk are essential factors in health inequality. Studies of a number of specific health problems highlight the cultural specificity of risk judgments that may conflict with health experts' views (see Luker 1975; Green and Sobo 2000). This point is evident in anthropological and sociological literature that addresses environmental health, environmental justice, and social inequalities in the distribution and management of risk (Bullard 1993, 1994; Szasz 1994; Kroll-Smith and Floyd 1997; Kroll-Smith, Brown, and Gunter 2000). Through a global and cross-cultural focus and with ethnographic depth, we argue that health risk is a particularly instructive lens for examining discourses and practices that contribute to and sustain differential access to "healthy" decision-making and to health care (cf. Gabe 1995). Several chapters (Hunt and de Voogd, Oaks, and Jerome) show that it is the moral value, not the truth value, of risk claims that is crucial in shaping perceptions of risk and influencing health behavior. Other chapters (Harthorn, Satterfield) show that individuals and groups disadvantaged by their socioeconomic conditions are systematically faced with greater risks—greater in terms of quantity and, especially, severity.

Globalization, both in the dispersal of technologies and in associated complex patterns of access, is argued to be a crucial force in changing distributions of health. Inhorn's chapter shows how the inequitable access to new reproductive technologies in Egypt leads to negative health consequences for some Egyptian women (and men), and chapters by Bray and Murphy-Lawless illustrate the health and food-safety inequities that result from global corporate forces whose agendas are, at root, not humanitarian. Finally, several chapters (Hunt and de Voogd, Jerome, Chua) provide evidence that around the globe, social control efforts—often in the guise of public health care—consistently trump the equitable delivery of health care.

ORGANIZATION OF THE BOOK

The book opens with an introductory essay by anthropologist Nichter, who argues on the basis of his own ethnographic studies and extensive international research experiences that harm reduction should be considered a core thematic area within medical anthropology. He examines how health-related harm-reduction practices are shaped by culturally embedded ideas about vulnerability, risk, and responsibility and calls for further ethnographic accounts of social risk that will capture the diversity of harm-reduction strategies selected by individuals as well as social groups. The chapters that follow Nichter's are organized into three additional Parts.

The chapters in the Part II, "The Cultivation of Fear," examine discourses and practices that incite fear about health risks produced through social, cultural, and biomedical processes. We argue that discourses and practices that aim to amplify social and individual fears offer critical insight into social processes of differentiation. This intrinsic tension is found throughout much public health discourse overtly aimed at increasing perception of risk as a technique to produce behavior change, often with unanticipated effects. Discourses of power and subjugation, within which perception of health risk is the point of struggle, provide clear evidence of other agendas and aims. Biomedical and public-health authorities and social movement activists, wittingly or not, define certain individuals and groups as "at risk." Those who are at risk are subject to social, cultural, medical, and moral control both by being defined by others as at risk and by defining themselves in this way (Gifford 1986; Furedi 1997; Press, Fishman, and Koenig 2000). Individuals who are labeled at risk may seek ways to prevent negative outcomes associated with risks and attempt to mitigate the stigma attached to being at risk. Thus, the process of the cultivation of fear—for example, through the marketing of risk-assessment technologies and authorities' health warning messages—functions as an apparatus of social control, potentially of both individuals' health practices and their risk subjectivities.

In the first chapter in Part II, anthropologists Hunt and de Voogd explore the consequences of being deemed at risk in their research on the experiences of low-income pregnant Latinas in Texas. They argue that the emotional burden of anxiety about the baby-to-be's health engendered by the clinical application of the at-risk label—and the moral dilemma of accepting that worry—have much more to do with women's decisions about pursuing further testing than the supposedly autonomous decision-making biomedicine and public health frameworks assume. Next, anthropologist and public health scholar Inhorn illustrates the multiplicity of fears and concerns attached to the perceived risks of newly imported in vitro fertilization (IVF) technologies in Egypt and argues that such feelings are essential to the reproductive decisions women (and men) make. Risks in this analysis include perceived risks to social, economic, and physical well-being; culturally complex risks related to moral fitness, religion, family, and age; and the hazardous negotiation of a chancy, global reproductive-technology delivery system. The final chapter in Part II, by anthropologist and women's studies scholar Oaks, focuses on how, in the absence of clear-cut scientific conclusions about specific health or safety risks, social movements' political agendas can be the driving force behind health advocacy campaigns. Oaks's analysis shows that antiabortion advocates use tactics of fear cultivation in media campaigns that masquerade as public health announcements claiming that abortion increases a woman's breast cancer risk to try to sway women to change their political views and their reproductive health practices.

Part III, "Perceptions of Health, Safety, and Hazard: Risk Makers and Risk Takers," focuses specifically on how health risks and safety are perceived by actors who have different positions of social and economic power. The chapters in this Part reveal the inadequacies in the pervasive imperative that individuals are responsible for reducing their exposures to risks. Individuals in communities that are socially and economically marginalized are constrained by structural forces that inhibit the possibility of risk avoidance. Yet, individuals do exert agency, attempting to safeguard their well-being despite their knowledge of ever-present hazards (Sobo 1995).

In the first chapter in Part III, anthropologist Jerome's analysis of the medicalization of indigenous medicines in northeastern Brazil examines how biomedical institutions adopt international development tools that assume control of women's indigenous knowledge of and access to medicinal plants. She demonstrates how public health officials have labeled traditional medicinal knowledge and practices as risky, recast herbal medicines from "food" into "drugs," and attempted to regulate both the cultivation and use of medicinal plants. Anthropologist Satterfield's chapter looks at the physical, psychological, and social consequences of an African American community's years-long exposure to environmental toxins in southern Georgia and the effects of the definition of the community as hazardous. She argues that community members felt both embodied and sociopolitical stigma, viewing their experience through racism, social marginalization, and the meaning of worthy and unworthy citizens. The actions that authorities took to "remedy" the pervasive hazards in this community exacerbated the experience of stigmas and heightened fears about personal, environmental, and sociopolitical risks. In a similar vein, anthropologist Harthorn's study of perception of risk from exposure to agricultural chemicals among California women and men farmworkers argues that pressing economic imperatives to accept hazardous work constrain the way farmworkers perceive their own health risks. In this study, immigrant low-income Latinas/-os are shown to choose unsafe agricultural work and to minimize the hazards to their own health while maintaining anxious concern for the health of their children, family, and community.

Part IV of the book, "Regulating Risk and the Public's Health," confronts contests over who regulates the public's health and how. The chapters in this Part emphasize the role of the state, via its regulatory agents, in protecting citizens and promoting healthy populations through institutional practices such as sponsoring public health programs and research task forces; measuring, defining, and surveilling public health problems; implementing legislation and policy; and allocating resources to risk prevention, education, and reduction. At the same time, globalization, the spread of diseases and disease threats across state borders, and global networks of scientists point to the inability of state authorities to act autonomously in the face of public health risks. This brings into question ultimately who has responsibility to regulate risk and where blame should be placed in cases in which state agencies neither effectively protect the public's health nor instill a sense of public trust in government health authorities. Further, it asks who within society is targeted as at risk (potential victims) and who are the agents producing risk (potential offenders). As global citizens are increasingly defined by their role as consumers, what stake do state or super-state governmental bodies have in limiting what is sold, by whom, and with what product-safety assurances? To what extent are consumers portrayed by the state as rational actors who have the responsibility to make healthy choices despite evidence that the choices available may entail hidden risks, particularly those resulting from the inability of the state to ensure safety in contexts of uncertainty?

In the first chapter in Part IV, sociologist Chua contributes a critical analysis of the social and political uses of HIV/AIDS health-risk campaigns in Southeast Asia. He examines researchers', states', and transnational entities' constructions of risk in "safer sex" strategies and programs aimed at women sex workers at international borders and their male clientele among international truck drivers. Chua argues that these practices of social regulation, focused on geographically peripheral and socially marginal groups, deflect concern away from urban elite sexual practices and serve to stigmatize and control specific groups. This chapter further shows that the unintended effects of these HIV/AIDS prevention efforts include the legitimization and normalization of women sex workers and an uncritical acceptance of transnational commodity flows. Next, anthropologist and historian of science Bray examines the controversial issue of the global safety of genetically modified (GM) foods for human consumption. Her analysis details the history of this technology and its uses and abuses by nation-state and corporate actors, documenting the development of corporate technology and capitalist or productivist efforts toward global domination of the GM market. Bray draws from Beck's notion of "shared risk" to examine the emergence of new social movements that have mobilized in opposition to corporate strategies to disseminate GM food crops. The final chapter, by Irish sociologist Murphy-Lawless, addresses the pivotal place of discussions of risk in mediating state and private concerns. The chapter explores the problem of living with uncertainty for a democratic citizenry in a world in which science is an enterprise of neoliberal capitalism and the political motivations of experts are clearly traceable in the construction of risk and the management of the social contract. The cases of the BSE (mad cow) and foot-and-mouth epidemics in Britain form the basis for Murphy-Lawless's discussion of the social construction of risk and crisis, analysis of the role of the state in managing food and health, and assessment of the components that enable effective citizen political action.

Taken together, the contributors to this book argue that the shifting valences of particular health risks index the socially constructed nature of all risks and that the concept of risk both produces and makes visible health inequalities. Risk provides social analysts a powerful lens for examining the politics of health and health care and the differential allocation of the conditions that produce morbidity and mortality. Critical cultural analysis of discourse, both public and private, illuminates the problems of agency and choice, danger and blame in risk-making and risk-taking. We must not lose sight of the seeming ever-escalating number, severity, and far-reaching transnational effects of health risks relating to issues ranging from food safety to the environment, new technologies to infectious disease. If we are to understand the fundamental social, cultural, economic, and political issues that represent the core of health inequalities and their attendant risks, our analyses of health-risk assessments, warnings, and controversies must fully consider how our perceptions of danger and blame are socially and culturally shaped.

REFERENCES

Balshem, Martha Levittan. 1993. *Cancer in the Community: Class and Medical Authority.* Washington: Smithsonian Institution Press.

Beck, Ulrich. 1992. *Risk Society: Towards a New Modernity.* Newbury Park, CA: Sage.

———. 1999. *World Risk Society.* Cambridge: Polity Press.

Bullard, Robert D., ed. 1993. *Confronting Environmental Racism: Voices from the Grassroots.* Boston: South End Press.

———. 1994. *Unequal Protection: Environmental Justice and Communities of Color.* San Francisco: Sierra Club Books.

Caplan, Pat, ed. 2000. *Risk Revisited.* London: Pluto Press.

Douglas, Mary. 1970. *Purity and Danger: An Analysis of Concepts of Pollution and Taboo.* Harmondworth: Penguin.

———.1992. *Risk and Blame: Essays in Cultural Theory.* New York: Routledge.

Farmer, Paul. 1999. *Infections and Inequalities: The Modern Plagues.* Berkeley and Los Angeles: University of California Press.

Freudenburg, William. 1988. "Perceived Risk, Real Risk: Social Science and the Art of Probabilistic Risk Assessment." *Science* 242: 44–49.

Furedi, Frank. 1997. *Culture of Fear: Risk-Taking and the Morality of Low Expectation.* London: Cassell.

Gabe, Jonathan, ed. 1995. *Health, Medicine and Risk: The Need for a Sociological Approach.* Oxford: Blackwell.

Giddens, Anthony. 1990. *The Consequences of Modernity.* Stanford: Stanford University Press.

Gifford, Sandra M. 1986. "The Meanings of Lumps: A Case Study of the Ambiguities of Risk." In *Anthropology and Epidemiology: Interdisciplinary Approaches to the Study of Health and Disease,* eds. Craig R. Janes, Ron Stall, and Sandra M. Gifford, 213–249. Dordrecht, The Netherlands: Reidel.

Green, Gil, and Elisa J. Sobo. 2000. *The Endangered Self: Managing the Social Risk of HIV.* New York: Routledge.

Hayes, Michael V. 1992. "On the Epistemology of Risk: Language, Logic and Social Science." *Social Science and Medicine* 35 (1): 401–407.

Kroll-Smith, Steve, and H. Hugh Floyd. 1997. *Bodies in Protest: Environmental Illness and the Struggle over Medical Knowledge.* New York: New York University Press.

Kroll-Smith, Steve, Phil Brown, and Valerie J. Gunter, eds. 2000. *Illness and the Environment: A Reader in Contested Medicine.* New York: New York University Press.

Lock, Margaret. 1998. "Breast Cancer: Reading the Omens." *Anthropology Today* 14 (4): 7–16.

Luker, Kristin. 1975. *Taking Chances: Abortion and the Decision Not to Contracept.* Berkeley and Los Angeles: University of California Press.

Lupton, Deborah. 1994. *Medicine as Culture: Illness, Disease and the Body in Western Societies.* London: Sage.

———. 1995. *The Imperative of Health: Public Health and the Regulated Body.* Thousand Oaks, CA: Sage.

———. 1999a. *Risk.* London: Routledge.

Lupton, Deborah, ed. 1999b. *Risk and Sociocultural Theory: New Directions and Perspectives.* New York: Cambridge University Press.

Nelkin, Dorothy. 1989. "Communicating Technological Risk: The Social Construction of Risk Perception." *Annual Review of Public Health* 10: 95–113.

———. [1987] 1995. *Selling Science: How the Press Covers Science and Technology.* New York: W.H. Freeman.

———. [1982] 2000. *The Creation Controversy: Science or Scripture in the Schools.* New York: Norton. Reprint, San Jose, CA: toExcel.

Nelkin, Dorothy, ed. [1979, 1984] 1992. *Controversy: Politics of Technical Decisions.* Newbury Park, CA: Sage.

———. 1985. *The Language of Risk: Conflicting Perspectives on Occupational Health.* Beverly Hills: Sage.

Nelkin, Dorothy, and Michael Stuart Brown. 1984. *Workers at Risk: Voices from the Workplace.* Chicago: University of Chicago Press.

Oaks, Laury. 2001. *Smoking and Pregnancy: The Politics of Fetal Protection.* New Brunswick, NJ: Rutgers University Press.

Petersen, Alan, and Deborah Lupton. 1996. *The New Public Health: Health and Self in This Age of Risk.* London: Sage.

Press, Nancy, Jennifer Fishman, and Barbara A. Koenig. 2000. "Collective Fear, Individualized Risk: The Social and Cultural Context of Genetic Testing for Breast Cancer." *Nursing Ethics* 2000 7(3): 237–249.

Rapp, Rayna. 1999. *Testing Women, Testing the Fetus: The Social Impact of Amniocentesis in America.* New York: Routledge.

Slovic, Paul. 1987. "Perception of Risk." *Science* 236 (4799): 280–285.

———. 1992. "Perception of Risk: Reflections on the Psychometric." In *Social Theories of Risk,* eds. Sheldon Krimsky and Dominic Golding, 117–152. Westport, CT: Praeger.

Slovic, Paul, Baruch Fischhoff, and Sarah Lichtenstein. 1982. "Facts versus Fears: Understanding Perceived Risk." In *Judgment under Uncertainty: Heuristics and Biases,* ed. Daniel Kahneman, Paul Slovic, and Amos Tversky, 463–489. New York: Cambridge University Press.

Slovic, Paul, ed. 2000. *The Perception of Risk.* Sterling, VA: Earthscan Publications.

Sobo, Elisa J. 1995. *Choosing Unsafe Sex: AIDS-Risk Denial among Disadvantaged Women.* Philadelphia: University of Pennsylvania Press.

Szasz, Andrew. 1994. *EcoPopulism: Toxic Waste and the Movement for Environmental Justice.* Minneapolis: University of Minnesota Press.

Chapter 1

Harm Reduction: A Core Concern for Medical Anthropology

Mark Nichter

One of the most important and least appreciated topics in medical anthropology is harm reduction. It is not only a practical logic that characterizes our age of risk, but a fundamental way people have approached preventive health within local health cultures. Using research I have conducted during the past 25 years in both international and national contexts, I first consider vulnerability and harm reduction in general to set the stage for a more detailed discussion of harm-reduction strategies. After reviewing longstanding and emergent harm-reduction strategies in South and Southeast Asia, I draw upon theories of reflexive modernity and risk society (Giddens 1991; Beck 1992, 1996) to discuss harm reduction as a way of life in the United States and end by highlighting a few areas of harm reduction that beg further inquiry to move the field forward.

VULNERABILITY AND RISK

The topic of harm reduction can be positioned within a larger thematic area in anthropology: the anthropology of vulnerability, risk, and responsibility. This thematic area encompasses the study of 1) layperson perceptions of vulnerability, 2) the production and representation of knowledge about risk, 3) the politics of responsibility associated with a knowledge of risk, 4) lay response to and trust of expert knowledge about risk, and 5) harm reduction as both an expression of agency and a form of manipulation.[1] As an expression of agency, harm-reduction practices are undertaken to reduce a sense of vulnerability and enhance a sense of self-control. As a form of manipulation, harm-reduction practices are fostered at the site of the individual body by parties who wish to deflect attention away from risk factors affecting a population's health. For example, attention may be deflected from labor conditions that expose people to environmental or occupational risk factors. Responsibility for maintaining health under adverse conditions allowed by lax state health policy may, for example, be placed onto individuals who are expected to monitor their health and adopt a healthy lifestyle. A harm-reduction industry may then capitalize on feelings of vulnerability fostered by information about risk. Such information is generated by health professionals and the media and by the proliferation of harm-reduction products and advertisements.

Vulnerability refers to the actual feeling of susceptibility to illness or misfortune. It is a state of weakness, fear, and worry. Risk has a broader meaning. In general parlance, risk indexes hazard, chance, and uncertainty. In epidemiology, risk refers to a calculated probability, the odds that something will occur (or not occur) within a given population exposed to specific risk (or protective) factors when compared to a reference population. However, members of a risk group may not see themselves as equally vulnerable to illness by way of comparative reasoning and consideration of cultural and personal factors outside the purview of those calculating the risk. When information about risk is presented to members of a group at risk, some members downplay the danger because they see others in their group as less diligent or more lax when it comes to factors that predispose or cause illness (e.g., diet, cleanliness, ritual protection, drinking, excessive sexual behavior). For other members of a risk group, exposure to risk data may trigger a sense of vulnerability, which then becomes a risk factor in its own right. For example, a seemingly objective population-based risk calculation may become a social fact that leads some people to assume a risk role that is unhealthy.

The same information can lead people to become fatalistic or dispassionate about a health issue just as easily as motivating them to engage in primary prevention or some form of harm reduction. Consider the impact of a newspaper headline that calls attention to the high prevalence of a disease (HIV, obesity, diabetes, hypertension) or some unhealthy behavior (smoking, drinking, eating fast food). Exposure to such headlines may either raise the consciousness of a population and trigger behavior change or make the problem or behavior appear normative, the dues one pays for living in a particular environment or being a member of a given social group.

TYPES OF VULNERABILITY

What leads people to feel vulnerable to a particular health problem? I outline five different ways people think about vulnerability that lead them to engage in harm-reduction practices and briefly illustrate these dimensions of vulnerability by using examples from my research in South and Southeast Asia.

Trait-Based Vulnerability

People may feel they have a weak constitution or predisposition to illness (in general or a specific illness) on the basis of a) physical signs and symptoms interpreted as traces of some underlying truth about the person, b) a past history of illness or poor health that leads them to be labeled as weak or susceptible, or c) some association with a hereditary predisposition that indexes familial or ethnic group histories of illness (addiction, for example), which in today's world extends to popular interpretations of genetics. Practitioners of humoral-based medical traditions (e.g., Ayurvedic and Chinese medicine) pay attention to body constitution (subject to age) when diagnosing illness as well as when prescribing health-enhancing and disease-prevention practices. Notions of body constitution also influence health-care-seeking behavior and resource allocation for young children perceived to be weak or strong in contexts of extreme poverty.[2]

Traits identifying a person as vulnerable may lead members of society to treat that person differently and the person to assume a risk role. For example, in a study of the condition *sema* in Sri Lanka (Nichter 1987), children from the middle class experiencing catarrh (sinusitis) were treated as fragile and socialized differently than other children. This study of a mundane condition shows that *sema anga* (phlegm body) people remind others in the society of indigenous health principles. Although most people break cultural health prescriptions much of the time, these individuals, along with infants, pregnant women, and elderly people, are the subject of public scrutiny and harm-reduction efforts. They remind others how one should ideally behave according to humoral reasoning.

Just as some people are deemed to have weak constitutions, others think of themselves as having strong constitutions (strong resistance to illness). Their sense of being less vulnerable than others likewise influences their health behavior. For example, the perception that they are strong leads some men in Thailand to think they can engage in riskier or more dangerous behavior than others, while taking fewer precautions. I have encountered men with a history of engaging in risky sex who interpret negative HIV tests as a measure of their strength. What else explains why they have not become ill? When I proposed to one informant that it was perhaps good fortune, he suggested to me that this in and of itself was a form of strength and not mere chance in a mathematical sense.

State-Based Vulnerability

A wide range of environmental factors is perceived to render people vulnerable to health problems. In South Asia, climatic conditions are thought to have a negative impact on constitutional proclivities triggering humoral imbalances. Sudden changes in climate are thought to render one vulnerable, as are particular types of winds. Different seasons are also associated with particular illnesses, and people engage in preventive health activities to minimize anticipated problems. In Southwest India, for example, a particular month during the rainy season is considered to be a time when impurities arise within the body and the earth. To counteract these perceived negative effects, people consume bitter herbal medicines and engage in special dietary precautions to remove internal toxins. This at once protects them against immediate threats to health and is a form of harm reduction that promotes health in the months to come.

Contact with spaces considered dangerous also renders one vulnerable. Negative attributes accrue to spaces for several reasons and include association with dangerous spirits, forms of impurity and pollution (including environmental toxins), endemic or epidemic diseases, and memories of violence or misfortune (toxic memories) embedded in landscapes and thought to exert an ongoing negative influence. When entering these spaces, precautions are taken and vigilance maintained.

Other state-dependent factors *widely* associated with vulnerability include transitional life stages such as pregnancy, infancy, and old age. These life stages are associated with states of openness, rapidly occurring transformation rendering one vulnerable, and states of weakness. The experience of negative emotional states (anger, sadness, jealousy) and shock are commonly thought to render one vulnerable to ill health as well as to exacerbate an existing illness by upsetting the afflicted individuals and opening them up to malevolent forces that prey off the weak. One reason friends and family gather around an ill person in Sri Lanka is to protect the person by warding off negative emotional states and spirits attracted to those who are vulnerable and ill. It is also a reason many Mexican families I have worked with on the wards in Arizona request that doctors not tell afflicted persons that their diagnosis is cancer. They fear the shock will negatively affect the prognosis of the afflicted person.

Vulnerability to Illness Transformation and Flare-Up

People who live in poverty and in a chronic state of ill health tend to view health as a relative state evaluated in relation to their ability to perform life tasks (functional health). For these people, preventive health largely entails harm reduction in the form of preventing preexisting health problems from becoming worse. Several types of behavior are recognized to cause preexisting health problems to flare up. These range from dietary habits to untimely bathing, sexual excess, and excessive consumption of alcohol, tobacco, or tea. These behaviors render one vulnerable to ill health in general, cause specific health problems, and exacerbate preexisting problems.

Anthropologists have long been aware that local ideas about causality are multidimensional and thought about in terms of instrumental, efficient, and ultimate causes (Glick 1967; Nichter 1987). However, it is not uncommon to lump together factors that render one vulnerable in general with factors thought to cause specific illnesses. In the Philippines, the term *pasma* is used to describe shocks to the body associated with hunger and untimely food consumption (*pasma sa guton*) as well as with shifts from hot to cold bodily (humoral) states. *Pasma* is commonly listed as a cause of illness in ethnographies of malaria and tuberculosis (TB). Does this mean informants do not believe mosquitoes or germs (*microbyo*) are the cause of these illnesses? Further investigation finds that *pasma* is viewed as the factor that has rendered one vulnerable to the illness in question and to mosquitoes and *microbyo*. After all, many people are exposed to bugs and germs all the time, yet only some become ill. Many people also have intermittent malaria. A key concern for these people is what causes their malaria to flare up, reemerge, or become more serious? In a context where they do not have a lot of control over environmental conditions, a sense of agency is gained through harm-reduction strategies that involve eating better, not shocking the body, taking medicines, and preventing existing illness from becoming worse.

Cumulative Sources of Negativity

Vulnerability is also associated with some negative entity accumulating within the body over time: impurities, residues, toxins, and germs. A common perception is that one can withstand some level of negative load, but that once a threshold level has been superseded, illness manifests.[3] Thresholds are generally thought to vary by person. Harm reduction may be followed to reduce one's relative load of negative accruement or to protect one from additional accumulation. In Thailand, donating blood is viewed as healthy for the donor (not just meritorious) because it removes old blood and allows the body to replenish itself with fresh blood. Saline drips containing vitamin cocktails also reduce the accumulation of negative residues in addition to making the body stronger. To reduce the harm of danger associated with sex, some Thai men consume medicines and soda water (attributed to have medicinal qualities such as hydrogen peroxide) before or after risky sex. They do so as a means of both killing germs while the germs are weak (not established in the body) and reducing cumulative loads of germs and impurity (Kanato 1994; Nichter 2001a).

Perceptions of illness latency add another dimension to cumulative vulnerability closely associated with concern about illness flare-up. It is not uncommon for those experiencing recurring illness to think that latent illness remains within their body, capable of flaring up when aroused or aggravated by some set of conditions. Harm reduction may entail protecting oneself from external threats (such as exposure to sources of heat or contamination) as well as regulating internal states through the consumption of medicines and the following of dietary practices.

Risk Information and Vulnerability

Exposure to information about risk can itself trigger a sense of vulnerability. In the Philippines (Cebu City), I observed that risky sexual behavior among commercial sex workers decreased following newspaper headlines about the threat of HIV. After these headlines disappeared for a few weeks, behavior tended to go back to the way it was before (Nichter 2001a). In this case, risk data increased a sense of vulnerability within the community, but the half-life of the impact was short. In other cases, the half-life of the information and its effect on the community was quite long but not what was anticipated by health officials. For example, in Northeast Thailand, screening tests for cervical cancer raised women's consciousness about the disease, but women imagined cervical cancer to be the final common pathway of uncured women's problems that transformed into this horrible disease (Boongmongkon, Pylypa, and Nichter 1999). Raising consciousness about a disease that may affect 20 to 30 women per 100,000 led to rising fear among women who imagined the disease to affect 3 out of every 10 women. I discuss an iatrogenic harm-reduction strategy followed by these women in the next section.

A sense of vulnerability may unintentionally be fostered by diagnostic tests at the individual as well as the community level (Kavanaugh and Broom 1998). Practitioners often recommend that a person undergo a diagnostic test to rule out a medical problem. However, the mere suggestion that someone should receive a test can inadvertently trigger a sense of vulnerability that remains even if the outcome of the test is negative. Diagnostic tests are responded to in a number of ways. Some people view tests as purely diagnostic, others think of them as curative, and still others see tests as opening up a Pandora's Box that invites illness. The way diagnostic tests are explained (and not explained) to people can also lead to a sense of vulnerability. Some practitioners in India do not explain to patients that their negative test results have ruled out an illness, because they feel it is too risky for them to do so. Practitioners worry that they might be held accountable later if the disease (or a related disease) manifests. These practitioners err on the side of caution (and profitability) by informing patients that they need to continue to monitor their condition, return for periodic tests, and often take medicines so the condition does not become worse. Notably, this provides the conditions under which a risk role may easily transform into a sick role. This is especially the case when somatic complaints take on meaning as an idiom of distress or concern by the "afflicted" person and concerned others. Diagnostic tests (and pseudo tests) may also be used to rationalize such decisions as to stop breastfeeding and give formula to a child (Mull 1992).

LONGSTANDING AND EMERGENT HARM-REDUCTION STRATEGIES IN SOUTH AND SOUTHEAST ASIA

Harm reduction involves a range of behaviors from managing factors that predispose illness to preventing illness from transforming into more serious problems. I highlight three types of preventive and promotive health behavior that may take place:

1. Upstream: Prior to a state of perceived heightened susceptibility
2. Midstream: During a state of perceived heightened susceptibility
3. Downstream: Following a state of perceived heightened susceptibility

Harm-reduction practices are an important part of popular health culture in Asia. Folk dietetic practices have long been followed to reduce humoral excess likely to occur in different seasons (Nichter 1986). Beyond a concern for hot and cold states, foods are or are not consumed to influence bodily states associated with routine bodily complaints ranging from gas and excess phlegm to the management of worm troubles. In rural South India (like many areas of Asia, Africa, and Latin America), a small number of intestinal worms are thought necessary for life. Problems occur when worm loads increase due to the consumption of too many sweets, the accumulation of undigested foods within the body, or the migration of the worms when disturbed. To prevent worm problems, diet is regulated as a means of enhancing digestion and removing undigested foods, and bitter medicines are taken to calm one's worms. Folk dietetic practices are also followed to prevent impurities and toxins in the blood (*nanju*) from building up and causing illness to manifest or wounds to turn septic. Great care is taken not to consume *nanju*-increasing foods such as eggplant, ladyfingers, or oily fish when one has a wound or skin disease. Indeed, more attention is paid to observing food restrictions than to applying topical medicines or keeping a wound clean. These practices are everyday forms of harm reduction.

In the same area of India, Ayurvedic preparations are consumed to purify the blood and enhance digestion, two of the primary causes of many illnesses. Medicines are taken to prevent illness associated with behavior thought to have a negative effect on the body. A rickshaw driver might ingest 100 ml of *dasamulla aristha* (an Ayurvedic tonic thought to enhance digestion) each day after work to reduce the harm of driving in congested traffic and breathing the fumes of vehicles. Other harm-reduction practices associated with occupational health include the consumption of vitamin tonics and vitamin B12 injections by beedie cigarette rollers. These medicines are thought to decrease weakness as well as protecting against diseases such as TB (Nichter and Vuckovic 1994).

Exposure to pesticides is well recognized to cause ill health among farmers. Harm-reduction practices are undertaken to minimize the negative health effects of dangerous chemicals in many Asian countries. For example, in India, plantation workers responsible for spraying areca trees demand coconut oil from their employers to place on their bodies after spraying. An oil bath is thought to cool and purify the body, reducing the harm of heat and toxic chemicals. In Northeast Thailand, farmers who spray rice fields with pesticides consume medicines such as alum to cause impurities in their body to settle ("like residue in a well") and other medicines to help them purge poisons. And in some areas of Southern Mexico, agricultural laborers consume Alka-seltzer because they believe the carbonation removes the harmful fumes trapped in the body (Cartwright, personal communication).

Notably, many Thai, Indian, and Sri Lankan farmers will not eat the vegetable crops they spray with pesticides and send to market. Separate plots are reserved for growing the foods the household will consume. In India, gastritis has emerged as a new illness category associated with the consumption of pesticide-laden foods (Nichter 2001b). Herbal medicines are taken to rid the body of toxins when forms of diarrhea treated with allopathic medicines do not subside. Ayurvedic doctors point out that the afflicted suffer from a condition caused by the buildup of toxins caused by both pesticide-laden foods and undigested medicines. For this reason, some people periodically take herbal medicines to reduce the harm of accumulated toxins in their bodies.

Like pesticides, strong allopathic (Western) medicines are thought to harm the body if one is exposed to them for an extended period of time. In India, there is a widespread belief that strong medicines, including antibiotics, are heating to the body and spoil the blood. Twenty years ago people consumed milk with antibiotics to reduce these side effects. Today, new herbal products are explicitly marketed to reduce the harm of allopathic medicines (Nichter and Vuckovic 1994). It is important to note that concerns about medicines have not reduced their popularity in South and Southeast Asia (India, Thailand, and the Philippines). The numbers of medicines have risen steadily until there are multiple pills for every ill. My point is that the very popularity of allopathic medicines has facilitated the growth of the harm-reduction market. Harm reduction is an important part of health-care transition in Asia (Nichter and Van Sickle 2002) as well as the rest of the world. A desire for fast relief, coupled with long-standing indigenous health concerns, has fostered the complementary use of modern and traditional medicines and the practice of integrated medicine. In India, allopathic medicines are taken to kill germs and for quick relief, while Ayurvedic and other herbal medicines are taken to reduce the harm of strong medicines and to restore the body's natural processes, humoral balance, and digestive power.

Medicines are widely used for harm reduction in Asia. Thresholds of symptom tolerance have dramatically reduced over the past two decades, and people turn to medicines much faster now than they used to for a wide variety of complaints. Medicines are consumed to reduce discomfort as well as to enable those living in polluted environments to cope with adversity. For many people living in a state of chronic ill health, medicines are purchased over the counter to get them through the day and night. Those living in polluted urban environments turn to medicines to manage recurrent abdominal complaints that they associate with everything from polluted water and adulterated foods to stress. In this case, medicines are often taken as harm reduction to prevent emergent symptoms from becoming worse.

Other medicines are taken to provide energy when strength is failing and to reduce pain when much work remains to be done. In Thailand, some agricultural employers provide stimulants and pain relievers to get harvest workers through the day. From a strictly functional health vantage point, workers view these as a form of harm reduction. For similar reasons, Valium is taken by manual laborers living in squalor to help them sleep so they can work the next day, and steroids are taken to reduce persistent body pain, skin diseases, or cough. Many users of these drugs whom I have interviewed recognize that these medicines are not solutions to their problems but only stop-gap measures. They are aware that they can become dependent on medicines and that taking medicines for too long may be harmful (Nichter 2001b). They recognize that temporary harm-reduction solutions may cause future problems. But what choice do they have? Is their medicine-taking a form of agency or a form of domination at the site of the body? This is not a simple and straightforward question to answer.

Let me now turn to another dimension of harm reduction, the appropriation of curative medicines for harm-reduction purposes. This emerging trend is important and an area of study I have dedicated several years to investigating. The first of three case studies involves medicines taken to manage latent women's illnesses in Northeast Thailand (Boonmongkon, Pylypa, and Nichter 1999; Boonmongkon, Nichter, and Pylypa 2001). The second case involves medicines taken to minimize the progression of lung problems to TB in the Philippines (Nichter 1994), and the third case involves medicines consumed as prophylactics to reduce the chances of getting a sexually transmitted disease in the Philippines and Thailand (Nichter 2001a). A fourth case illustrates how vaccinations are understood as a form of harm reduction by a population that has little understanding of the immune system.

Mot Luuk Problems: Keeping Latent Illness in Check

In Thailand, a wide array of symptoms broadly associated with the reproductive tract, abdominal and pelvic regions, and sometimes the urinary tract are linked to the uterus *(mot luuk)* through cultural reasoning. *Mot luuk* problems are associated with childbearing and inadequate postpartum care, menstruation and forms of contraception that interfere with menstruation, hard manual labor and accidents, and exposure to impurity and sexually transmitted infections. Both past events and current exposures to these risk factors are thought to render a woman vulnerable to *mot luuk* problems. Many women with recurrent symptoms view their problems as ultimately resulting from some earlier life event such as an injury experienced during youth, a complication during a past pregnancy or abortion, or an inadequate period of *yuu fai. Yuu fai* is the postpartum practice of "staying by the fire" for 10 to 15 days following childbirth to reposition and dry out the *mot luuk*. A proper *yuu fai* is considered to be an investment in a woman's future health, and it is clearly related to harm reduction. A uterus that remains damp constitutes an internal environment in which troubles related to impurity more readily occur and internal wounds are more difficult to heal.

Various forms of impurities are sources of *mot luuk* problems. Symptoms are spoken of as resulting from *seua laa [cheua raa]*, a term that literally translates as "fungus" but is also more broadly associated with dirtiness or germs. Women are particularly susceptible to *seua laa* because the vagina is open to *seua laa* from the exterior world, in contrast to men's genitals, which are more closed. Particularly relevant here is that women with recurrent or chronic symptoms often see their illness as latent. Disease or germs remain in their bodies because a "wound" *(phee [phlee])* in the uterus persists without ever entirely healing. *Look lop nai [rook lop nai]* refers to such illness that "hides" in the body and emerges at times of vulnerability. Some women interpret vaginal discharge experienced before menses as a latent illness emerging. Others speak of *seua laa* accumulating in the body as a result of poor hygiene or sexual transmission. At times of vulnerability, the *seua laa* emerges as disease.

Many women fear that recurrent or chronic symptoms will transform into more severe illnesses, their greatest concern being cervical cancer (*maleng paak mot luuk*, or simply *maleng*). To keep latent disease in check, women commonly treat their *mot luuk* problems, regardless of perceived etiology, with two popular brands of tetracycline (Kaanoo® and Hero®). Notably, these brands of tetracycline are widely believed to be good for *mot luuk* problems in general and both curative and harm-reduction properties are attributed to them.[4] They are at once taken for symptomatic relief, to prevent *mot luuk* problems from becoming worse, and as a prophylactic against the recurrence of problems experienced in the past. Just as some agricultural workers swallow painkillers during harvest season to enable them to work harder and longer, some women swallow antibiotics to prevent pain and to reduce the negative impact hard work might have on their *mot luuk*.

Preventing Weak Lungs from Becoming TB

In popular Filipino health culture, *weak lungs* is a specific ambiguous term used to describe states of ill health in which a child experiences recurrent or prolonged cough and cold, loss of weight and lack of appetite, fatigue and restlessness, and low-grade "inside fever" *(nangingilalim ang lagnat)*. Under such conditions it is often imagined that either the lungs have become coated with mucus *(plema)* as a result of previous illnesses (usually associated with acute respiratory illness) or a child is predisposed to weak lungs as a result of signs such as wheezing *(hapo)* or a history of TB in the family. Among adults, if a person is unable to work hard, weak lungs are suspected.

Weak lungs are recognized as a common condition by the lay population, who believe that many children suffering from weak lungs will develop TB when they get older if their condition is not cured. Practitioners contribute to local perceptions of weak lungs. To avoid stigmatizing patients, doctors commonly talk about weak lungs in cases of both primary complex (TB among children) and TB without dramatic signs such as spitting blood. Patients are given TB medication and told to take it so they do not become TB patients. This contributes to the belief that coughs transform into weak lungs that may then become TB.

Medicines taken to strengthen weak lungs are commonly referred to as *vitamin sa baga*, vitamins for the lungs, and anti-TB drugs such as INH are perceived to strengthen the lungs.[5] Consequently, poor patients on TB regimens sometimes share *vitamin sa baga* with family members and neighbors as a harm-reduction resource when they have a long-standing cough or wheeze. I have documented INH being purchased over the counter for this purpose in both the Philippines and South India.

Taking Prophylactic Antibiotics to Prevent STDs

While conducting in-depth interviews with female commercial-sex workers in Cebu City, Philippines, I found that most engaged in some form of harm-reduction practice besides the use of condoms as a means of reducing the chance of becoming infected with a sexually transmitted disease (STD). Their harm-reduction practices ranged from urinating after sex to douching with shampoo, toothpaste, or Coca Cola; swallowing laundry detergent after sex; or using antibiotics as a prophylactic (Nichter 2001a).

The practice of taking antibiotics as a means of harm reduction proved to be quite popular. Out of a random sample of 160 women who had had sex for money in the past two weeks, 20 percent reported that they took antibiotics to reduce their chances of getting an STD occasionally and another 18 percent stated they did so routinely.[6] Among occasional and routine users, 24 percent reported using prophylactic antibiotics after having sex with each customer, 9 percent before having sex, and 4 percent before and after having sex. Fifteen percent reported taking antibiotics for prophylaxis two or three times a week, 6 percent once a month, and 31 percent when they felt that some illness might be developing in their body.

Why were these medicines taken? While some commercial-sex workers (CSWs) used a combination of condoms and antibiotics to play it safe, the most common users of antibiotics were freelance CSWs in the weakest position to negotiate condom use with their clientele. They had the lowest condom use and were the most inclined to take antibiotics as both a routine harm-reduction practice and a way to enhance their sense of personal control. Notably, many thought antibiotics might protect them against AIDS.

Prophylactic use of antibiotics as a form of harm reduction following risky sex is also common in Thailand. Before visiting prostitutes, some men take antibiotics to render themselves less vulnerable to illness; others take antibiotics or purifying medicines (*ya lang tai, ya kap lum klung*—which often contain diuretics and antibiotics) after sex to kill germs while they are weak. Notably, many Thai men have stopped going to brothels since government health-education programs began demonizing prostitutes as the source of AIDS. Many men now have sex with pick-up girls working in restaurants, and although the rate of condom use in brothels is presently quite high, the rate of condom use with pick-up girls is quite low. Men feel they are less likely to get AIDS from these women and rely on antibiotics as a form of harm reduction against STDs. Some men interviewed spoke of this behavior as harm reduction for their wives, who might pick up impurities and germs from them but have less resistance to disease. Men commonly waited a few days after extramarital sex to see if symptoms would manifest or took special foods to hasten symptoms, enabling them to treat disease before it became established and before any germ could infect their wives.

Measles Vaccinations As Harm Reduction

The popular interpretation of measles vaccine in rural India provides a final lesson for us to consider in this section as it raises the issue that in some contexts harm reduction may be a more culturally acceptable concept than total prevention. How does one explain how vaccinations work to a group of people having minimal knowledge of germs and immunity? Although this is difficult in general, explaining the purpose of measles vaccinations in India is particularly challenging for three reasons: a) the disease is associated with the wrath of various deities, b) other diseases share symptoms with measles and are thought to be variations of the same illness complex, and c) people fear adult measles to such an extent that childhood measles seems less a threat. Explanations to Indians that measles vaccinations prevented the disease did not sit well with many informants, who were much more comfortable with the message that the vaccination prevented their children from developing a serious life-threatening case of measles (Nichter 1995; Bishat and Coutinho 2000). Total protection was not seen as possible nor did it match local experience, which was colored by ineffective vaccinations and the occurrence of rashes caused by other diseases. Harm reduction in the form of protection, on the other hand, was appreciated because it was a concept familiar to local populations.

HARM REDUCTION AS A WAY OF LIFE IN THE UNITED STATES

My discussion of harm reduction as a way of life in the United States is informed by theories of "risk society" proposed by social theorists such as Beck (1992, 1996) and Giddens (1991). Emerging during late modernity and superseding industrial, class-based society, risk society is characterized by an individualized response to risk at a time when confidence in the state is lagging, the future appears uncertain, and mistrust of the corporate scientific enterprise is increasing.[7] According to risk society theorists, people experience information overload and maintain some measure of doubt about the motives of information brokers who are recognized to be stakeholders. In this context, people construct risk biographies and exercise agency by choosing courses of action based on those facts they choose to acknowledge at any given time. Harm-reduction practices take on new meaning in this environment in relation to 1) a rising sense of risk and vulnerability fostered by science, the media, and a burgeoning risk industry; 2) decreasing optimism that scientific discovery will be able to solve pressing health problems in short measure; and 3) growing pressure to assume personal responsibility for health fostered by the state, business interests, and a long-standing Jacksonian self-help ethic.

Three topics provide unique perspectives into the meaning of harm-reduction practices in the United States. One is the importance of token harm-reduction gestures in an environment saturated with fast-fix opportunities that appeal to a population on the run. Another is the manner in which the U.S. political economy has forced workers to take up harm-reduction practices to stay on the job. The final topic covers harm-reduction products that create the illusion that we can indulge in unhealthy but enjoyable behavior while acting responsibly; smoking safer cigarettes is one example.

Harm Reduction: Token Gestures

Returning to America after research in a developing country is always sobering to me. Thankful to be able to drink water from the tap, I am struck by people's increasing mistrust of public water and willingness to purchase water from exotic places where life is pure. Then there is the rising concern about food. A read of the best-selling book *Fast Food Nation* (Schlosser 2001) is enough to make anyone insecure about much of what they eat. Add to this newspaper headlines and journal articles about "resistant pathogens" found in the meat of animals dosed with prophylactic antibiotics (Gorbach 2001), and one cannot help but consider becoming a vegetarian. But then again, are vegetables safe, given pesticide use and genetic engineering (Reidar 1999; Bray, this volume)?

A quick trip to any U.S. supermarket might suggest to a foreign visitor that people in the United States are obsessively concerned about the safety of their food. After all, where else in the world are products sold more by what they do not contain (calories, cholesterol, sodium, caffeine, "chemicals") than by what they actually have in them? Given this apparent health consciousness, one might expect to see consumer citizens cautiously reading food labels and engaged in defensive shopping. Although some people do so, many people are in a hurry, purchase familiar products, and pay little attention to food labels.[8] In response to information overload about what is and is not in foods, it is likely that as many Americans assume a fatalistic attitude toward risk as buying into biopower (heightened health consciousness) and engage in personal surveillance.[9] Where one falls on a risk-concern continuum depends largely on one's immediate sense of strength and vulnerability. One thing that is fairly certain, however, is that most people engage in some form of token harm-reduction gesture at some time—if not for themselves, then for concerned others.

Token harm-reduction gestures provide people with a sense of control and enable them to feel they are acting responsibly. If people cannot take major steps toward promoting their health or reducing harm due to cost, time, or inclination, they can at least do something token and beneficial, such as using low-sodium salt, drinking 1-percent milk, or consuming chips with 30 percent less fat. An entire harm-reduction industry caters to the psychosocial as well as physical needs of Americans who attempt to balance some measure of control and release in their lives (Crawford 1984). The provision of NutraSweet, "lite," and organic solutions for the problems of modern living is big business and fosters as much hype as it offers promise (Nichter and Nichter 1991).

Vitamins As a Quick Fix

Vitamins are a case in point. Vitamins were a $6-billion business in the United States in 1996[10] and the harm-reduction resource of choice for millions of Americans (Apple 1996). Vitamins are marketed to the masses as a means of addressing a wide variety of health concerns in the present as well as avoiding health problems in the future. As a form of harm reduction, vitamins are taken when people do not feel that their fast-paced lifestyles are conducive to healthy eating and as insurance against environmental hazards, life stresses, compromised immune systems, and potential deficiencies (Vuckovic and Nichter 1997). At a time when the quality of the American diet is being questioned, vitamin pills are taken as an antidote for fast-food deficiencies and to remove antioxidants that accumulate from poor eating habits. Taking one's vitamins, like the eating of health foods, allows one to balance out an otherwise unhealthy diet (Backett 1992), reduce the harm of a drinking binge, minimize the ill effects of too little sleep, or reduce the chances of getting cancer. Vitamins are thought to help one compensate for suboptimal behavior and buy time to engage in healthy behavior later.

Vitamins are popular worldwide. Is the meaning of vitamin-taking in the United States any different from vitamin-taking elsewhere? The answer is both no and yes. In all countries, vitamins are taken to enhance strength, promote health, and protect against illness. In the United States, however, taking vitamin pills is associated with a new secular moral identity (Conrad 1993) in which health actions such as harm reduction are valorized. In taking vitamins, acts of appropriate consumption produce a health identity by what they signify (Baudrillard 1981; Ito Hardenbergh 2001). Even people who don't exercise or eat fruits and vegetables can at least take their vitamins. In an environment where corporeal transgression in the form of indulgence is commonplace (Williams 1998) and where people are expected to promote health and engage in harm reduction, taking vitamins is a basic minimal act of responsibility.

Vitamins are also a food drug (Jankowiak and Bradburd 1996) that fits the ideology of our times, an ideology of flexible accumulation (Martin 1991) wherein adaptability, multitasking, and robustness are valued by a society experiencing economic change that is constantly in flux. Vitamins are sold as a resource to increase vitality and enhance one's immune system in an uncertain world full of new challenges. Vitamins are marketed as giving one an edge, and in an era of "flexible specialization," there appears to be a vitamin combination specially designed for every health challenge.

Practicing Harm Reduction to Stay Employed

We live in an age of "time famine" when there just doesn't seem to be enough time to get all the things done we need to do. This is as true (if not more true) for poor people as for the middle class. In her research on self-medication in American households, Vuckovic (1999) found that self-medication was often used as a means of coping with time famine. Her female informants expressed that they did not have time to be sick and thus used over-the-counter medicines for themselves or their children so they could continue being productive despite their illness.

What I would call attention to here is the necessity of working mothers to engage in harm reduction as a means of staying employed. In today's insecure work environment, many people worry about losing their jobs due to sickness. Two complementary patterns of harm-reduction behavior emerge.

The first behavior pattern involves mothers who cannot afford to stay home for fear of losing their jobs when their young children are ill. Mothers send their children to day care centers, knowing this is the easiest place for a child to pick up an illness. Many remain vigilant about their children's health and practice many forms of harm reduction. They may wash their children with antibacterial soap, give their children vitamins every day, give their children leftover antibiotics at the first sign of illness, or give them cough medicines to mask symptoms so they can attend day care the next day. Mothers attempt to buy time with these medicines, enabling them to make it through the week until the weekend when they will have time to tend to the child during the day.

The second complementary pattern of behavior involves workers who mask the symptoms of illness on the job to keep the job. Workers often self-treat illnesses during the week and attempt to make it through until the weekend. Going to work while ill and contagious leads to the spread of disease among coworkers. Aware of this, coworkers are compelled to engage in forms of harm reduction that typically involve the taking of medicines, be they antibiotics or herbal remedies.

Harm Reduction As Illusion: Cigarettes

Many of the things we find enjoyable we later learn place us at considerable risk for ill health. This knowledge creates a demand for some way to reduce the harm of a valued but risky behavior as an alternative to having to give it up entirely. In many instances a safer way of doing or consuming something can be identified (using sunscreen lotion, for example). In other cases, the illusion of harm reduction is sold to a public all too willing to be deluded. The story of safer cigarettes is a prime example. It is beyond the scope of this essay to go into a detailed history of the tobacco industry's attempts to sell the illusion of a healthier cigarette (see Stratton et al. 2001 for a review), but let me list five strategies the industry has used:

1. The introduction of various types of filters, leading one to believe that the harmful elements of tobacco smoke are removed
2. Creating milder light and ultra-light brands
3. Adding menthol to tobacco, making deep "cool" inhalation easier due to menthol's anesthetic properties
4. Engaging in the tar and numbers game and feeding comparative reasoning and the belief that there are safer cigarettes
5. Advertising cigarettes as containing no "bull" and being a natural product devoid of harmful chemicals

The tobacco industry has worked hard to popularize the idea that safe smoking is possible, even though cigarettes are one of the few products freely available in the marketplace that, if used as directed, will harm you. Many people smoke light or ultra-light cigarettes as an act of harm reduction, thinking that smoking 10 of these cigarettes could not be as unhealthy or addictive as smoking 10 regulars. Studies of smoking topography suggest this is not true. It has been well demonstrated that humans have the capacity to adjust their smoking behavior (self-regulating the rate and depth of inhalation) to adjust to the quantity of nicotine in a cigarette. Other smokers engage in harm-reduction strategies based on the impression that only smoking at particular levels is harmful (e.g., more than five a day), and still others don't see smoking as unhealthy in the short term because they view the risk of smoking as cumulative (Slovic 2000). They, of course, plan to quit before the cumulative harm is great and talk about quitting later. Their "quit talk" serves as a means of establishing a positive health identity (Tesler 2000). It is at once a response to biopower ("I should quit") and a harm-reduction strategy aimed at protecting one's identity as a responsible person who "knows when to say when."[11]

FUTURE RESEARCH

Let me identify what I see as productive avenues of future research in the anthropology of vulnerability, risk, and harm reduction. The literature on risk, especially risk society, is often painted with very broad brush strokes. For medical anthropologists, it is diversity in the experience and response to risk that are important. We need finer-grain assessments of how individuals actually cope with states of vulnerability and perceptions of risk (Lupton 1999: 102–103). Called for are studies of "clever citizens" (Giddens 1994) coping with partial and often contradictory information about protective and risk factors affecting their health. How do these people respond to information about risk and to what extent is their response influenced by the form and content of information versus the credibility of the person delivering it? When vulnerability is experienced or risk is recognized, who chooses which types of harm-reduction strategies, in what circumstances, and with what ramifications for themselves and others?

To understand the harm-reduction actions of individuals, we need to better appreciate the social relations of risk and vulnerability. Needed are ethnographies of risk management within households and communities that pay attention to social risk (that is, risk to social relations/identity) and existing and potential social relations. Concern about social risk often eclipses concern about physical risk (Connors 1992; Sobo 1994, 1995; Campbell 1995; Heise and Elias 1995; Nichter 2002). Understanding when this happens may give us insights into why preventive health measures are and are not adopted and when downstream harm reduction (such as taking antibiotics after risky sex) is preferred to upstream prevention (such as using a condom).

Finally, we need to move beyond a focus on utilitarian individualism and consider the response of social networks to risk as well as examples of how risk may mobilize community in the name of mutual protection and healing. Future research on harm reduction needs to pay as much attention to collective efficacy as to personal efficacy.

Harm reduction is a subject that invites anthropologists to consider diversity in the way people experience and respond to risk individually and within social groups. It leads us to ponder the great balancing act between short-term gain and potential long-term consequences.

NOTES

1. Another domain of research within this thematic area is formative research with the purpose of developing harm-reduction strategies in public health. An example would be research facilitating needle-exchange programs to reduce HIV and hepatitis transmission.

2. Perceptions of weak and strong children influence patterns of behavior referred to by various scholars as selective survival (Howard 1994) and selective neglect (Scheper-Hughes 1985).

3. See the work of Slovic (2000) on cumulative risk thinking and how it affects smoking behavior in the United States.

4. In Thailand, tetracycline products are wrongly marketed as good for women's problems (Boongmongkon, Nichter, and Pylypa 2001).

5. The impression that TB medicines are vitamins for weak lungs is fostered by the marketing strategies of manufacturers of INH. Some brands of INH prominently display the word "vitamin" on the label of the product (e.g., odinah). In other cases, product names are suggestive (e.g., Trisovit).

6. The median number of antibiotic pills or capsules taken for prophylactic purposes was one per treatment event, and the most common antibiotics used were ampicillin (55 percent), rifampicin (16 percent), and amoxicillin (15 percent). Rifampicin misuse is cause for alarm as it is the most important of all TB drugs.

7. Beck and Gidden's theories of reflexive modernization draw a distinction between early and late modernity. Early modernity is characterized by the invention of the concept of risk, which transformed a radically indeterminate cosmos into a manageable one through the myth of calculability (Reddy 1996). The late period is characterized by a growing sense of uncertainty and ambivalence, distrust of rapidly changing and contradictory expert knowledge, and the globalization of doubt. In late modernity, risk is not easily calculable, and the politics of responsibility become more, not less, complex. Scientific skepticism turns inward, risk factors are contested, and progress is questioned in the wake of experiments in modernity gone awry. Fear mongers also depict would-be perils as imminent disasters (Glassner 1999).

8. The health claims used to market foods are often misleading if not spurious.

9. Foucault (1980) uses the term "biopower" to describe how knowledge and power relations are closely aligned. For example, once people are informed about risk, they feel compelled to act accordingly; they change their practices and engage in personal surveillance. Knowledge about risk makes social institutions as well as individuals accountable.

10. The vitamin industry grossed over $6 billion in 1996, doubling its sales from 1992. According to vitamin retailer GNC, the total retail value for the market for vitamins and supplements in 1998 was $8.9 billion, and it is projected to reach $16.5 billion by 2003. Growth is driven mostly by demographics. Adults over the age of 45, already the heaviest vitamin users by far, are also the fastest-growing population segment (Apple 1996).

11. My reference here is to a Budweiser advertisement for responsible drinking.

REFERENCES

Apple, Rima. 1996. *Vitamania: Vitamins in American Culture.* New Brunswick, NJ: Rutgers University Press.

Backett, Kathryn. 1992. "Taboos and Excesses: Lay Health Moralities in Middle Class Families." *Sociology of Health and Illness* 14(2): 255–274.

Baudrillard, Jean. 1981. *For a Critique of the Political Economy of the Sign.* St. Louis, Mo: Telos Press.

Beck, Ulrich. 1992. *Risk Society: Towards a New Modernity.* London: Sage Publications.

———. 1996. "World Risk Society as Cosmopolitan Society? Ecological Question in a Framework of Manufactured Uncertainties." *Theory, Culture and Society* 13(4): 1–32.

Bishat, Suman, and Lester Coutinho. 2000. "When Cure is Better Than Prevention: Immunity and Preventive Care of Measles." *Economic and Political Weekly* 35(8–9): 697–708.

Boonmongkon, Pimpawun, Mark Nichter, and Jen Pylypa. 2001. "Women's 'Mot Luuk' Problems in Northeast Thailand: Why Women's Own Health Concerns Matter as Much as Disease Rates." *Social Science and Medicine.* 53(8): 1095–1112.

Boonmongkon, Pimpawun, Jen Pylypa, and Mark Nichter. 1999. "Emerging Fears of Cervical Cancer in Northeast Thailand." *Anthropology in Medicine* 6(3): 359–380.

Campbell, Carole A. 1995. "Male Gender Roles and Sexuality: Implications for Women's AIDS Risk and Prevention." *Social Science and Medicine* 41(2): 197–201.

Cartwright, Liz. Personal communication. November 1, 2000.

Conners, Margaret M. 1992. "Risk Perception, Risk Taking, and Risk Management among Intravenous Drug Users: Implications for AIDS Prevention." *Social Science and Medicine* 34(6): 591–601.

Conrad, Peter. 1993. "Wellness as Virtue: Morality and the Pursuit of Health." *Culture, Medicine, and Psychiatry* 18(3): 385–401.

Crawford, Robert. 1984. "A Cultural Account of 'Health': Control, Release, and the Social Body." In *Issues in the Political Economy of Health Care,* ed. John McKinlay, 60–101. New York: Tavistock Publications.

Foucault, Michel. 1980. *The History of Sexuality.* Vol. 1. New York: Vintage Books. Translated from the French by Robert Hurley.

Giddens, Anthony. 1991. *Modernity and Self-Identity: Self and Society in the Late Modern Age.* Cambridge: Polity Press.

———. 1994. *Beyond the Left and the Right: The Future of Radical Politics.* Cambridge: Polity Press.

Glassner, Barry. 1999. *The Culture of Fear: Why Americans Are Afraid of the Wrong Things.* New York: Basic Books.

Glick, Leonard B. 1967. "Medicine as Ethnographic Category: The Gimi of the New Guinea Highlands." *Ethnology* 6(1): 31–56.

Gorbach, Sherwood L. 2001. "Antimicrobial Use in Animal Feed—Time to Stop." *The New England Journal of Medicine* 345(16): 1202–1203.

Heise, Lori L., and Christopher Elias. 1995. "Transforming AIDS Prevention to Meet Women's Needs: A Focus on Developing Countries." *Social Science and Medicine* 40(7): 931–943.

Howard, Mary. 1994. "Socio-economic Causes and Cultural Explanations of Childhood: Malnutrition among the Chagga of Tanzania." *Social Science and Medicine* 38(2): 239–251.

Ito Hardenbergh, Loren. 2001. Swallowing Health Ideology: Vitamin Consumption among University Students in the Contemporary United States. Master's thesis, Department of Anthropology, University of Arizona.

Jankowiak, William, and Dan Bradburd. 1996. "Using Drug Foods to Capture and Enhance Labor Performance: A Cross Cultural Perspective." *Current Anthropology* 37(4): 717–720.

Kanato, Manop. 1994. An Ethnographic-Participatory Study of Commercial Sex Workers Responding to the Problem of HIV/AIDS in Khan Kaen, Thailand. Doctoral dissertation, McMaster University.

Kavanaugh, Anne M., and Dorothy H. Broom. 1998. "Embodied Risk: My Body, Myself?" *Social Science and Medicine* 46(3): 437–444.

Lupton, Deborah. 1999. *Risk.* New York: Routledge.

Martin, Emily. 1991. "The End of the Body?" *American Ethnologist* 19(1): 121–140.

Mull, Dorothy S. 1992. "Mother's Milk and Pseudoscientific Breast Milk Testing in Pakistan." *Social Science and Medicine* 34(11): 1277–1290.

Nichter, Mark. 1986. "Modes of Food Classification and the Diet-Health Contingency: A South Indian Case Study." In *Modes of Food Classification in South Asia*, eds. R. Khare and K. Ishvaran, 185–221. Durham, N.C.: Carolina Academic Press.

———. 1987. "Cultural Dimensions of Hot-Cold and *Sema* in the Sri Lankan Health Culture." In *Hot-Cold Conceptualization: A Reassessment*, ed. Lenore Manderson, 377–387. *Social Science and Medicine* (special edition).

———. 1994. "Illness Semantics and International Health: The Weak Lungs/TB Complex in the Philippines." *Social Science and Medicine* 38(5): 649–663.

———. 1995. "Vaccinations in the Third World: A Consideration of Community Demand." *Social Science and Medicine* 41(5): 617–632.

———. 2001a. "Vulnerability, Prophylactic Antibiotic Use, Harm Reduction and the Misguided Appropriation of Medical Resources: The Case of STD's in Southeast Asia." In *Culture and Reproductive Health*, ed. Carla Obermeyer, 101–127. Oxford University Press.

———. 2001b. "India and the Political Ecology of Health: Indigestion as Sign and Symptom of Defective Modernization." In *Healing Powers: Traditional Medicine, Shamanism and Science in Contemporary Asia*, eds. Linda Connor and Geoffrey Samuel, 85–108. New York: Greenwood Press.

———. 2002. "Social Relations of Therapy Management." *New Horizons in Medical Anthropology*, eds. Mark Nichter and Margaret Lock, 81–110. New York: Routledge.

Nichter, Mark, and Mimi Nichter. 1991. "Hype and Weight." *Medical Anthropology* 13(3): 249–284.

Nichter, Mark, and David Van Sickle. 2002. "The Challenges of India's Health and Health Care Transition." In *India Briefing: Quicken the Pace of Change*, eds. Alyssa Ayres and Philip Oldenburg. Armonk, N.Y.: Asia Society Publication.

Nichter, Mark, and Nancy Vuckovic. 1994. "Agenda for an Anthropology of Pharmaceutical Practice." *Social Science and Medicine* 39(11): 1509–1525.

Reddy, Sanjay. 1996. "Claims to Expert Knowledge and the Subversion of Democracy: The Triumph of Risk over Uncertainty." *Economy and Society* 25(2): 222–254.

Reidar, Almas. 1999. "Food Trust, Ethics, and Safety in Risk Society." *Sociological Research Online* 4(3): U282-U291.

Scheper-Hughes, Nancy. 1985. "Culture, Scarcity, and Maternal Thinking: Maternal Detachment and Infant Survival in a Brazilian Shantytown." *Ethos* 13(4): 291–317.

Schlosser, Eric. 2001. *Fast Food Nation: The Dark Side of the All-American Meal.* Boston: Houghton Mifflin.

Slovic, Paul. 2000. "What Does It Mean to Know a Cumulative Risk? Adolescents' Perceptions of Short-term and Long-term Consequences of Smoking." *Journal of Behavioral Decision Making* 13(2): 259–266.

Sobo, Elisa J. 1994. "Inner-City Women and AIDS: The Psychosocial Benefits of Unsafe Sex." *Culture, Medicine and Psychiatry* 17(4): 455–485.

———. 1995. *Choosing Unsafe Sex: AIDS-Risk Denial among Disadvantaged Women.* Philadelphia: University of Pennsylvania Press.

Stratton, Kathleen, Padma Shetty, Robert Wallace, and Stuart Bondurant, eds. 2001. *Clearing the Smoke: Assessing the Scientific Base for Tobacco Harm Reduction.* Washington, D.C.: Institute of Medicine, National Academy Press.

Tesler, Laura. 2000. Locations of Self in Smoking Discourses and Practices: An Ethnog-
    raphy of Smoking among Adolescents and Young Adults in the United States.
    Master's thesis, Department of Anthropology, University of Arizona.
Vuckovic, Nancy. 1999. "Fast Relief: Buying Time with Medications." *Medical Anthro-
    pology Quarterly* 13(1): 15–68.
Vuckovic, Nancy, and Mark Nichter. 1997. "Pharmaceutical Practice in the U.S.: Re-
    search Agenda for the Next Decade." *Social Science and Medicine* 44(9):
    1285–1302.
Williams, Simon. 1998. "Health as Moral Performance: Ritual, Transgression and
    Taboo." *Health* 2(4): 435–457.

Part II

The Cultivation of Fear

Chapter 2

Autonomy, Danger, and Choice: The Moral Imperative of an "At Risk" Pregnancy for a Group of Low-Income Latinas in Texas

Linda M. Hunt and Katherine B. de Voogd

INTRODUCTION

It is increasingly common in clinical medicine to assess the risk status of individual patients for various diseases or health outcomes and recommend treatments or other behaviors based on that assessment. The probability that an individual will develop a given condition is calculated based on epidemiological observations of characteristics associated with the distribution of the condition in the general population. Once classified as having an at-risk health status, the individual encounters an implicit social imperative to modify risk-related attributes or behaviors, for example, by avoiding or consuming certain substances or by accepting certain tests or services (Handwerker 1994; Kenen 1996; Rockhill 2001).

Risk assessment is particularly salient in the burgeoning field of genetic diagnosis. At present, clinical applications of our growing genetic knowledge are limited to risk-modeling of the statistical likelihood that an individual having a particular genetic profile will develop a given condition. There are currently no specific clinical interventions for modifying the genetic risk status of an individual, but only techniques designed to assess the likelihood of a gene's manifestation or reproduction.

We wish to thank the San Antonio Area Foundation for a generous grant in support of this project. Julia Sargent made many important contributions to the data analysis and interpretations presented in this chapter. Elizabeth Cameron and Holly Dygert also assisted with data analysis. Many thanks to Carole Browner, who was integrally involved in conceptualizing the research we report here and generously shared her research instruments with us. Dr. Browner also provided thoughtful comments on an earlier draft of this chapter. We also wish to thank the staff and patients of the Prenatal Genetics Clinic, whose kind cooperation made this project possible.

One field in which assessment of genetic risk status has moved into the mainstream and is affecting a wide cross section of the population is prenatal genetic testing. Screening for certain genetic and chromosomal conditions is now a routine part of prenatal care in the United States (Rothman 1986; Press and Browner 1994; Rapp 1998, 2000). It is now standard obstetric practice to assess the risk of all pregnant women for carrying a fetus affected by common genetic anomalies, including Down Syndrome and neural tube defects. Women with pregnancies found to be at risk, based on their age, family history, or blood test results, are offered further testing to determine whether a birth anomaly in fact exists.

It is the condition of being at risk and the woman's perception of what she can and should do in responding to that risk status that we will examine in this chapter. We report on a study of low-income Latinas in Texas whose pregnancies were determined to be at risk based on abnormal blood tests. For most of these women, being classified as at risk was completely unexpected due to the routine nature of the blood test. By considering their experiences, we have an opportunity to explore how women may perceive and respond to the at-risk label per se in the absence of preconceived expectations about the risk status of their pregnancy.

Until recently, it was primarily educated, white, middle-class women who were being offered prenatal genetic screening and diagnostic tests. However, as these tests have become routine in prenatal care, large numbers of low-income and working-class ethnic minority women are being asked to make decisions about their desire to be tested. Many women now being offered these tests may hold values, goals, and understandings different from those of mainstream clinical culture (Browner, Preloran, and Cox 1999; Rapp 2000). Although a handful of studies have considered some socioeconomic correlates of minority women's prenatal testing behavior (Sokal et al. 1980; Swerts 1987; Evans et al. 1993; Pryde et al. 1993), little is known about the way such patients might make these decisions. In a study of amniocentesis decision-making, Browner and Preloran (1999) found that the Latina women they studied were often unprepared for making the choice they were offered and accepted the test not so much out of an interest in having the diagnostic information but as a way to resolve the doubts about the pregnancy introduced by the screening results.

To further explore these questions, we have replicated Browner and Preloran's methodology with a group of low-income Latina women who, in the course of routine prenatal care at a public clinic in Texas, were told that their blood-screening test indicated they were at risk for carrying a fetus with a genetic anomaly. Our analysis of their experiences and perceptions indicates that such women may not perceive the offer of further testing in morally neutral terms but rather as carrying an implicit responsibility. Having their pregnancies classified as at risk was experienced by many of these women as a moral imperative to take action "for the good of the baby" (cf. Press and Browner

1997). Many accepted further testing not so much because they valued the knowledge it would produce but simply because they felt compelled to remove the pregnancy from the quasi-disease state of being classified as at risk. We contend that many women experienced the unsolicited knowledge provided by prenatal genetic screening not as an opportunity to make an autonomous decision about their desire to have a definitive diagnosis but as a moral mandate to accept further testing to restore their pregnancies to a normal, healthful status.

CONTEXT AND BACKGROUND

Assessing risk status for Down Syndrome, neural tube defects, and Trisomy 18[1] is currently a standard practice in prenatal care in the United States. Based on epidemiological trends, if a pregnant woman is over 35 years of age or has a family history of these conditions, her fetus is considered to be at increased risk. Additionally, pregnant women are routinely offered the Triple Screen blood test, to further assess risk status for these conditions. The Triple Screen test, which is usually performed between the 15th and 20th weeks of pregnancy, evaluates levels of three marker chemicals in the mother's blood. If any of these chemicals are found at concentrations outside the range determined to be normal for the given gestational age of the fetus, the pregnancy is classified as being at increased risk for these conditions (Hodges 1997).

When a pregnancy is classified as at risk, the woman is offered a diagnostic test called an amniocentesis. Amniocentesis consists of withdrawing fluid from the amniotic sac with a large needle and then culturing the cells. Examination of the cultured cells can determine with great accuracy whether certain genetic or chromosomal abnormalities are in fact present. Although amniocentesis is a highly accurate test, it is an invasive procedure that is accompanied by a number of important risks. Performing an amniocentesis may induce infection or leakage of amniotic fluid, and in about 1 in 200 cases, this may result in miscarriage.

The protocol of combining the Triple Screen test with a subsequent amniocentesis has proven capable of identifying 60–80 percent of cases where Down Syndrome, neural tube defect, or Trisomy 18 is present (National Institute of Child Health and Human Development 1996). However, one notable disadvantage of the Triple Screen is that it has a very high false-positive rate. Out of every 1,000 women who are tested, up to 100 will have an abnormal test result, but of those 100 abnormal results, only 1 or 2 will actually have a fetus with a birth anomaly (Evans et al. 1992; Alteneder et al. 1998). In other words, as many as 99 percent of the pregnancies classified as at risk by the Triple Screen test are in fact free of the three anomalies the test is designed to detect. Still, in the eyes of the pregnant woman, once her pregnancy has been classified as at risk, she is confronted by the problem of a pregnancy with an ambiguous health status. What had been a "normal" experience is transformed into a pathologized one, that is, one whose healthful outcome is in doubt (Lippman 1993).

Kenen (1996) has argued that being classified as having an at-risk health status calls for carrying out a set of prescribed normative roles. The at-risk individual encounters social expectations about performance of specific health behaviors and actions. In the case of genetic screening, these prescribed behaviors would consist of accepting what Kenen has termed a diagnostic invitation to receive the gift of knowing. She argues that in prenatal testing, the invitation for a definitive diagnosis presupposes that having this knowledge will be intrinsically good and empowering, ignoring the fact that knowledge is empowering only if it is beneficial.

Because there are no treatments for the birth anomalies identified through routine prenatal genetic diagnosis, the value of producing such information is controversial, raising a plethora of ethical issues ranging from debates about reproductive choice to questions about the rights of disabled people (Gillam 1999; Parens and Asch 1999). In the absence of effective therapies, the benefits of this gift of knowing are limited. The only recourse, once one of these conditions is identified in a developing fetus, is to prepare for the birth of an affected child or to terminate the pregnancy (Markel 1997). Although providing women with such knowledge about their pregnancies does indeed have the potential benefit of informing their reproductive decisions or forewarning them about the baby's health, knowledge is not always power. Having this information may be highly anxiety provoking. The woman is then confronted with difficult choices embedded with morally charged issues such as the acceptability of abortion, the value of a disabled child, and whether mothering such a child should be viewed as discretionary (Rothman 1986; Rapp 2000).

Because of the highly controversial nature of the decisions that must be made in responding to this knowledge, parental autonomy has surfaced as a hallmark ethical principle in prenatal genetic testing. Respect for autonomy is a central ethical construct in clinical medicine and has long been defined as a basic requirement for obtaining informed consent. An autonomous individual is one who is free to choose according to his or her own vision of "the good." In quite general terms, then, autonomous decision-making requires that the individual be both free from controlling influences and capable of intentional action. In the clinical context, autonomous choice would therefore require that patients have sufficient understanding of the options before them to effectively analyze the good they might expect to come from a particular decision (Beauchamp and Childress 1994; Headings 1997).

In the interest of assuring informed, autonomous decision-making, clinicians are to provide relevant information in a genetics counseling session before asking a woman with an at-risk pregnancy to choose whether or not she wants an amniocentesis. Typically, the information included in these sessions focuses not only on the technical details about the risks and benefits of the procedure to be performed but also on the nature and relative risks of the anomalies it might diagnose (Chadwick 1993; Dunne and Warren 1998). Genetic counseling protocols emphasize that clinicians be nondirective and morally neutral when offering genetic testing. This is meant to protect patients' self-determination, to assure that parental decision-making is autonomous and based solely on the patient's own moral values (Chadwick 1993; Wertz and Fletcher 1993; Dailey et al. 1995).

The nondirective genetic counseling model has been criticized for being unrealistic regarding the providers' proper role in assuring informed patient decision-making. Critics have argued that, by its very nature, the act of offering prenatal testing is morally biased toward acceptance, intrinsically putting forth that possession of this knowledge will promote health and be empowering (Chadwick 1993; Dunne and Warren 1998; Browner, Preloran, and Cox 1999). Headings (1997) has further argued that, in the context of genetic counseling, strict application of the principle of nondirectiveness may actually undermine autonomy. He proposes that in operational terms, autonomous decisions require the individual to be capable of informed analytical work, such as reality-testing of the possible outcomes of alternative choices. The appropriate role of the genetic counselor interested in promoting autonomous choice, he argues, would therefore extend to developing the patient's skills for moral deliberation rather than merely taking a stance of moral neutrality.

Huibers and van 't Spijker (1998) have raised an even more basic set of issues regarding the role of autonomy in prenatal genetic testing. They ask whether offering testing to women classified as having an at-risk pregnancy may be inherently incompatible with the basic requirements of autonomous choice. They argue that autonomy requires much more than simply the absence of coercion. For a choice to be truly autonomous, it requires voluntariness (the ability to choose according to one's own values), alternativity (the existence of two or more options), competence (the capacity for rational decision-making), and adequate information (information sufficient for rational choice). They posit that assuring these requirements are met is particularly problematic when a person is confronted with an at-risk health status. In this situation, autonomy may be threatened by the nature of the experience itself, wherein patients may feel they lack authority and alternatives. They may be responding to fear and uncertainty rather than acting out of a full understanding of what it means to be classified as at risk. Once this first step has been taken, that is, once the patient is told her pregnancy is at risk, she may feel she has no choice but to accept the offer of genetic testing (Browner and Press 1996).

Responding to being classified as at risk is made even more complicated by the broad and imprecise ways the term "risk" is used in clinical discussions about prenatal genetic testing. Risk has multiple meanings in this context, but the standard form of these discussions obscures this multiplicity, leaving it to the patient to navigate these various meanings to reach an informed decision. In addition to the general notion that the pregnancy is at risk, the clinician typically presents the patient with a variety of specific risk statistics. The patient is told the percent risk that there is an anomaly, based on epidemiological trends for her age or the values of the marker chemicals in her blood test. She is encouraged to contrast this figure against the percent risk that the procedure will provoke a miscarriage. Although the evaluation of each of these figures may require a different calculus and a different mind-set, they are commonly presented to the patient as equivalent constructs that must be weighed according to her own moral values.

Adding yet another layer of complication to this already potentially baffling array of risk concepts is the important but often unexamined difference between epidemiological and personal notions of risk (Gifford 1986; Rose 1992; Kaufert and O'Neil 1993; Rockhill 2001). Risk factors refer to aggregates of individuals, not to individual cases. This distinction is generally left out of discussions of risk assessment in clinical settings, perhaps in part because the clinicians themselves are not taught to appreciate the implications of these distinctions. Rockhill (2001) has pointed out that few rules exist for translating this aggregate-level concept of risk into a language that makes sense in terms of individualized concerns about health outcomes and strategies. This, she argues, has resulted in a widespread but erroneous notion that risk is an intrinsic property of an individual, subject to manipulation through modification of individual behaviors. In fact, on an individual level, risk factors are poor predictors of who will actually develop a condition or disease (Rockhill 2001).

The information provided in genetic counseling sessions, although intended to enable patients to weigh expected risks and benefits, was not designed to assist patients in understanding the various nuances of meaning and interpretation that risk assessment entails. Although some previous research has focused on patients' evaluations of clinically relevant risks, such as the risk associated with the testing procedure or the likelihood that a fetal anomaly is present (Wertz, Sorenson, and Heeren 1986; Kolker and Burke 1993; Markens, Browner, and Press 1999), these studies have not considered how patients understand and respond to the more generic notion that they are at risk. There is some evidence that the at-risk health status itself, more than these specific clinically relevant risks, may be central to patients' deliberations about prenatal testing (cf. Kenen 1996; Baillie et al. 2000).

Our research has led us to consider what role the at-risk health status might play in patients' acceptance of prenatal genetic testing. Rather than acting out of an autonomous desire to know the health status of their pregnancy, some patients may be seeking a therapeutic measure intended to take their pregnancy out of the ambiguous state of being at risk. This may be especially true for women who have not sought out this information but instead are suddenly and unexpectedly confronted with an ambiguous health status as part of routine prenatal care. For them, being given the opportunity to share in the gift of knowing may be a distinctly disempowering experience (Davis 2000).

SETTING

The study was conducted in the outpatient clinic facility of a large university teaching hospital in south Texas. They serve an indigent and very low-income clientele who are more than 90 percent Latino. A variety of obstetric and gynecology services are provided, staffed by medical school faculty and students.

All the Ob/Gyn clinical services are provided in one wing of the clinic facility. The Ob/Gyn clinic is a very busy place, and the environment is quite different from what one might encounter in a private doctor's office. The waiting room is often crowded, and waits can exceed four and five hours. Reflecting the demographic mix of the region, most of the patients are Latina, and one is as likely to overhear conversations in Spanish as in English. Many patients come accompanied by their husbands, children, or other family members. Family members are usually permitted to accompany patients into the consultation rooms, and about a third of the women have a husband, a boyfriend, or an adult female relative with them during the consultation.

One half-day per week, along with other ongoing Ob/Gyn services, a Prenatal Genetics Clinic (PGC)[2] is held. The PGC provides a variety of services related to prenatal genetics diagnosis, including genetic counseling and diagnostic testing, with on-site facilities for both ultrasound and amniocentesis.

Services at the PGC are provided mostly by medical students and residents and are overseen by an attending physician. The usual PGC team consists of an attending physician, two residents, a fourth-year medical student, an ultrasound technician, and a clerk who manages patient flow and paperwork. The residents and medical students rotate every four to six weeks, so the only consistent staff are the attending physician, the technician, and the clerk. Although the PGC has a policy of promoting continuity of care whenever possible, in practice, heavy reliance on residents and medical students results in an ever-changing medical staff. Patients often do not have the opportunity to develop an ongoing relationship with a single clinician. Instead, they may see a different provider at each visit.

Patients whose pregnancies have been classified as at risk based on their age, family history, or an abnormal Triple Screen blood test are referred to the PGC from a variety of public prenatal clinics throughout the city. Gestational age is an important factor in calculating Triple Screen test results, so verifying the age of the fetus is the first step for a woman referred to the PGC due to an abnormal Triple Screen. This is done by taking a set of measurements during an ultrasound. If the fetal age is determined to be different from that which had initially been used to interpret the test, the results are recalculated. At this point, many women are told that their blood test was not abnormal but only appeared so due to "wrong dates," and they are sent home.

Those women whose risk status is confirmed after checking fetal age are offered diagnostic tests, most commonly an amniocentesis or sometimes, as a less reliable alternative, a high-resolution ultrasound.[3] If a woman accepts an amniocentesis, it is performed at the PGC, often on the same day. Women at this clinic are encouraged to decide on the spot whether they want an amniocentesis so that there is no need to schedule another appointment for the procedure. The staff preference for same-day testing is based on the difficulty of scheduling the procedure in a timely fashion, given that this clinic is held only once per week. The staff also feel that many patients won't return for a second appointment, so they try to provide all their services in a single appointment, if at all possible.

It is important to note that because the Triple Screen test is offered as a routine part of prenatal care, quite commonly women coming to the PGC are unaware that they have had such a test. Many arrive with no clear idea of why they have been sent to the PGC, with no prior knowledge of the kind of testing they have undergone, and without having had the chance to consider its implications for their pregnancy. As a result, for many of the patients at the PGC, the only information they have about the decision they are being asked to make is that which is discussed during the prenatal genetics counseling session. However, because of reliance on inexperienced residents and medical students and the very limited time available for each consultation, genetic counseling at the PGC is often done in a rather cursory way, giving women not only very little time but also little information for making this difficult decision.

In a typical genetic counseling session at the PGC, the clinicians usually begin by asking the patient if she knows why she has been sent there, and then respond by using the same terms the patient has suggested: "Yes, you had a bad blood test," "Yes, your baby might have Down Syndrome." Next they briefly discuss the fetal abnormality in question. They usually note that the blood test result doesn't say the baby *has* the condition, but only that it might, and often name the specific percent risk indicated by the test. They then tell the patient further testing is necessary to know for certain whether the baby has the condition. This is usually followed by briefly describing the amniocentesis procedure itself and mentioning the numeric risk that the procedure may cause infection or a miscarriage. At this point, the clinicians sometimes interject interpretive statements, saying that amniocentesis is relatively safe and that the percent risk of miscarriage is very low. The entire discussion is usually completed within five to ten minutes, often concluding with a summary statement and a request for a decision, such as, "Okay. You understand that your risk for Down Syndrome is 1 in 86 and your risk of losing the baby because of the amnio is 1 in 200. Do you have any questions? [Pause.] So, what do you think? Do you want to go ahead and have the amnio today?"

It is also important to note that, although as many as 40 percent of the patients at the clinic facility speak Spanish as a first language, no formal translation services are available there. Many of the PGC clinicians speak some basic Spanish and attempt to conduct consultations in Spanish as well as they can. When communication becomes too difficult, they look for a clerk or a nurse's aide to assist with translation. Although these staff members may be conver-

sant in Spanish, most do not have the training and background to fully understand the concepts involved. When the clinicians sense that the translator is
having difficulty with the concepts, they often simplify the information being
given to the patient to even more rudimentary terms than those just described.

METHODS

Women were eligible to be interviewed for this study if they were self-
identified Latinas, had been referred to the clinic due to an abnormal Triple
Screen test, and were subsequently offered amniocentesis. Reflecting the overall clientele served by the clinic, those interviewed were all low income as well.
Over the course of nine months, we attended the PGC each week to recruit patients to participate in the study. In the course of patient recruitment, we took
detailed fieldnotes of our observations of clinic consultations and of day-to-
day clinic life.

We arranged to interview 29 women in their homes or other locations of
their choice. Interviews were conducted by Katherine B. de Voogd in Spanish or
English as the women preferred. Interviews were tape recorded, transcribed,
and then summarized in English.

The interviews focused on the woman's reproductive history, current pregnancy experience, what she understood about fetal abnormalities and testing
procedures, how she made her decision about amniocentesis, and her general
experience and satisfaction with the genetics consultation.

The interviews followed an interview guide composed of both open-ended
and structured-response questions. Examples of the open-ended questions include

Do you know why you were sent to the Prenatal Genetics Clinic?

Tell me what happened when you were there?

What did they tell you? What did you think about that?

Did you decide to have the amniocentesis?

How did you decide? What kinds of things did you take into consideration?

The structured-response questions consisted of an instrument developed by
Browner, Preloran, and Cox (1999) for assessing the importance of various factors in parental decision-making about amniocentesis. The instrument consists
of a list of 30 items the women were asked to rate according to how much they
had considered each in their decision to accept or decline the amniocentesis: not
at all, a little, somewhat, or a lot. The list included items such as: "Wanted
what's best for the baby," "Wanted reassurance," "Would want the child regardless of health problems," and "Didn't want to risk a miscarriage."

All fieldnotes and transcripts were indexed by topic. We created a database whose variables were grounded in both open-ended and structured responses to relevant questions in the interviews. We also developed a database for coding selected material from the observation fieldnotes. These databases were later analyzed by using Statistical Package for the Social Sciences (SPSS for Windows 10.0).[4]

Interview transcripts were coded and their content analyzed for primary categories of meaning, as described by Miles and Huberman (1994). First we established a series of provisional categories and a filing and retrieval system. Then we displayed blocks of text in matrixes according to subject content, for example, focusing on the women's reasoning for accepting or declining the amniocentesis, their comments about the expected costs and benefits, their concepts of risk and of perceived dangers, and their experiences of anxiety or relief. The matrixes were then reviewed for emergent patterns and themes, and text material was further abstracted. New, higher level matrixes were then built, organized around thematic categories such as their stated goals and the types of decisions they described making.

All phases of data analysis were cross-checked in conference sessions in which the research team discussed specific cases and reached consensus about how coding categories should be applied and interpreted. We checked for consistency by having a second researcher code case material for all subjects and then compared the results to verify consistency in coding and classification procedures among all the data analysts. Any anomalies or discrepancies in coding procedures were addressed and resolved during these sessions.

FINDINGS

Of the 29 women we interviewed, two-thirds were born in Mexico, and a little more than half chose to be interviewed in Spanish. They ranged in age from 15 to 40, with a mean age of 26. The majority had a high school education or less, were not formally employed, were married, and had an annual household income of less than $16,000. According to clinic staff, these characteristics are typical of the women attending the clinic from which they were recruited.[5] (See Table 2.1.)

For most of the women in our study, finding that their pregnancies were considered at risk came as a shock. Only 8 of the 29 (28 percent) said they had been told by their referring clinic that the reason they were being sent to another clinic was the possibility of a birth defect or so that they might have an amniocentesis. Nearly three-fourths (21/29, 72 percent) said they either were told nothing and came to the PGC thinking it was for a routine prenatal check-up or were only told they had an abnormal blood test.

Despite the notably vague way in which these referrals were often made, 90 percent of the women (26/29, 83 percent) reported that they had understood from the outset that something might be wrong with their pregnancies, and

Table 2.1
Selected Characteristics of 29 Latina Patients

Place of Birth	Mexico	19
	U.S.	10
Language of Interview	Spanish	16
	English	13
Age	15-18	5
	19-25	9
	26-30	10
	31+	5
Education	5-8 yrs.	6
	9-11 yrs.	8
	H.S. graduate	8
	Some college/tech	6
	College graduate	1
Employment Status	Homemaker	11
	Student	4
	Unemployed	4
	Employed	10
Marital Status	Single	10
	Married	18
	Divorced	1
Annual Household Income	< $16,000	16
	> $16,000	10
	Missing	3
Number of Children	0	15
	1-2	10
	3-4	4
Screening Result "At-Risk For"	Down Syndrome	21
	Neural Tube Defects	6
	Trisomy 18	2
Amniocentesis Decision	Accepted	21
	Declined	8

nearly all (24/29) reported feeling very anxious and frightened at finding that out. They consistently described feeling fear and sadness, with many recounting a moment of shock followed by crying, prayer, and loss of sleep.

Interestingly, in their overall discussion of their experiences, the at-risk concept was framed in a very personal and embodied way, as a sense of something actually being wrong and needing to be set right. It should be noted that all the interviews were conducted *after* the women had received their amniocentesis results, and all but one were given a clean bill of health for the fetus, so they already knew the screening-test result had been a false alarm. Still, the language they used to describe how they had felt when they found out something *could be* wrong indicates that many remembered this as finding out something *was* wrong.[6] Comments like these were common: "I found out that the baby was probably sick," "I felt very sad that something was wrong with the baby," "I was very alarmed and thought the baby would probably come out with a defect," and "The Triple Screen test came up that my baby was sick—I think they said he had Down Syndrome."

Thus, for many, an abnormal screening test produced an alarming sense that their baby was in danger. It seems the idea of being at risk in itself was perceived as a disorder. As one woman explained it, "I thought once you were called to be 'at risk' that there was for sure something wrong in some way—that's how I was thinking . . . I thought maybe the doctor saw some abnormality somewhere that I didn't know about."

After being told that their pregnancies were at risk, the women were offered the opportunity to have an amniocentesis to confirm whether there was in fact an abnormality. In principle, the purpose of prenatal diagnosis is to enable the woman to terminate the pregnancy or prepare for the birth of an affected child. If these considerations were indeed the reasons women accept, one would expect to find that women who would not consider an abortion and those who are prepared to care for any child they may have would be unwilling to take the risk of an amniocentesis. However, we did not find this to be the case.

Table 2.2 summarizes issues the women raised in response to open-ended questions, and Table 2.3 shows responses to relevant items from the structured-response instrument. It is noteworthy that of the 21 women in our study who *did* accept the amniocentesis, most said they would not consider an abortion (13/21, 62 percent) and that they would want the child regardless of the outcome of the test (19/21, 90 percent). Only a handful said they wanted to be prepared for such a birth (5/21, 24 percent), and fewer still said they accepted the amniocentesis so they might choose to terminate an affected pregnancy (3/21, 14 percent). Clearly, most of these women cannot be presumed to be motivated by the supposed goals of informing termination decisions or preparing for the birth of an affected child. What then might better explain their decision to accept a test that could potentially harm their pregnancy?

Nearly all said that until receiving the blood-screening result they had felt their pregnancy was normal and healthy (26/29, 90 percent), but that being told their pregnancy was at risk made them very anxious (24/29, 83 percent), leaving them with a sense that their baby was in danger. Once this sense of disruption was introduced, accepting the amniocentesis became the only way they could know that the baby was all right and return to a sense that they were having a normal pregnancy (cf. Browner and Preloran 1999). As one woman explained it, "It was the most effective way to stop being as frightened as I was, to have something more concrete, an answer." Another commented, "I said to myself, if I don't do this, I'll have this doubt over me the whole time I'm waiting for the birth, and that would be a heavy burden, really; that's why I did it."

The women who accepted amniocentesis were almost unanimous in saying that they wanted to know for sure what was going on, as a way to get rid of the worry (19/21, 90 percent) and to be reassured of the health of their baby

Table 2.2
Reasons Accept/Decline Amniocentesis (Open-Ended Responses) Reported by 29 Latina Patients

	Accepted (n=21)	Declined (n=8)	Total (n=29)
Would not consider abortion	13 (62%)	7 (88%)	20 (69%)
To choose an abortion	3 (14%)	3 (38%)	6 (21%)
To be prepared	5 (24%)	0 (0%)	5 (17%)
To know; to dispel worry	19 (90%)	1 (12%)	20 (69%)

Table 2.3
Considerations in Making Decision (Closed-Question Responses) Reported by 29 Latina Patients

	Accepted (n=21)	Declined (n=8)	Total (n=29)
What's best for the baby	20 (95%)	7 (88%)	27 (93%)
Wants child regardless	19 (90%)	7 (88%)	26 (90%)
Our families are all in good health	18 (86%)	8 (100%)	26 (90%)
Can harm the baby	18 (86%)	7 (88%)	25 (86%)
Wanted reassurance	18 (86%)	5 (62%)	23 (79%)
Doctor advised	18 (86%)	4 (50%)	22 (76%)
Had "feeling" baby was fine	13 (62%)	8 (100%)	21 (72%)
Miscarriage risk	12 (57%)	8 (100%)	20 (69%)
Abortion not an option	11 (52%)	7 (88%)	18 (62%)

(18/21, 86 percent). The comments of a 30-year-old Mexican-born mother of three illustrate this point.

Well, I decided to do it because I wanted to know if in reality the baby really was fine ... to feel more at ease and to know for sure ... It's better to do the amnio, so that you can get rid of the burden, the trauma that you've got in your head. If you don't do the amnio you're left in doubt.

In responding to the sense of malady that the at-risk status had engendered, many viewed accepting the amniocentesis as the only means of promoting the welfare of the pregnancy. Nearly all (20/21, 95 percent) who had accepted amniocentesis expressed the idea that it was in their baby's best interest to do so. Comments like the following were common: "I was doing it for the good of the baby." "The doctor said it was good for me and good for the baby." "I did it for my own sake, and for the baby's sake."

During the time they waited for the amniocentesis results, which took a minimum of two weeks and sometimes longer, most of the women continued to feel anxious (18/21, 86 percent). But at the end of the whole experience, once they had received the results, they all said they were no longer anxious and felt a return to a sense of well-being about their pregnancy (20/20, 100 percent, one missing data). Two women's comments indicate the extent of the disruption they experienced due to the at-risk health status. One noted that she didn't tell people she was pregnant until after finding out the results of the amniocentesis; the other said she waited to choose a name for the baby and decide where the baby's room would be until after the amniocentesis came back normal. Interestingly, the one woman who had received a positive diagnosis of Down Syndrome also reported feeling relief once the result was confirmed because she no longer was left with the anxiety of wondering about the condition of her baby.

It would seem that for all of these women, the quasi-disease state of having been assigned the at-risk health status was effectively dispelled by proceeding with the amniocentesis. The disruption engendered by the abnormal blood test was resolved once the pregnancy was moved out of a state of ambiguity.

DISCUSSION

In prevailing ethical standards for the offer of prenatal genetic testing, the protection of parental autonomy has been a primary goal. To allow patients to make autonomous informed choices, the genetic counseling model calls for presenting appropriate information to patients in morally neutral terms (Yarborough, Scott, and Dixon 1989; Headings 1997; Dunne and Warren 1998). The information thought pertinent to patient decision-making includes the nature of the potential disorder, the likelihood that the fetus may have the disorder, and the risk that the procedure may provoke a miscarriage. This emphasis presumes that patients' acceptance of the tests would be based on their weighing their willingness to risk a miscarriage against their desire to either be able to terminate an affected pregnancy or be prepared for the birth of an affected child.

Our study of the perceptions and responses to abnormal Triple Screen results among a group of low-income Latinas leads us to question whether, given the circumstances under which they are asked to make this choice, they can be considered to be making an autonomous decision at all. These women did not seek out this information, but instead, in the course of routine prenatal care, were abruptly confronted with the news that their pregnancy could be at risk. Then, after receiving only a brief overview of pertinent information about the amniocentesis procedure and the birth anomaly in question, they were asked to decide on the spot whether they wanted the diagnostic test. Under these conditions, can a woman's decision about the procedure be reasonably assumed to reflect her autonomous assessment of how her own vision of the "good" will be best served?

The women we interviewed who accepted amniocentesis did not report making their decision based on the considerations presumed pertinent in the professional model for offering prenatal genetics testing. Although the risk of miscarriage was indeed important to all those refusing amniocentesis, most who accepted the test did not report doing so to consider abortion or to be prepared for an affected birth. Instead, they chose to proceed with the amniocentesis to dispel the worry of having their pregnancy classified as at risk.

Previous research by Browner and colleagues on the amniocentesis decisions of a group of Latinas in California (Browner and Preloran 1999; Browner, Preloran, and Cox 1999; Markens, Browner, and Press 1999; Browner and Preloran 2000) report similar findings. They found that patients' attitudes toward abortion and their interest in knowing the condition of the baby did not predict whether they accepted amniocentesis. Instead, many of the women felt an implicit pressure to accept the test, and those women having more confidence in doctors and medical science were more likely to accept the test. As in our study, they report that many accepted amniocentesis because they perceived it as the only way to resolve the worry and doubt prompted by the offer of the test itself.

In considering the meaning of being classified as at risk, Gifford has argued that, for the patient, the ambiguity of an at-risk health status "results in the creation of a new state of being ... that is somewhere between health and disease" (Gifford 1986:215). Many of the women we spoke with found themselves suddenly and unexpectedly in such a gray area. For them, being classified as at risk seems to have had an iatrogenic effect. The at-risk label essentially transformed what had been until then a normal, healthy pregnancy into a state of quasi-disease that required action to reinstate a sense of well-being (Lippman 1993), and accepting the test was perceived as the only means available for restoring the pregnancy to a state of normalcy.

In the nascent field of prenatal genetic diagnosis, one is led to wonder if the patient's right to know is counterbalanced by a "right not to know" (Press and Browner 1995). Does the notion of informed consent have any real salience for women who are abruptly confronted with an unsolicited choice about accepting a test when that test presents the only avenue for resolving this imposed ambiguity?

Under these circumstances, assuring that the basic requirements of autonomy (Huibers and van 't Spijker 1998) are met seems highly problematic. By its very nature, being at risk implies that the woman should take action to improve her risk status (Kenen 1996; Rockhill 2001). Thus, rather than acting out of voluntariness, according to her own values, a patient may feel she lacks the authority to decline testing and is instead compelled to accept "for the good of the baby." She may also lack a sense of alternativity; that is, she may not feel there are two or more options but instead perceive that accepting the test is the *only* way to restore her pregnancy to a state of health. Finally, rather than making a competent, informed decision based on rational review of pertinent information, she may be responding to the fear and uncertainty intrinsic in the ambiguous state of being classified as at risk. Once the pregnancy has been classified as at risk, regardless of the neutrality and adequacy of the information she receives, the patient's autonomy may be inherently undermined. In clinics like the PGC, where information is provided in a cursory fashion and patients are encouraged to make a decision on the spot, the assurance of autonomous choice would seem even more doubtful.

The socioeconomic status of low-income minority patients, such as those in our study, may also undermine the possibility of autonomous decision-making. Their low-income status, low educational levels, and limited English skills may seriously circumscribe their ability and confidence in making an independent assessment of their preferences about prenatal diagnosis. Even if the clinical and statistical concepts underlying the at-risk label were fully explained, the patients may be ill-equipped to understand the concepts sufficiently to make a truly informed choice.

Furthermore, due to the already compromised social status of such patients, it is likely that they are unaccustomed to a clinical situation in which they are asked to assess information and exercise autonomous choices rather than simply urged to comply with medical advice. The ideology of neutrality and nondirectiveness in genetic counseling is unique among clinical encounters in its insistence that the clinician not indicate a recommended course to the patient but instead allow the patient to choose based on her own values and goals. But can it be reasonably expected that an uneducated, socially disempowered patient might emerge from the genetics counseling session as a sudden expert of sorts, confident and capable of making an independent, informed decision regarding her moral assessment about the value of such testing?

Although, of course, our findings from a very small convenience sample taken at a single clinic cannot be generalized to a broader population, our analysis raises some important questions about the moral implications of having one's pregnancy classified as at risk. For the women in our study, at least, it seems inappropriate to think of them as autonomously accepting or refusing neutral offers of amniocentesis. From their point of view, being classified as at risk for fetal disorders invoked an earnest struggle to comprehend and respond to an ambiguous threat to the well-being of the pregnancy. Rather than acting out of an autonomous desire to have more information, many were instead responding to the sense of danger engendered by the at-risk label itself and felt compelled to accept further testing for the protection of the pregnancy.

It should not be overlooked that 99 percent of abnormal Triple Screen test results are false-positive, forcing large numbers of women with normal pregnancies to unnecessarily grapple with this difficult decision (Evans et al. 1992; Alteneder et al. 1998). We question the routine use of such an unreliable screening test, particularly given that it is not clear all women who accept further genetic testing are indeed acting autonomously.

Assuring the autonomous decision-making of low-income minority women whose pregnancies have been classified as at risk is especially challenging. This would require the development of genetic counseling programs that are capable of addressing the special limitations these women face in this situation. Such programs would need to assure that the women have complete and nuanced understanding of the meaning of being classified as at risk and of the capacities and limitations of the screening test as well as of the diagnostic tests and a realistic appreciation for the lack of clinical options for acting on such information. Such a program would also need to be at a literacy level and in language that is fully accessible to the women and presented within a time frame sufficient to allow them to fully process and respond to the information. In the absence of these features, programs that routinely offer prenatal diagnosis to low-income minority women may seriously compromise the women's autonomy.

NOTES

1. An extra gene at the 21st chromosome causes Down Syndrome, resulting in mild to severe mental retardation, slow physical development, and characteristic physical features sometimes known as mongolism. Neural tube defects result from failure of the neural tube to close during early gestation and can result in negligible to severe neurological impairment such as anencephaly or spina bifida. Trisomy 18 is caused by an extra gene at chromosome 18, resulting in severe mental and physical deformity and usually fatal within the first year. Down Syndrome and neural tube defects each affect about 1 in 1,000 births; Trisomy 18 is less common, affecting about 1 in 8,000 births (Thomas 1997).

2. This is a pseudonym.

3. The high-resolution ultrasound is preferred by some women because it is noninvasive and there is no danger of its provoking a miscarriage. However, because the ultrasound cannot provide definitive diagnosis to the extent possible through amniocentesis, it is generally presented as a less desirable, secondary option.

4. Statistical Package for the Social Sciences (SPSS for Windows 10.0. SPSS, Inc., 1999).

5. There was a high concentration of very young women with first pregnancies in our sample, as is the case for the Ob/Gyn clinic overall. This may be because women who are more experienced with pregnancy and with the health care system don't use this public clinic but instead have found ways to access other, more attractive sources of care that are available in the city to women who qualify for Medicaid coverage.

6. Others have reported similar findings among women confronted with abnormal results in prenatal screening for chromosomal abnormalities. See, for example, Gekas et al. (1999) and Baillie et al. (2000).

REFERENCES

Alteneder, Ruth R., Carole Kenner, Diane Greene, and Sharon Pohorecki. 1998. "The Lived Experience of Women Who Undergo Prenatal Diagnostic Testing." *MCN American Journal of Maternal Child Nursing* 23(4): 180–186.

Baillie, C., J. Smith, J. Hewison, and G. Mason. 2000. "Ultrasound Screening for Chromosomal Abnormality: Women's Reactions to False Positive Results." *British Journal of Health Psychology* 5(4): 377–394.

Beauchamp, Tom L., and James F. Childress. 1994. *Principles of Biomedical Ethics.* 4th ed. New York: Oxford University Press.

Browner, Carole H., and H. Mabel Preloran. 1999. "Para Sacarse la Espina (To Get Rid of the Doubt): Mexican Immigrant Couples and Amniocentesis." In *Localizing and Globalizing Reproductive Technologies*, eds., Ann R. Saetnan, Nelly Oudshoorn, and Marta Kirejczyk, 368–383. Columbus: Ohio State University Press.

———. 2000. "Latinas, Amniocentesis and the Discourse of Choice." *Culture, Medicine and Psychiatry* 24(3): 353–375.

Browner, Carole H., H. Mabel Preloran, and Simon J. Cox. 1999. "Ethnicity, Bioethics, and Prenatal Diagnosis: The Amniocentesis Decisions of Mexican-Origin Women and Their Partners." *American Journal of Public Health* 89(11): 1658–1666.

Browner, Carole H., and Nancy Press. 1996. "The Production of Authoritative Knowledge in American Prenatal Care." *Medical Anthropology Quarterly* 10(2): 141–156.

Chadwick, Ruth F. 1993. "What Counts as Success in Genetic Counseling?" *Journal of Medical Ethics* 19(1): 43–46.

Dailey, J. V., M. A. Pagnotto, S. Fontana-Bitton, and S. J. Brewster. 1995. "Role of the Genetic Counselor: An Overview." *Journal of Perinatal and Neonatal Nursing* 9(3): 32–44.

Davis, Dena. 2000. *Genetic Dilemmas: Reproductive Technology, Parental Choices, and Children's Futures.* New York: Routledge Press.

Dunne, Cara, and Catherine Warren. 1998. "Lethal Autonomy: The Malfunction of the Informed Consent Mechanism within the Context of Prenatal Diagnosis of Genetic Variants." *Issues in Law and Medicine* 14(2): 165–202.

Evans, M. I., J. E. O'Brien, J. L. Moody, and A. Drogan. 1992. "Alpha-Fetoprotein and Bio-Chemical Screening." In *Reproductive Risks and Prenatal Diagnosis*, ed. Mark I. Evans, 223–236. Norwalk, CT: Appleton and Lange.

Evans, M. I., P. G. Pryde, W. J. Evans, and M. P. Johnson. 1993. "The Choices Women Make about Prenatal Diagnosis." *Fetal Diagnosis and Therapy* 8 (Supplement): 170–180.

Gekas, J., J. Gondry, S. Mazure, P. Cesbron, and F. Thepot. 1999. "Informed Consent to Serum Screening for Down Syndrome: Are Women Given Adequate Information?" *Prenatal Diagnosis* 19(1): 1–7.

Gifford, Sandra. 1986. "The Meaning of Lumps: A Study of the Ambiguity of Risk." In *Anthropology and Epidemiology,* eds. Craig R. James, Ron Stall, and Sandra Gifford, 213–246. Dordrecht, The Netherlands: D. Reidel Publishing Co.

Gillam, Lynn. 1999. "Prenatal Diagnosis and Discrimination against the Disabled." *Journal of Medical Ethics* 25(2): 163–171.

Handwerker, Lisa. 1994. "Medical Risk: Implicating Poor Pregnant Women." *Social Science & Medicine* 38(5): 665–675.

Headings, V. E. 1997. "Revisiting Foundations of Autonomy and Beneficence in Genetic Counseling." *Genetic Counseling* 8(4): 291–294.

Hodges, Walter J. 1997. *Alpha-Fetoprotein and the Obstetric Triple Screen.* [Online publication. Retrieved Aug. 29, 2002.] Available from www.novaobgyn.com/Sept97 .html.

Huibers, Alex K. and Adriaan van 't Spijker. 1998. "The Autonomy Paradox: Predictive Genetic Testing and Autonomy: Three Essential Problems." *Patient Education and Counseling* 35(1): 53–62.

Kaufert, Patricia A., and John O'Neil. 1993. "Analysis of a Dialogue on Risks in Childbirth: Clinicians, Epidemiologists, and Inuit Women." In *Knowledge, Power and Practice: The Anthropology of Medicine in Everyday Life,* eds. Shirley Lindenbaum and Margaret Lock, 32–54. Berkeley and Los Angeles: University of California Press.

Kenen, Regina H. 1996. "The At-Risk Health Status and Technology: A Diagnostic Invitation and the 'Gift' of Knowing." *Social Science and Medicine* 42(11):1545–553.

Kolker, Aliza and B. Meredith Burke. 1993. "Deciding about the Unknown: Perceptions of Risk of Women Who Have Prenatal Diagnosis." *Women and Health* 20(4): 37–57.

Lippman, Abby. 1993. "Prenatal Genetic Testing and Geneticization: Mother Matters for All." *Fetal Diagnosis and Therapy* 8 (Supplement): 1175–188.

Markel, Howard. 1997. *Scientific Advances and Social Risks: Historical Perspectives of Genetic Screening Programs for Sickle Cell Disease, Tay-Sachs Disease, Neural Tube Defects and Down Syndrome, 1970–1997.* [Online publication. Retrieved Nov. 7, 2000.] Available from www.nhgri.nih.gov/ELSI/TFGT_final /appendix6.html.

Markens, Susan, C. H. Browner, and Nancy Press. 1999. "'Because of the Risks': How US Pregnant Women Account for Refusing Prenatal Screening." *Social Science and Medicine* 49(3): 359–369.

Miles, Matthew, and A. Michael Huberman. 1994. *Qualitative Data Analysis: An Expanded Source Book.* 2nd ed. Thousand Oaks, CA: Sage Publications.

National Institute of Child Health and Human Development. 1996. *Prenatal Diagnosis.* [Online publication. Retrieved Nov. 7, 2000.] Available from www.nichd.nih.gov /publications/pubs/mrdd/sub10.htm.

Parens, Erick, and Adrienne Asch. 1999. "The Disability Rights Critique of Prenatal Genetic Testing. Reflections and Recommendations." *Hastings Center Report* 29(5): S1-S22.

Press, Nancy, and C. H. Browner. 1994. "Collective Silences, Collective Fictions: How Prenatal Diagnostic Testing Became Part of Routine Prenatal Care." In *Women and Prenatal Testing: Facing the Challenges of Genetic Technology,* eds. Karen H. Rothenberg and Elizabeth J. Thomson, 201–218. Columbus: Ohio State University Press.

———. 1995. "Risk, Autonomy, and Responsibility. Informed Consent for Prenatal Testing." *Hastings Center Report* 25(3): S9-S12.

———. 1997. "Why Women Say Yes to Prenatal Diagnosis." *Social Science and Medicine* 45(7): 979–989.

Pryde, Peter G., Arie Drugan, Mark P. Johnson, Nelson B. Isada, and Mort I. Evans. 1993. "Prenatal Diagnosis: Choices Women Make about Pursuing Testing and Acting on Abnormal Results." *Clinical Obstetrics and Gynecology* 36(3): 496–509.

Rapp, Rayna. 1998. "Refusing Prenatal Diagnosis: The Meanings of Bioscience in a Multicultural World." *Science, Technology and Human Values* 23(1): 45–70.

———. 2000. *Testing Women, Testing the Fetus: The Social Impact of Amniocentesis in America.* New York: Routledge Press.

Rockhill, Beverly. 2001. "The Privatization of Risk." *American Journal of Public Health* 91(3): 365–368.

Rose, Geoffrey. 1992. *The Strategy of Preventive Medicine.* New York: Oxford University Press.

Rothman, Barbara K. 1986. *The Tentative Pregnancy: Prenatal Diagnosis and the Future of Motherhood.* New York: Viking.

Sokal, D.C., J.R. Byrd, A.T. Chen, M.F. Goldberg, and G.P. Oakley, Jr. 1980. "Prenatal Chromosomal Diagnosis. Racial and Geographic Variation for Older Women in Georgia." *JAMA* 244(12): 1355–1357.

Swerts, A. 1987. "Impact of Genetic Counseling and Prenatal Diagnosis for Down Syndrome and Neural Tube Defects." *Birth Defects: Original Article Series* 23(2): 61–83.

Thomas, Clayton L. 1997. *Taber's Cyclopedic Medical Dictionary.* 18th ed. Philadelphia: F.A. Davis Co.

Wertz, Dorothy C., and John C. Fletcher. 1993. "Feminist Criticism of Prenatal Diagnosis: A Response." *Clinical Obstetrics and Gynecology* 36(3): 541–567.

Wertz, Dorothy C., James R. Sorenson, and Timothy C. Heeren. 1986. "Clients' Interpretation of Risks Provided in Genetic Counseling." *American Journal of Human Genetics* 39(2): 253–264.

Yarborough, Mark, Joan A. Scott, and Linda K. Dixon. 1989. "The Role of Beneficence in Clinical Genetics: Non-Directive Counseling Reconsidered." *Theoretical Medicine* 10(2): 139–149.

Chapter 3

The Risks of Test-Tube Baby Making in Egypt

Marcia C. Inhorn

Since 1978, when the world's first "test-tube baby," Louise Brown, was born in England, new reproductive technologies (NRTs)—particularly in vitro fertilization (IVF)—have rapidly gained acceptance in the Western world and are now routinely employed in most "developed" countries to overcome otherwise intractable infertility. Clearly, NRTs—and particularly the more controversial or sensational aspects of their deployment, including high-order multiple births, third-party gamete donation practices, and pregnancies in postmenopausal women—have attracted both media and scholarly attention in the West. Although the media have tended to glorify the successes of NRTs—including the "miracle babies" born to "desperate" infertile couples (Condit 1994; Franklin 1997)—many scholars, including feminist theorists, bioethicists, technoscience studies scholars, anthropologists, and even some health care practitioners engaged in the provision of NRTs, have been less sanguine, revealing how these technologies are both a blessing and a curse. Feminist scholars in particular have described in great detail all that is "wrong" with the NRTs,[1] often focusing on the risks of these technologies to women's bodies and to women's status when motherhood is pursued "at all costs," thereby upholding traditional patriarchal family forms (Thompson 2001).

My deepest gratitude goes to the many Egyptians—infertile women and their husbands, physicians specializing in infertility and NRTs, research assistants, Al-Azhar University faculty members, and staff of the Binational Fulbright Commission—who have participated in or in other ways facilitated my research over the past two decades. I am also grateful for the financial support provided by the U.S. Department of Education's Fulbright-Hays fellowship programs, the Fulbright Institute for International Education, and the National Science Foundation. My thanks go to Barbara Herr Harthorn and Laury Oaks for their insightful editorial comments on this chapter.

However, something important has been missing from these discussions, focusing as they do almost exclusively on EuroAmerican settings. Namely, neither the media nor scholars themselves have recognized the now massive global spread of NRTs to the "developing" societies of the non-Western world. Yet limited reports show that NRTs are swiftly but silently globalizing—moving from Western sites of global production (mainly the United States, Western Europe, and Australia) to non-Western sites of global consumption on the continents of Asia, Africa, and Latin America (Nicholson and Nicholson 1994; Okonofua 1996; Kahn 2000; Bharadwaj 2001; Handwerker 2001; Kahn 2001). The scholarly erasure of this global phenomenon is quite remarkable, considering the now voluminous literature on NRTs in the West. However, in this particular case, Western scholars themselves may be contributing in unfortunate ways to "stratified reproduction" (Ginsburg and Rapp 1995); they do so by privileging the experiences of white, Western (mostly middle- to upper-class) infertile women, who are often able to achieve their reproductive desires through the use of reproductive technologies (Sandelowski and de Lacey 2001), over the experiences of those in other global locations who are disempowered and even despised as reproducers.

Nonetheless, infertility is clearly a global health phenomenon; in fact, the risks of becoming infertile are much greater in parts of the developing world than they are in the West (Sciarra 1994; Hamberger and Janson 1997; Van Balen and Gerrits 2001; Inhorn 2002). Reproductive tract infection (RTI) leading to infertility is the world's leading cause of *preventable* infertility, affecting nearly two-thirds of all infertile women in Africa and approximately 40 percent in Latin America (Cates, Farley, and Rowe 1985; World Health Organization 1987; Sciarra 1994, 1997). Africa, in fact, has the dubious distinction of having an "infertility belt" wrapped around its center, with nearly one-fifth to one-third of all couples in some populations unable to conceive after at least one year of trying (Collet et al. 1988; Larsen 1994; Ericksen and Brunette 1996; Larson 2000; Leonard 2001). Given the significant prevalence of infertility outside the West, it is not surprising that many Third World societies provide ready markets for NRTs,[2] even in the face of other more pressing health problems such as HIV/AIDS. NRTs are, in fact, the only solution for overcoming tubal infertility caused by RTIs and male infertility, the latter of which contributes to half of all cases of infertility and is often untreatable by any other means (Howards 1995; Devroey et al. 1998; Kamischke and Nieschlag 1998).

However, NRTs are accompanied by significant risks—risks that spread with the technologies themselves—and these risks may be exacerbated in Third World settings, where assisted reproduction centers operate under very different structural conditions. To date, no studies from the Third World have asked infertile individuals or couples to identify their concerns and worries regarding these technologies. Thus, local views of NRT risk—from the perspective of NRT users themselves—have yet to emerge from India, Egypt, Nigeria, Ecuador, China, and the many other global sites where IVF is now being regularly practiced.

NRTs are not transferred into cultural voids when they reach Third World sites. Local concerns—having to do with factors that may be biological, social, cultural, economic, or even political in nature—shape and sometimes curtail the ways in which these Western-generated technologies are both offered to and received by non-Western subjects. Examining the perceived risks and constraints facing IVF consumers wherever these technologies spread clearly serves to deconstruct the myth that NRTs are some sort of panacea, a miracle cure for infertility everywhere it occurs.

This is where an anthropological perspective—informed by recent developments in globalization theory—becomes extremely useful. Globalization theory suggests that we should ask how Third World recipients of global technologies, including health technologies, resist their application or at least reconfigure the ways they are to be adopted in local cultural contexts (Ginsburg and Rapp 1995; Freeman 1999). In other words, globalization is not enacted in a uniform manner around the world, nor is it simply homogenizing—necessarily "Westernizing" or even "Americanizing"—in its effects (Appadurai 1996; Hannerz 1996). The global is always imbued with local meaning, and local actors mold the very form global processes take, doing so in ways that highlight the dialectics of gender and class, production and consumption, and local and global cultures (Freeman 1999). Moreover, anthropology—with its methodological tools of in-depth, field-based ethnography, its central concept of culture, and its attention to *la vie quotidienne,* or the everyday, lived experiences of others—represents a unique realm for examining these tensions and constraints, thereby revealing how local actors in specific cultural contexts confront, experience, and give shape to the forms of globalization.

THE RISKS OF TEST-TUBE BABY MAKING: EGYPTIAN PERSPECTIVES

This chapter focuses on the experiences and concerns of those who, by virtue of their intractable infertility, must "consume" and embody NRTs in the Middle Eastern Muslim country of Egypt. This chapter asks, What do infertile Egyptians themselves regard as the risks of NRTs? And how might these risks act as constraints on infertile Egyptian couples' desires to make a test-tube baby? As we shall see, Egyptians' notions of risk are not about risk per se but rather about many dimensions of treatment-seeking that make infertile Egyptians feel uncertain, worried, and afraid. Thus, in Egypt, at least, fear—as the emotional component of perceived risk—is what infertile women and men relate as they describe the tortuous "medical and emotional road of trials" on which they journey in search of a test-tube baby (Sandelowski, Harris, and Black 1992). As I will argue, in the case of Egypt, infertile women and men willing to consider the use of NRTs are confronted with numerous arenas of constraint, or structural, ideological, social relational, and practical obstacles and apprehensions surrounding the use of these technologies. Some of these, such as the physical risks and low success rates associated with IVF, are similar to those faced by Western users of NRTs. However, many of the dilemmas and perceived risks of test-tube baby making experienced by infertile Egyptians themselves have little to do with Western discourses of risk; instead, Egyptian views of NRT risk are deeply embedded in local cultural understandings and practices.

Indeed, Egyptians themselves do not deploy the language of risk in the epidemiological sense of that term. Perhaps because epidemiology (as a basic public health discipline) is in an inchoate stage of development in Egypt,[3] Egyptians are not confronted with daily messages about the many risks to their health and thus do not seem to view themselves as living in a threatening "risk society" (Beck 1992). Whereas some authors have suggested that Westerners now live in "cultures of fear" (Furedi 1997), where the media have helped promote an obsessional focus on health, safety, and survival leading, in turn, to many anxious and self-destructive individual behaviors and social effects (Freudenburg 1988), this sort of preoccupation with health and safety risks is much less evident in Egypt. To take but a few examples, seat belts are never worn; children do not ride in car seats; condoms are rarely used, and not for the practice of safe sex; most men smoke; "fitness fanaticism" has yet to take hold, even among elites;[4] and, hence, urbanites are increasingly overweight, diabetic, and hypertensive (Amin 2001). Instead, in this predominantly Muslim setting, concepts of pervasive health risk are supplanted by indigenous notions of *rizq*, or beliefs in God's grace and sustenance of every individual He brings onto this earth. Indeed, for most Egyptian Muslims—and Middle Easterners in general—proof of God's generous sustenance is manifest in the very lifestyles (e.g., smoking, heavy meat consumption, lack of physical activity) that are now seen in the West as health-demoting and dangerous.

This does not mean, however, that Egyptians do not perceive dangers to their health and well-being, and this is especially true of those who are confronted, head on, with a significant health problem such as infertility. In fact, in the case of infertility, the Egyptian media have been heavily involved in increasing public awareness of this health and social problem and its potential "solution" through NRTs (Inhorn, forthcoming 2003). However, media publicity has had a dual and contradictory effect: On the one hand, the media have glorified the NRTs by spotlighting the "miraculous" births of Egyptian IVF triplets and even higher-order multiple births to long-term infertile couples. On the other hand, the Egyptian media have aroused public fear and anxiety surrounding the potential immorality of the test-tube baby making enterprise, largely by highlighting some of the most "notorious" cases in the West—including IVF doctors impregnating scores of patients with their own sperm, grandmothers bearing the test-tube babies of their own daughters, and the birth of test-tube twins of different races due to careless sperm admixtures in Western IVF laboratories. These signal events—all of which happen to be true and have subsequently been dramatized in some cases on Egyptian television—have led to what some theorists in the West have called the "social amplification of risk" (Kasperson 1992; Slovic 1992), or far-reaching effects in Egypt on the perception of heightened risk surrounding these new technologies (Freudenburg 1988).

Indeed, in interviews I conducted among nearly 200 infertile women and men in two separate studies (in 1988–89 and 1996),[5] I learned of the many fears and concerns confronting Egyptians who, by virtue of their failure to conceive, were contemplating treatment or had actually undertaken IVF or a related reproductive technology. Couching their concerns in the language of emotion, infertile women and men talked about what aspects of the NRTs frightened them, made them upset, or were suspected of posing dangers to their bodies or their IVF offspring. Although some individuals had only one or two major concerns, many women in Egyptian IVF centers could reel off lists of fears, or dimensions of IVF that made them or their husbands anxious and worried. Furthermore, as we shall see, numerous social and cultural forces, including indigenous views of reproductive biology, religious institutions and mores, gender relations and family politics, class structures, the culture of biomedicine and the pharmaceutical industry, and even the intimate politics of envy, influence the affective and cognitive dimensions of risk assessment regarding test-tube baby making in Egypt. Despite the high hope placed in these technologies by most infertile Egyptian couples and their IVF physicians, negative emotions—including worry, anxiety, fear, and pessimism—seem almost inevitable when one considers the socially and culturally regnant "dangers" of embarking on this particular line of therapy. Indeed, following Douglas (1992:46), who argues that "the very word 'risk' could well be dropped from politics" to make room for the more experience-near term "danger," I would argue that test-tube baby making is perceived as an inherently dangerous enterprise, eliciting numerous fears and concerns on the part of potential Egyptian IVF consumers. But what are these fears, and how are they produced?

Fears of Impoverishment

Although the prohibitive expenses of NRTs are typically recognized as a major constraint on their utilization, these high costs are "lived" by infertile Egyptians who must muster the financial resources to undergo IVF. In Egypt, the exorbitant expenses associated with IVF lead to very class-stratified access: Most poor and even middle-class infertile Egyptians are absolutely excluded from undertaking IVF by virtue of its expense—roughly $2,500 to $3,000 per treatment cycle in a country where the average per capita annual income in 1996 was only $1,200 (Population Reference Bureau 1999). With only one exception (the University of Alexandria's Shatby Hospital, where I conducted my initial research), all Egyptian IVF centers today are private businesses, charging high prices for the procedures and drugs that patients pay for out of pocket. Health insurance is new and not widespread, and the Egyptian government has little interest in subsidizing NRTs in the country.

As a result, the only patients who can truly afford to utilize these technologies are Egyptian elites drawn from the upper-middle to upper classes. In a society where the majority of women remain illiterate and do not work in the formal sector, the women patients who present to IVF clinics today tend to be highly educated professionals who are employed as doctors, lawyers, architects, engineers, accountants, bankers, professors, tourism officials, and even movie stars. Furthermore, many of these women and their husbands are members of the Egyptian "brain drain" generation; namely, they move themselves from middle to upper-middle-class status by working in the petro-rich Arab Gulf countries, returning home annually on monthlong summer vacations to undertake one trial of IVF.

Many elites argue that they would never be able to afford IVF—and particularly not repeated trials of IVF—if they could not work as labor migrants outside the country. This "no labor migration = no IVF" equation is experienced as very stressful, given that it forces many infertile professionals to maintain residency outside Egypt for extended periods of time, thereby limiting access to IVF (and relatives) "back home." Furthermore, with the exception of the truly wealthy, most IVF patients worry about their ability to pay for repeated trials of IVF and fear that the expenses associated with repetition will literally bankrupt them over time. Indeed, in some cases, doctors, lawyers, engineers, and others of similar status end up depleting their savings and selling off personal possessions (such as gold jewelry, pieces of land, cars) to finance their infertility treatments. Thus, infertile Egyptians typically equate IVF with gambling, as both involve the expenditure of large amounts of money for very uncertain rewards. Whereas the truly wealthy, who represent only about 1 percent of Egyptian society, can afford to "play the game," as they put it, IVF is experienced by everyone else as a financially risky treatment that can destroy one's financial future and literally lead to downward social mobility in a society where most people are barely clinging to their current class positions. Thus, in a society where few can afford to "make" a test-tube baby, the financial risks of IVF are experienced as *the* major arena of constraint, keeping most infertile Egyptians out of the test-tube baby making business and depleting the resources of those who venture in.

Fears of Unnatural Procreation

Furthermore, for many infertile Egyptians, particularly those of the lesser-educated lower classes, NRTs are clearly cognitively disruptive, given that they challenge deeply held notions of how babies are to be made "naturally," according to God-given plans. NRTs require men to ejaculate their sperm into plastic containers and women to take powerful hormonal medications to stimulate their egg production for the purposes of harvesting. The embryos then formed through in vitro fertilization in a laboratory are placed back inside a woman's body after a brief period of extracorporeal development.

As such, this technology challenges the most basic beliefs about baby making held among lower-class Egyptians, who subscribe to what Delaney (1991) has called a "monogenetic" view of procreation. Namely, men are thought to be the sole procreators, carrying preformed fetuses in their sperm, or "worms," as sperm are called among the Egyptian poor. As the gestational nurturers of these man-made fetuses, women are not deemed to contribute biogenetic substance to their offspring—and particularly not eggs, which would make human females the equivalents of chickens. Thus, NRTs are profoundly challenging to deeply held beliefs about the nature of the human reproductive body and reproductive physiology in Egypt. Among lower-class individuals who are unfamiliar with the Western notions of duogenetic procreation that undergird these technologies, these technologies cause considerable confusion and profound disbelief that human scientists could be "playing God" by creating children in such an unnatural manner. These concerns—coupled with lingering questions about what happens to test-tube babies during the period in which they are in vitro (and perceived to be floating in giant test tubes or aquariums)—are deeply troubling to Egyptians of all social classes, keeping many dubious infertile couples from pursuing IVF treatment altogether.

Fears of Immorality

Fears of procreating unnaturally are coupled in the minds of many Egyptians with fears of going against the explicit teachings of Islam. As early as 1980, Islamic religious scholars at Egypt's world-renowned Al-Azhar University condemned the NRT practices of third-party donation involving donor sperm, eggs, embryos, or surrogate uteruses (Serour 1992, 1996). This religious view, which has been upheld since then throughout the Muslim world (Meirow and Schenker 1997; Blank 1998),[6] considers third-party donation to lead to a morally illicit "mixture of relations" whereby blood ties between parents and their offspring are severed, issues of paternity, descent, and inheritance are hopelessly confused, and half-siblings from the same anonymous donor are likely to enter into unwitting incestuous relationships. Furthermore, surrogacy is believed to tamper with the God-given "natural maternal instinct" that emanates from a single mother to her biological offspring.

For Egyptian Muslims, then—as well as for Egyptian Coptic Christians, who make up between 6 and 10 percent of the total Egyptian population and whose church has followed the Muslim lead on this issue—the thought of using donor sperm, eggs, or embryos from a bank is simply reprehensible and is tantamount in their minds to committing *zina*, or adultery. Although most Egyptians believe that IVF physicians are good Muslims who would never practice third-party donation intentionally, many infertile patients who are considering IVF spend long hours worrying about accidental donation—namely, unintentional laboratory mix-ups of sperm, ova, or embryos. These fears and suspicions prevent some couples from undertaking IVF altogether, because once the products of conception leave one's body, it is virtually impossible to know for sure whether these products will be returned untainted—as has happened now in several infamous cases of Western laboratory negligence that have been widely publicized in the Egyptian media (Robertson 1996). Although most Egyptian IVF physicians take elaborate measures to guard against this eventuality—as well as every opportunity to reassure patients about their own religiosity and vigilance—patients' fears of unknowingly doing something profoundly immoral "according to the religion" certainly keep some of them away from NRTs. Indeed, in public opinion, NRTs are widely construed as going against Islam, with test-tube babies themselves being viewed as "children of sin." Thus, few IVF patients in Egypt disclose their treatment status for fear of being viewed—no matter how unjustly—as participating in practices that are inherently immoral.

Fears of Physicians' Characters

Given these moral anxieties, infertile Egyptians undergoing IVF must trust their physicians absolutely. But finding a sympathetic and trustworthy physician—and particularly one who is religious—can be a major challenge. Just as IVF patients spend hours worrying about potential mistakes being made in IVF laboratories, they spend many hours considering their physicians' characters—trying to assess whether the man is honest, devout, scrupulous, vigilant, technically competent, and ultimately caring for his patients.[7] Because this is the man who will literally facilitate the creation of life, he must be seen as a servant of God as well as a brilliant technician who is savvy about the latest Western technologies. In other words, Egyptian IVF physicians themselves are expected to manage a delicate balancing act as both providers of high-tech global technologies and upholders of local religious and cultural traditions.

Some IVF physicians realize this and spend considerable time in patient counseling and rapport building (where they often accentuate their Muslim religiosity). Such physicians tend to develop "saint-like" reputations and, not surprisingly, attract large patient followings. However, some IVF physicians are less concerned with upholding their images than with their ability to move patients swiftly through the complicated IVF treatment system, thereby making large amounts of money for their clinics.

Encountering such a "greedy" physician is considered one of the major risks of undertaking IVF in Egypt. Many Egyptian IVF patients report bad experiences suffered at the hands of physicians who are perceived as "uncaring" and "only in it for the money." Brusque communication styles, insensitive comments, frank technical incompetence, and outright rejection of clients who are seen as poor risks for the improvement of clinic success rates are experienced as profoundly demoralizing by patients already made emotionally fragile by years of intractable infertility. Such experiences—remarkably common in a country fraught with ongoing medical paternalism and characteristic authoritarian physician-patient communication styles (El-Mehairy 1984; Inhorn 1994)—lead to considerable "doctor-shopping" between IVF clinics as infertile couples seek a physician who makes them feel "comfortable" and "confident" in his abilities. In short, the inability to find a moral, competent, and caring physician—to whom an infertile couple can literally entrust their most precious gametes—continues to be one of the major risks of test-tube baby making in Egypt.

Fears of Divorce

For couples who find a good physician, one of the major risks of undertaking IVF is the effects of treatment on marital dynamics. Generally, infertile Egyptian women of all social classes live in fear that their marriages will collapse because Islamic personal status laws consider a wife's barrenness to be a major ground for divorce (Inhorn 1996).[8] Although most husbands of infertile Egyptian women do not divorce their wives, thereby resisting tremendous family pressure, some men would rather "replace" their infertile wives than undergo the trials, tribulations, and expenses surrounding IVF.[9] Furthermore, during the IVF treatment process, marriages sometimes come unglued under the intense physical and psychological pressures that this therapy typically exacts on couples—a social sequela of NRTs that has also been reported in the West (Greil, Leitko, and Porter 1988; Abbey, Andrews, and Halman 1991).

Perhaps the saddest new twist in marital politics in Egypt has occurred as a result of the recent introduction of intracytoplasmic sperm injection (ICSI), the newest of the new reproductive technologies. Since its introduction in the early 1990s, ICSI—which is a variant of IVF and involves microscopically guided "injection" of a single spermatozoon directly into an oocyte—has heralded a revolution in the treatment of *male* infertility. With ICSI, men with very poor semen profiles are now able to produce a biological child of their own as long as a single viable spermatozoon can be retrieved from their bodies, even through harvesting from the testis, which is required in the 15 percent of men who are azoospermic, or lacking sperm in the ejaculate (Hamberger and Janson 1997).

Unfortunately, for many of the wives of these infertile Egyptian men, the presence of ICSI poses new marital risks. Most middle-age women, who have stood by their infertile husbands for years, even decades in some cases, have grown too old to produce viable ova for the ICSI procedure. Because contemporary Islamic opinion in Egypt forbids both donor eggs and surrogacy, couples with a "reproductively elderly" wife face four difficult options: first, to remain together permanently without children; second, to legally foster an orphan, which is rarely viewed as a tenable option by Egyptians; third, to remain together in a polygamous marriage, which is rarely accepted these days by Egyptian women; or finally, to divorce so that the husband can remarry a younger, potentially more fertile woman. Unfortunately, more and more highly educated Egyptian men are choosing the final option of divorce—believing that their own reproductive destinies may lie with younger, more fecund wives allowed to men under Islam's personal status laws. In short, the recent introduction of ICSI—coupled with ongoing personal status legislation in Egypt—places infertile Egyptian women and the "old" wives of infertile Egyptian men in an extremely precarious position vis-à-vis their reproductive and marital futures.

Fears of "Aging Out"

Many women at Egyptian IVF centers desperately fear the passage of time and the possibility that they will "age out" of IVF or ICSI treatment. For Egyptian women, the age of 40 marks a key watershed, because ovulatory function typically begins to decline precipitously at this point. Because many women in their forties do not respond well to ovulation induction as they enter the perimenopausal period, they are less likely to be successful with NRTs of all kinds. As a result, many Egyptian IVF centers—concerned about boosting their own success rates for presentation to other prospective clients—refuse to take female patients above the age of 40, arguing to them that they are wasting their time and money on probably futile efforts to become pregnant.[10]

Although some Egyptian IVF physicians justify this exclusion of older women as a compassionate restriction, women in their late thirties live in fear of this eventuality and often see themselves as engaging in a "race against time." Given that NRT technologies are viewed as a last resort in Egypt, it is not surprising that most women do not reach IVF centers until many years of marriage and many failed treatment attempts have already passed. Thus, women on the cusp of turning 40 are extremely prevalent in Egyptian IVF centers, where their angst about aging is palpable. In the context of NRTs, fears of aging in general and "aging out" of treatment in particular are pronounced in a society where IVF physicians turn away older women from their clinics and where donor egg technology and surrogacy are both strictly prohibited on religious grounds.

Fears of Hormonally Induced Weakness

Egyptian women who do not face these age restrictions are often fundamentally ambivalent about taking the powerful hormonal agents required before any trial of IVF or ICSI. Their fears have to do with culturally entrenched beliefs about the bodily "weakness" produced by hormones of any kind. "Weakness" is a common cultural illness idiom in Egypt (DeClerque et al. 1986; Early 1993) and is rife in popular Egyptian reproductive imagery. The medications women are given prior to an IVF or ICSI cycle are generally viewed as "strengtheners," capable of stimulating ovarian function even in the "weakest" ovaries. However, the paradoxical problem with these agents is that they may overcome weakness in the ovaries only to produce a more generalized bodily "weakness" apparent in the noticeable list of side effects that they produce. These include generalized enervation, muscular weakness, loss of appetite, and even fainting. Furthermore, women receiving pre-IVF hormonal injections often experience more immediate debilitating side effects, such as pain, bruising, and swelling at the site of injections; abdominal bloating, fluid retention, and weight gain; breast enlargement and tenderness; nausea and vomiting; headaches, dizziness, lightheadedness; and general feelings of moodiness and depression.

Women are understandably concerned about whether such bodily weakness is temporary, lasting, or even permanent, and many of them worry that even worse problems, such as grave diseases like cancer, may be produced by these agents in the long term. Such concerns are especially pronounced for women who have experienced literally years of hormonal therapies for their infertility and are now faced with repeated cycles of ovulation induction prior to IVF. Thus, the hormones that are part and parcel of the IVF experience are of great concern to Egyptian women. This is particularly true given deeply entrenched beliefs that hormones of any kind (including the oral contraceptives, Depo-Provera injections, and Norplant contraceptives that have been "pushed" on Egyptian women by Western-backed population control programs) cause powerful, debilitating, and lasting side effects that are best to be avoided (De-Clerque et al. 1986).

Fears of Drug Shortages

In addition to these concerns about the weakening effects of hormones on their bodies, Egyptian women have faced ongoing concerns about their ability to obtain these hormonal agents before they embark on scheduled trials of IVF or ICSI. Although Egypt has a well-developed pharmaceutical industry, with pharmacies appearing on virtually every city block, the hormonal agents used with the NRTs have never been widely available in Egyptian pharmacies and have often been limited to particular "specialty" pharmacies whose owners make occasional drug-purchasing trips to foreign markets, usually in Europe (Inhorn 1994). Furthermore, because many of these agents are imported to Egypt, the Egyptian NRT drug market has been, at times, at the mercy of global fluctuations in drug availability, resulting in chronic shortages of some of the most important hormonal agents.

Many Egyptian patients whose IVF/ICSI cycles have been scheduled literally scour the pharmacies of Egypt in sometimes futile efforts to obtain the prescribed medications. In other cases, patients must resort to a kind of transnational "suitcase trading," whereby family members, friends, and even flight attendants are enjoined to obtain these agents abroad and fly the drugs back to Egypt in special refrigerated coolers (although they are rarely apprised of the exact uses of these drugs, for reasons I will describe later). These extraordinary efforts to obtain NRT medications create levels of uncertainty, frustration, and despair among infertile Egyptian couples that have rarely been described in

Western treatment settings. This is particularly true among couples whose scheduled trials of IVF or ICSI are cancelled due to lack of medication, and who must then watch from the sidelines as other patients with the required drugs move up on the clinic's waiting list.

Fears of Failure

Given the great lengths to which many Egyptians must go to access hormonal medications and NRTs themselves, they are clearly concerned about whether their efforts will be fruitful—whether placing one's body at risk and enduring periods of forced income-generating exile from the country will lead, ultimately, to a successful pregnancy and birth of a precious "baby of the tubes." Consequently, patients are keen to know percentages of success, and they spend long hours worrying about whether undergoing IVF or ICSI is worth the price, monetary and otherwise, of failure. Unfortunately, because of the various technical obstacles and lack of training and technique in many Egyptian IVF centers (Inhorn 2002, forthcoming 2003), local success rates in Egypt—except in the very best centers—may be comparatively diminished; yet they are rarely presented as such to patients. Instead, patients are routinely quoted inflated success rates—generally in the 30 to 40 percent range—to maintain their hope and willingness to undergo NRT procedures (cf. Becker 2000). Such percentages are high, even by Western standards, a fact that is suspected by some savvy Egyptian IVF patients who are conscious of their position in the global arena.

Furthermore, many patients are given false hope that a first trial of IVF or ICSI will be successful. Given all the hardships described, it is not surprising that patients ardently hope to avoid repeated trials of IVF and are usually devastated when pregnancy is not achieved on the first trial. With very few exceptions, most Egyptian patients hope that the first trial of IVF will lead to multiple births, ideally twins or even triplets. Because of the cultural unacceptability of a one-child family, low-order multiple births mean the "ideal" Egyptian family size of at least two but not more than three children can be achieved without having to resort to future IVF or ICSI trials. Thus, among Egyptian IVF hopefuls, multiple births are considered one of the great benefits of IVF—a true embarrassment of riches and of God's *rizq*—rather than one of the most serious risks of the procedure as argued by medical experts (Okonofua 1996; Scholz et al. 1999).

Fears of Losing a Pregnancy

Even if Egyptian IVF patients welcome, rather than fear, multiple-order pregnancies, the state of pregnancy achieved by some IVF patients is not necessarily experienced as overwhelmingly joyous. Instead, from the moment of embryo transfer, many IVF patients live in fear of losing the pregnancy and take extraordinary measures to guard against this possibility. Egyptian women who have undergone embryo transfer tend to immobilize themselves, barely moving from bed during the two-week period until the pregnancy test is performed. Women hope that by remaining "still" and inactive, the embryo will "stick" or "hang" (i.e., implant) and will not "fall." Those days in bed are rarely restful for women, who tend to brood excessively about whether the IVF trial has been successful.

The lucky few who do become pregnant may spend the rest of their pregnancy on bed rest—rarely reflecting doctors' orders but rather following widely held Egyptian injunctions about avoiding pregnancy loss through overexertion. Western warnings about the need for healthful diets and exercise during pregnancy are rarely if ever heeded in Egypt. Rather, the opposite injunctions—to move as little as possible and to eat rich foods and gain weight to take care of oneself and one's test-tube baby—are much more likely to be followed. In other words, pregnancy, if achieved through NRTs, engenders a particular local form of bodily discipline—one marked by self-enforced and socially reinforced inactivity, immobilization, and inertia. More than anything, Egyptian women who have succeeded in conceiving through IVF or ICSI fear losing their precious "baby of the tubes" through physical activity that could have been avoided. So, to the extent that they can, they and their husbands pamper their bodies through prolonged rest and inactivity. That such bodily restriction may actually produce pregnancy complications is an open question but one that points to potential conflicts between local Egyptian cultural logics of well-being and the actual embodiment of Western-generated reproductive technologies.

Fears of Envy

Moreover, widespread cultural notions of *hasad*, or "envy"—resulting in harm to the pregnancy or to the test-tube baby itself—come into play even among educated Egyptian elites. Egyptians of all social backgrounds abide by the notion that those who covet one's success, including in pregnancy, may direct an envious glance (the so-called evil eye), thereby harming or "ruining" another's good fortune. As a result, most Egyptians are never boastful—even hiding or lying about particular accomplishments, good health, and good fortune.

As has been widely documented throughout the Middle East, *hasad* is considered to be a major etiological factor in childhood illness, and covetous infertile women are considered to be major perpetrators of the evil eye (Inhorn 1996). Although they may not intend to harm a child, these women are seen as incapable of controlling their feelings of envy and are sometimes accused of causing childhood misfortunes. As a result, infertile women are often avoided by others with children, and infertile women themselves are often sensitive about attending rituals and celebrations where many children are present.

Given that infertile Egyptian women know all too well how society views them, they are likewise concerned about revealing their own good fortune when they eventually become pregnant through IVF or ICSI. Many infertile women who achieve pregnancies tell no one and attempt to hide their pregnancies for as long as possible, fearing that envious others who know about the pregnancy might harm them. In practical terms, this means that pregnant IVF patients often fear attending IVF centers, where high numbers of potentially covetous infertile patients are to be found. As a result, some ask to see their IVF physicians for prenatal care at their private Ob/Gyn offices, and others are simply "lost to follow-up" after pregnancy is achieved—leaving behind unpleasant memories of IVF clinics and the envy of the not-yet-pregnant.

Fears of Weak Offspring

Whereas Egyptian women worry about losing the pregnancy either through overexertion or envy, Egyptian men, and particularly those with severe forms of male infertility, worry about the physical health of the offspring conceived through ICSI. Because male infertility problems are glossed as weakness of the sperm (or, among the lower class, "weak worms"), many infertile Egyptian men seem to take this cultural idiom to heart, feeling that they themselves are somehow weak, defective, and even unworthy as biological progenitors (Inhorn 2003). Indeed, many men in Egyptian IVF centers are openly concerned about whether they will "pass their weakness" on to their children, and this is particularly pronounced among men with spermatic deformities, who wonder if their children will suffer from congenital malformations and other genetic defects. These fears, furthermore, are not abated by prenatal genetic testing in Egypt, which is essentially absent in the country. Although this lack of prenatal testing appears rather ironic, given the enthusiasm for other forms of "high-tech" reproductive medicine, it clearly reflects cultural ambivalence about and the continuing criminalization of abortion in the country (Lane 1997).

However, given the growing evidence that ICSI offspring are just as normal as any other population of children conceived through NRTs, Egyptian physicians who perform ICSI often attempt to reassure their male patients that their offspring will be healthy and normal. Nonetheless, these lingering doubts about the general health and well-being of offspring conceived "from weakness" plague many men—up to and even beyond the birth of their own evidently physically normal ICSI babies.

Fears of Social Ridicule and Disclosure

Even when test-tube babies are born physically normal, they arrive in the world with an "abnormal" social status—not as socially valorized "miracle babies," but rather as stigmatized oddities, fashioned in test tubes with unknown and perhaps immorally mixed biogenetic substances. Thus, test-tube baby making continues to engender wild speculation and moral uncertainty in Egypt, casting doubt on the very humanity of such children.

Egyptian parents of test-tube babies are well aware of this social reception and therefore are extremely concerned about future social ridicule and stigmatization of their children. Although some hope that views of NRTs may "become better," normalizing over time, they realize that this day has yet to come in Egypt. Thus, to protect their children's futures—sparing them from the taunts of schoolmates and even lack of future marriageability—parents of test-tube babies engage in extraordinary measures to guarantee the privacy of this procedure, usually disclosing to no one or to only the closest family members that IVF is being undertaken. Indeed, test-tube baby making in Egypt is shrouded in mystery, with patients themselves describing the entire affair as "top secret."

In this local world marked by fear, envy, and the paranoia of being found out, infertile couples who attempt NRT procedures must go it alone in both social and emotional isolation. Fears of disclosure and envy clearly militate against the formation of patient-run support groups (such as RESOLVE in the United States). Although many Egyptian IVF patients admit that self-help groups would be extremely beneficial for the purposes of information-sharing and alleviating many of the fears described in this chapter, they are quick to point out that these will "never happen" in Egypt, where fears of social stigmatization render test-tube baby making—and test-tube babies themselves—socially invisible.

CONCLUSION

This chapter has asked how the risks of test-tube baby making are lived by Egyptian users of NRTs. By entering the "local moral worlds" of infertile Egyptians (Kleinman 1992), it becomes clear that what Egyptians themselves fear about NRTs may or may not accord with Western notions of risk. Rather, the landscape of fear surrounding test-tube baby making in Egypt is a unique terrain, marked by cultural logics and practices that are deeply locally embedded.

These findings suggest that the global spread of NRTs to new local sites in non-Western societies such as Egypt requires careful investigation. As this chapter has shown, the utilization of these technologies is highly dependent upon local considerations, including indigenous perceptions of what makes these technologies inherently risky and frightening. To take the case of Egypt, the perceived risks of test-tube baby making are manifold, probably preventing many infertile couples from availing themselves of these technologies and worrying those who do. Indeed, in the course of my research, I never found an infertile woman or her husband who did not express at least one of these fears.

Although the main worries were clearly religious and financial in nature, most Egyptian IVF patients had multiple concerns that varied in specific configuration from informant to informant. In other words, each woman I met in an Egyptian IVF clinic could tell me her particular story of fear and suffering, stories that were often different from one another. Ultimately, I came to conclude that the very presence of these women and their husbands in Egyptian IVF clinics was a remarkable sign of courage, involving a giant leap of faith into the brave new world of Egyptian test-tube baby making.

In closing, since the birth of Louise Brown more than two decades ago, there have been many critics of NRTs, who have argued that these technologies should not be used at all and especially not in the "overpopulated" Third World. Yet the rapid globalization of these technologies to countries far from the producing nations of the West bespeaks the powerful desire of Third World infertile couples in places such as Egypt to overcome their childlessness through, in many cases, the only available technological means. To deny infertile people access to such technologies based on their social location in the global hierarchy of rich and poor nations seems, in my view, patently unfair and even bespeaks a kind of neo-Malthusian rationing of reproductive rights. Clearly, there is a need for these technologies in parts of the world where tubal infertility—and, increasingly, male infertility—take their extraordinary tolls on both physical and social reproduction. There are many costs inherent in this global transfer of NRTs, and one of these is the social and cultural amplification of risk in places such as Egypt. As seen in this chapter, the world of test-tube baby making in Egypt is an inherently risky cultural terrain, where only the bold dare to venture.

NOTES

1. For examples of this feminist literature, see Corea et al. (1987); Spallone and Steinberg (1987); Stanworth (1987); Klein (1989); Overall (1989); Ratcliff (1989); Rothman (1989); McNeil, Varcoe, and Yearley (1990); Scutt (1990); Rowland (1992); Raymond (1993); Squier (1994); Van Dyck (1995); Farquhar (1996); Hartouni (1997); Lublin (1998); and Andrews (1999).

2. I use the term "Third World" here interchangeably with "developing," as in "developing country." Third World bespeaks the global politics of difference and hierarchy whereby nations such as Egypt become located on the global periphery in relation to wealthy "First World" nations. "Developing," on the other hand, bespeaks evolutionary discourses of modernization whereby resource-poor countries are expected to be developing toward the superior example set by the "modern, developed" countries. Such development discourses have been heavily criticized in anthropology, including by scholars of Egypt (Mitchell 1991).

3. There is only one school of public health in Egypt (one of two in the entire Middle Eastern region) and only a few departments of community medicine where epi-

demiology is taught. Because of the dearth of trained epidemiologists in the country, the Centers for Disease Control and Prevention (CDC) in Atlanta has entered into a cooperative arrangement with the Egyptian Ministry of Health to offer a Field Epidemiology Training Program (FETP), teaching Egyptian physicians how to engage in disease investigation and surveillance.

4. However, diet clinics catering to elites are increasingly prevalent in urban areas of Egypt (Basyouny 1997).

5. In 1988–89 during the "early period" of IVF in Egypt, I conducted 15 months of anthropological fieldwork on the problem of infertility in Egypt, basing my research in the University of Alexandria's large public Ob/Gyn teaching hospital, which was initiating the only public IVF program in the country. There I conducted in-depth semistructured interviews in the Egyptian colloquial dialect of Arabic with 100 infertile women and a comparison group of 90 fertile ones, the vast majority of whom were poor, uneducated, illiterate housewives (Inhorn 1994, 1996). Returning to Egypt in the mid-1990s during the IVF "boom period," I spent the summer of 1996 conducting semistructured interviews with 66 mostly middle- to upper-class, highly educated professional women in two of the most well-established private IVF centers in Cairo. In 40 percent of these interviews (in marked contrast to my earlier research), husbands were present and participated often enthusiastically in interviews, half of which were in Arabic and half in English (Inhorn 2003).

6. Only recently, the minority Shi'a branch of Islam, found in Iran, parts of Lebanon, and the Arab Gulf, has approved the use of donor egg technology (Dr. Michael Fakih, personal communication 2002). However, in all branches of Islam, the use of donor sperm is strictly forbidden.

7. The male pronoun is used here because virtually all Egyptian IVF physicians (with the exception of some laboratory personnel) are male, reflecting the ongoing male domination of obstetrics and gynecology in Egypt.

8. Although Islamic personal status laws in Egypt also allow women to divorce if male infertility can be proven, a woman's initiation of a divorce continues to be so stigmatizing in Egypt that women rarely choose this option unless their marriages are truly unbearable. In Egypt, such personal status laws cover issues of marriage and divorce, child custody and fosterage, and rights of inheritance, which, when in dispute, are taken to religious (as opposed to civil) courts to be heard.

9. Although patterns of divorce have, to my knowledge, never been systematically studied in Egypt, divorce can occur among Muslim couples of any social class, urban versus rural background, degree of educational attainment, or level of religiosity. However, divorces are usually initiated by the husband, for the reason cited in footnote 8. Only among Egyptian Coptic Christians is divorce explicitly forbidden. For that reason, infertile Coptic couples with adequate financial resources are particularly avid users of NRTs, given that divorce and remarriage to a fertile partner are never viable options.

10. The turning away of older infertile women, with women's ensuing "panic" over becoming forty and "aging out" of NRT treatments, occurs in other global sites as well, including the United States, as recently described by Becker (2000).

REFERENCES

Abbey, Antonia, Frank M. Andrews, and L. Jill Halman. 1991. "Gender's Role in Responses to Infertility." *Psychology of Women Quarterly* 15(2): 295–316.

Amin, Ezzat. 2001. "The Epidemiologic Transition in Egypt." Paper presented at the pre-conference workshop on "The Epidemiologic Transition among Arab Populations: Local-Global Connections." University of Michigan, Ann Arbor, May 10.

Andrews, Lori B. 1999. *The Clone Age: Adventures in the New World of Reproductive Technology.* New York: Henry Holt and Company.

Appadurai, Arjun. 1996. *Modernity at Large: Cultural Dimensions of Globalization.* Minneapolis: University of Minnesota Press.

Basyouny, Iman Farid. 1997. *Just a Gaze—Female Clientele of Diet Clinics in Cairo: An Ethnomedical Study.* Cairo: The American University in Cairo Press.

Beck, Ulrich. 1992. *Risk Society: Towards a New Modernity.* London: Sage Publications.

Becker, Gaylene. 2000. *The Elusive Embryo: How Women and Men Approach New Reproductive Technologies.* Berkeley and Los Angeles: University of California Press.

Bharadwaj, Aditya. 2001. "Conception Politics: Medical Egos, Media Spotlights, and the Contest over Testtube Firsts in India." In *Infertility around the Globe: New Thinking on Childlessness, Gender, and Reproductive Technologies,* eds. Marcia C. Inhorn and Frank van Balen, 315–333. Berkeley and Los Angeles: University of California Press.

Blank, Robert. 1998. "Regulation of Donor Insemination." In *Donor Insemination: International Social Science Perspectives,* eds. Ken Daniels and Erica Haimes 131–150. Cambridge: Cambridge University Press.

Cates, W., Timothy M. M. Farley, and Patrick J. Rowe. 1985. "Worldwide Patterns of Infertility: Is Africa Different?" *The Lancet* 2(8455): 596–598.

Collet, M., J. Reniers, E. Frost, R. Gass, F. Yvert, A. Leclerc, C. Roth-Meyer, B. Ivanoff, and A. Meheus. 1988. "Infertility in Central Africa: Infection Is the Cause." *International Journal of Gynecology and Obstetrics* 26(3): 423–428.

Condit, Celeste Michelle. 1994. "Hegemony in a Mass-Mediated Society: Concordance about Reproductive Technologies." *Critical Studies in Mass Communication* 11(3): 205–230.

Corea, Gena, Renate Duelli Klein, Jalna Hanmer, Helen B. Holmes, Betty Hoskings, Madhu Kishwar, Janice Raymond, Robyn Rowland, and Roberta Steinbacher. 1987. *Man-Made Women: How New Reproductive Technologies Affect Women.* Bloomington: Indiana University Press.

DeClerque, Julia, Amy Ong Tsui, Mohammed Futuah Abul-Ata, and Delia Barcelona. 1986. "Rumor, Misinformation and Oral Contraceptive Use in Egypt." *Social Science & Medicine* 23(1): 83–92.

Delaney, Carol. 1991. *The Seed and the Soil: Gender and Cosmology in Turkish Village Society.* Berkeley and Los Angeles: University of California Press.

Devroey, Paul, M. Vandervorst, Peter Nagy, and Andre Van Steirteghem. 1998. "Do We Treat the Male or His Gamete?" *Human Reproduction* 13 (Supplement 1): 178–185.

Douglas, Mary. 1992. *Risk and Blame: Essays in Cultural Theory.* London: Routledge Press.

Early, Evelyn A. 1993. *Baladi Women of Cairo: Playing with an Egg and a Stone.* Boulder, CO: Lynne Rienner.

El-Mehairy, Theresa. 1984. *Medical Doctors: A Study of Role Concept and Job Satisfaction, the Egyptian Case.* Leiden, The Netherlands: E. J. Brill.

Ericksen, Karen, and Tracy Brunette. 1996. "Patterns and Predictors of Infertility among African Women: A Cross-national Survey of Twenty-seven Nations." *Social Science & Medicine* 42(2): 209–220.

Fakih, Dr. Michael. Personal communication. June 19, 2002.

Farquhar, Dion. 1996. *The Other Machine: Discourse and Reproductive Technologies.* New York: Routledge Press.

Franklin, Sarah. 1997. *Embodied Progress: A Cultural Account of Assisted Conception.* New York: Routledge Press.

Freeman, Carla. 1999. *High Tech and High Heels in the Global Economy: Women, Work, and Pink-collar Identities in the Caribbean.* Durham, NC: Duke University Press.

Freudenburg, William R. 1988. "Perceived Risk, Real Risk." *Science* 242(4875): 44–49.

Furedi, Frank. 1997. *Culture of Fear: Risk-taking and the Morality of Low Expectation.* London: Cassell.

Ginsburg, Faye D., and Rayna Rapp. 1995. "Introduction: Conceiving the New World Order." In *Conceiving the New World Order: The Global Politics of Reproduction,* eds. Faye D. Ginsburg and Rayna Rapp, 1–17. Berkeley and Los Angeles: University of California Press.

Greil, Arthur L., Thomas M. Leitko, and Karen L. Porter. 1988. "Infertility: His and Hers." *Gender & Society* 2(2): 172–199.

Hamberger, L., and P. O. Janson. 1997. "Global Importance of Infertility and Its Treatment: Role of Fertility Technologies." *International Journal of Gynecology & Obstetrics* 58(1): 149–158.

Handwerker, Lisa. 2001. "The Politics of Making Modern Babies in China: Reproductive Technologies and the 'New' Eugenics." In *Infertility around the Globe: New Thinking on Childlessness, Gender, and Reproductive Technologies,* eds. Marcia C. Inhorn and Frank van Balen, 298–314. Berkeley and Los Angeles: University of California Press.

Hannerz, Ulf. 1996. *Transnational Connections: Culture, People, Places.* London: Routledge Press.

Hartouni, Valerie. 1997. *Cultural Conceptions: On Reproductive Technologies and the Remaking of Life.* Minneapolis: University of Minnesota Press.

Howards, Stuart S. 1995. "Treatment of Male Infertility." *The New England Journal of Medicine* 332(5): 311–317.

Inhorn, Marcia C. 1994. *Quest for Conception: Gender, Infertility, and Egyptian Medical Traditions.* Philadelphia: University of Pennsylvania Press.

———. 1996. *Infertility and Patriarchy: The Cultural Politics of Gender and Family Life.* Philadelphia: University of Pennsylvania Press.

———. 2002. "Global Infertility and the Globalization of New Reproductive Technologies: Illustrations from Egypt." *Social Science & Medicine.*

———. 2003. "'The Worms Are Weak': Male Infertility and Patriarchal Paradoxes in Egypt." *Men & Masculinities* 5: 238–258.

———. Forthcoming, 2003. *Local Babies, Global Science: Gender, Religion, and In Vitro Fertilization in Egypt.* New York: Routledge Press.

Kahn, Susan Martha. 2000. *Reproducing Jews: A Cultural Account of Assisted Conception in Israel.* Durham, NC: Duke University Press.

———. 2001. "Rabbis and Reproduction: The Uses of New Reproductive Technologies among Ultraorthodox Jews in Israel." In *Infertility around the Globe: New Thinking on Childlessness, Gender, and Reproductive Technologies,* eds. Marcia C. Inhorn and Frank van Balen, 283–297. Berkeley and Los Angeles: University of California Press.

Kamischke, Axel, and Eberhard Nieschlag. 1998. "Conventional Treatments of Male Infertility in the Age of Evidence-Based Andrology." *Human Reproduction* 13 (Supplement 1): 62–75.

Kasperson, Roger E. 1992. "The Social Amplification of Risk: Progress in Developing an Integrative Framework." In *Social Theories of Risk,* eds. Sheldon Krimsky and Dominic Golding, 153–178. Westport, CT: Praeger.

Klein, Renate. 1989. *Infertility: Women Speak Out about Their Experiences of Reproductive Medicine.* London: Pandora Press.

Kleinman, Arthur M. 1992. "Local Worlds of Suffering: An Interpersonal Focus for Ethnographies of Illness Experience." *Qualitative Health Research* 2(2): 127–134.

Lane, Sandra D. 1997. "Gender and Health: Abortion in Urban Egypt." In *Population, Poverty, and Politics in Middle East Cities,* ed. Michael E. Bonine, 208–234. Gainesville: University Press of Florida.

Larsen, Ulla. 1994. "Sterility in Sub-Saharan Africa." *Population Studies* 48(3): 459–474.

———. 2000. "Primary and Secondary Infertility in Sub-Saharan Africa." *International Journal of Epidemiology* 29(2): 285–291.

Leonard, Lori. 2001. "Problematizing Fertility: 'Scientific' Accounts and Chadian Women's Narratives." In *Infertility around the Globe: New Thinking on Childlessness, Gender, and Reproductive Technologies,* eds. Marcia C. Inhorn and Frank van Balen, 193–214. Berkeley and Los Angeles: University of California Press.

Lublin, Nancy. 1998. *Pandora's Box: Feminism Confronts Reproductive Technology.* Lanham, MD: Rowman and Littlefield.

McNeil, Maureen, Ian Varcoe, and Steven Yearley, eds. 1990. *The New Reproductive Technologies.* London: Macmillan.

Meirow, Dror, and Joseph G. Schenker. 1997. "The Current Status of Sperm Donation in Assisted Reproduction Technology: Ethical and Legal Considerations." *Journal of Assisted Reproduction and Genetics* 14(3): 133–138.

Mitchell, Tim. 1991. "America's Egypt: Discourse of the Development Industry." *Middle East Report* 21(2): 18–36.

Nicholson, Roberto F., and Roberto E. Nicholson. 1994. "Assisted Reproduction in Latin America." *Journal of Assisted Reproduction and Genetics* 11(9): 438–444.

Okonofua, Friday. 1996. "The Case against New Reproductive Technologies in Developing Countries." *British Journal of Obstetrics and Gynaecology* 103(10): 957–962.

Overall, Christine, ed. 1989. *The Future of Human Reproduction.* Toronto, Ontario: The Women's Press.

Population Reference Bureau. 1999. *World Population Data Sheet: Demographic Data and Estimates for the Countries and Regions of the World.* Washington, DC: Population Reference Bureau.

Ratcliff, Kathryn Strother, ed. 1989. *Healing Technology: Feminist Perspectives.* Ann Arbor: University of Michigan Press.

Raymond, Janice G. 1993. *Women as Wombs: Reproductive Technologies and the Battle Over Women's Freedom.* San Francisco: Harper.

Robertson, John A. 1996. "Legal Troublespots in Assisted Reproduction." *Fertility and Sterility* 65(1): 11–12.

Rothman, Barbara Katz. 1989. *Recreating Motherhood: Ideology and Technology in a Patriarchal Society.* New York: W. W. Norton.

Rowland, Robyn. 1992. *Living Laboratories: Women and Reproductive Technology.* London: Octopus Publishing.

Sandelowski, Margarete, and Sheryl de Lacey. 2001. "The Uses of a 'Disease': Infertility as Rhetorical Vehicle." In *Infertility around the Globe: New Thinking on Childlessness, Gender, and Reproductive Technologies,* eds. Marcia C. Inhorn and Frank van Balen, 33–51. Berkeley and Los Angeles: University of California Press.

Sandelowski, Margarete, Betty G. Harris, and Beth Perry Black. 1992. "Relinquishing Infertility: The Work of Pregnancy for Infertile Couples." *Qualitative Health Research* 2(3): 282–301.

Scholz, T., S. Bartholomaus, I. Grimmer, H. Kentenich, and M. Obladen. 1999. "Problems of Multiple Births After ART: Medical, Psychological, Social and Financial Aspects." *Human Reproduction* 14(12): 2932–2937.

Sciarra, J. 1994. "Infertility: An International Health Problem." *International Journal of Gynecology and Obstetrics* 46(2): 155–163.

———. 1997. "Sexually Transmitted Diseases: Global Importance." *International Journal of Gynecology and Obstetrics* 58(1): 107–119.

Scutt, Jocelynne A., ed. 1990. *The Baby Machine: Reproductive Technology and the Commercialisation of Motherhood.* London: Merlin Press.

Serour, Gamal I. 1992. "Medically Assisted Conception: Dilemma of Practice and Research—Islamic Views." In *Proceedings of the First International Conference on "Bioethics in Human Reproduction Research in the Muslim World," 10–13 December, 1991,* ed. Gamal I. Serour, 234–242. Cairo: International Islamic Center for Population Studies and Research, Al-Azhar University.

———. 1996. "Bioethics in Reproductive Health: A Muslim's Perspective." *Middle East Fertility Society Journal* 1(1): 30–35.

Slovic, Paul. 1992. "Perception of Risk: Reflections on the Psychometric Paradigm." In *Social Theories of Risk,* eds. Sheldon Krimsky and Dominic Golding, 117–152. Westport, CT: Praeger.

Spallone, Patricia, and Deborah Lynn Steinberg, eds. 1987. *Made to Order: The Myth of Reproductive and Genetic Progress.* Oxford: Pergamon.

Squier, Susan Merrill. 1994. *Babies in Bottles: Twentieth-Century Visions of Reproductive Technology.* New Brunswick, NJ: Rutgers University Press.

Stanworth, Michelle, ed. 1987. *Reproductive Technologies: Gender, Motherhood and Medicine.* Cambridge: Polity Press.

Thompson, Charis M. 2001. "Fertile Ground: Feminists Theorize Infertility." In *Infertility around the Globe: New Thinking on Childlessness, Gender, and Reproductive Technologies,* eds. Marcia C. Inhorn and Frank van Balen, 52–78. Berkeley and Los Angeles: University of California Press.

Van Balen, Frank, and Trudie Gerrits. 2001. "Quality of Infertility Care in Poor-Resource Areas and the Introduction of New Reproductive Technologies." *Human Reproduction* 16(2): 215–219.

Van Dyck, Jose. 1995. *Manufacturing Babies and Public Consent: Debating the New Reproductive Technologies.* London: Macmillan.

World Health Organization. 1987. "Infections, Pregnancies, and Infertility: Perspectives on Prevention." *Fertility and Sterility* 47(6): 964–968.

Chapter 4

The Politics of Health Risk Warnings: Social Movements and Controversy over the Link between Abortion and Breast Cancer

Laury Oaks

INTRODUCTION

This chapter examines controversy in the United States over antiabortion advocates' efforts to link abortion with another highly visible, politicized, and emotionally laden women's health issue: breast cancer. Drawing on scholarship that emphasizes the politics of risk perception, assessment, and communication, I analyze both how antiabortion activists have supported their claims and how women's health and abortion rights advocates have responded to antiabortion campaigns that publicize the putative "fact" that abortion increases a woman's risk of subsequently contracting breast cancer. Whether abortion and breast cancer are linked in this way has been labeled by some medical professionals as "one of the most controversial and important questions in women's health today" (Bartholomew and Grimes 1998:708) and identified by others as "scientifically complex and politically charged" (Gammon, Bertin, and Terry 1996).[1] Health professionals and advocates who represent both sides of the abortion debate have analyzed evidence of the risk of breast cancer associated with abortion on both scientific and political terms. Controversy over antiabortion advocates' campaign to publicize the "scientific fact" that abortion increases a

I would like to thank Jo Murphy-Lawless, Jessica Jerome, and Francesca Bray for their feedback on an early version of this chapter, which was presented at the 2000 American Anthropological Association meetings. Talia Walsmith and Alena Donovan provided valuable, detailed research assistance, and the Institute for Social, Economic, and Behavioral Research at the University of California, Santa Barbara, provided funding support. The chapter has benefited enormously due to close readings of its several iterations by Doug English and Barbara Herr Harthorn. I owe an abundance of thanks to Barbara, whose vision and energy have sustained our collaborative work on this volume from its inception as a conference panel to its completion as a book manuscript.

woman's risk of contracting breast cancer demonstrates how advocates on either side of the abortion debate deploy scientific knowledge and the concept of
risk in support of their position.

Through billboard campaigns and pressure on some states' legislatures to institute breast cancer risk warnings in informed-consent abortion laws, antiabortion activists have sought to dissuade women from opting for abortion on
the grounds that they are putting their health and lives at risk. In 2001, 17
states enforced laws that require abortion providers to deliver state-scripted literature about abortion procedures and risks, fetal development, and abortion
alternatives as part of the medical informed-consent process and to require a
waiting period of at least 24 hours before a woman can consent to abortion after
receiving this information (see NARAL 2002:11).

Antiabortion advocates refer to such legislation as "women's right to know"
laws, and contend that access to knowledge about the risks of abortion empow-
ers women. Responding to the charge that such laws restrict women's abortion
rights, one antiabortion advocate pointedly asks, "But what choice do women
really have if they do not know the facts?" (Hughes 2001:7). I argue that the
antiabortion argument describing "right to know" legislation as in women's
best interest invokes the concepts of choice and rights in ways that attempt to
undermine the logic and validity of a pro-choice or abortion rights position.
The informed-consent laws and public information campaign supported by antiabortion activists are premised on the belief that women's fears of breast cancer
are so high that if a woman has the "facts" about the health risks allegedly associated with abortion, she will choose not to have an abortion. This position ignores that the facts available on abortion are partial and that women's abortion
decision-making is based on social and emotional dynamics and not simply on
"scientific facts."

Antiabortion advocates' attention to the abortion-breast cancer risk
(abortion-BCR) link has followed their efforts since the late 1980s to reshape
the social and political debate over abortion by publicizing the contention that
abortion causes mental distress (so-called post-abortion stress syndrome) and
serious long-term physical problems, primarily infertility and future pregnancy complications (see Wilmoth 1992; Miller 1996a, 1996b; Major et al.
2000; Elliot Institute 2001). Abortion-BCR warnings challenge women's health
advocates and abortion rights supporters to publicly discredit antiabortion advocates' representation of "scientific facts" about the health risks related to
abortion. To understand these dynamics, I systematically collected and analyzed national and local media reports, materials produced by advocacy organizations, public health officials' statements, and medical research articles.

As acknowledged by scholars and, as this chapter demonstrates, for health
professionals and political activists alike, understandings of risk are not simply
based on scientific evidence but also on the social and political evaluation of
what is deemed dangerous. Foremost scholars of risk, including Nelkin, Giddens, Douglas, and Beck, demonstrate that dispute over the meaning of risk re-

flects disagreement over social, cultural, and political values and power (see Lupton 1999a, 1999b). Health controversies, writes Nelkin, are characterized by conflict over a series of claims, including the "significance of risk, the adequacy of evidence, the methodologies for evaluating and measuring risk, the severity of health effects, and the appropriate standards to guide regulation" (Nelkin 1989:98). Each of these factors is salient in the abortion-BCR controversy. The data that proponents and opponents of the link between abortion and breast cancer cite as the grounds for their arguments are framed simultaneously as objectively scientific and politically biased as antiabortion and abortion rights advocates invoke the authority of science, medicine, and statistics to legitimize their positions (see Best 2001). Further, risk communication is an increasingly complex area of the scholarly study of risk and scientific uncertainty, with a focus on understanding individuals' and groups' perceptions of—and responses to—risk messages (Wilkins and Patterson 1991; Bennett and Calman 1999; Slovic 1999). Public announcements about risk communicate ideas about trust, fear, and blame and include explicit and implicit directives about how risk should be perceived and acted upon.

The perceived certainty or uncertainty of the evidence supporting risk claims is crucial to risk communication. Currently, medical and scientific data provide inconclusive and contradictory evidence about whether abortion increases a woman's risk of having breast cancer, yet the data have been used by advocates on both sides of the debate in ways that obscure this uncertainty. The downplaying of uncertainty strengthens assertions about the actions that ought to be taken by individual women, as well as by public health officials and state legislators, in line with advocates' interpretations of the scientific evidence. Therefore, the abortion-BCR issue provides a particularly useful case for examining contestations over risk.

Breast cancer risk campaigns capitalize on the pervasive moral imperative embedded in health risk warnings that instruct individuals to take steps to protect themselves from disease by making "healthy choices" to avoid or reduce risk (Crawford 1980; Balshem 1993; Lupton 1995; Petersen and Lupton 1996; Oaks 2001). Antiabortion activists' claims about the risks of breast cancer associated with abortion assert that all women can—and should—choose to act in ways that will decrease their risk of contracting breast cancer. Warnings about a link between abortion and breast cancer heighten an already ever-present and powerful discourse of fear around breast cancer that has been produced by women's health activists, medical professionals, and the media (Lock 1998; Kaufert 1999; Press, Fishman, and Koenig 2000; Lerner 2001). Risk messages gain power not only when based on claims of certainty but also when based on those of uncertainty.

Abortion-BCR warnings may compound the effects of women's feelings of living in an "at risk" state in which risk itself becomes an illness to be treated. Anthropologist Gifford's (1986:234) analysis of how doctors and women view benign breast condition as a risk factor for breast cancer concludes, "Being diagnosed at risk is itself a risk factor. It represents the risk of medicalization and the risk of losing control over the definition of one's own health." The irony of the identification of breast cancer risk factors and the promotion of risk assessments and screening is that medical professionals can offer no assurance that any action will prevent a woman from being diagnosed with breast cancer. Prophylactic mastectomy (the removal of the at-risk breast) represents an extreme measure and dramatically captures the attempts of some women (and their doctors) to control uncertainty (see Gifford 1986; Lerner 2001). Highly visible public and medical concern about the prevention and cure of breast cancer provided a context within which antiabortion advocates' warnings could gain significant attention, beginning in the early 1990s. Antiabortion advocates have worked to identify abortion as a dangerous medical procedure that women should both fear and blame in relation to breast cancer.

FRAMEWORKS THAT SUPPORT ANTIABORTION ADVOCATES' BREAST CANCER RISK CLAIMS

Although research on the link between abortion and breast cancer risk dates back to a 1957 Japanese study (Segi, Fukushima, and Kurihara 1957), the first public statements suggesting a connection between abortion and breast cancer in the United States were made by an antiabortion advocate during a political campaign. For two weeks in 1993 during a Virginia race for lieutenant governor, Republican candidate Michael Farris stated in interviews that part of his opposition to abortion was that it increased a woman's risk of breast cancer (Goodstein 1993:A1). Although Farris subsequently dropped his attention to the issue, members of the antiabortion movement have continued to pressure government officials to tell the "truth" about this "risk" and have threatened class-action lawsuits against abortion providers and clinics on behalf of women who consented to abortion without being told that it carried a risk of breast cancer.

Antiabortion advocates charge the mainstream medical establishment with intentionally covering up what they refer to as the ABC link (a term that seems strategically designed to connote a simple relationship). Antiabortion lobbyists contend that public health officials, and the medical field in general, have led the public to mistakenly believe that abortion is a safe procedure that does not pose long-term health risks. To right this perceived wrong, opponents of abortion contend that informed-consent procedures should include information about various psychological and physical risks, including the risk of breast cancer. Despite contradictory scientific findings on the association between abortion and breast cancer risk, which I explore later, 24 measures were introduced in 18 states in 2001 to include breast cancer risk warnings in informed-consent procedures (NARAL 2002:2). A so-called public education campaign, however, has been the most highly visible public aspect of the breast cancer warning efforts.

On billboards near highways, on bus sideboards, and on kiosks in mass transit systems in a number of cities across the country, antiabortion organizations have sponsored warnings about the risk of breast cancer "caused" by abortion.

The arguments that the antiabortion movement rely on to frame their warnings have been generated primarily by two activists: Sommerville, a lawyer with a Harvard degree, and Brind, a professor of biology and endocrinology at Baruch College, City University of New York. Sommerville and Brind have collaborated by speaking about the issue on Christian radio, contributing articles to church and antiabortion publications, and selling Sommerville's 1993 pamphlet "The Link between Abortion and Breast Cancer" (Goodstein 1993:A4). While conducting breast cancer research in 1992, Brind reportedly "stumbled onto the link" with abortion (Sommerville 1993:11), and following a 1996 research publication by Brind and colleagues, the scientist Brind's name rather than the lawyer Sommerville's has been repeated in media coverage on the theory that abortion is linked to breast cancer risk.[2] Brind et al.'s (1996) review and meta-analysis of 23 studies conducted in 11 countries reported a 30-percent increase in the risk of breast cancer attributable to a woman's having one or more abortions.

It is notable that the mainstream news press has identified Brind's status in contradictory ways. Although a *Newsweek* article begins, "Joel Brind is a scientist, not an activist" (Cowley and Hager 1996), *U.S News & World Report* on the same date included Brind's statement, "It's fine with me to help women to choose not to have an abortion" (Rubin 1996:96). Brind has written for the *National Right-to-Life News* (1998), presented his views at antiabortion conferences, including Human Life International's 17th World conference held in 1998, and served on the board of the Coalition on Abortion/Breast Cancer. Such activities make clear that Brind is both a scientist and an activist. Antiabortion advocates repeatedly cite Brind's meta-analysis as providing indisputable evidence for their campaign to publicize the abortion-BCR link.

Sommerville's 1993 self-published pamphlet stresses the political use of science as he divides the research studies conducted on abortion and breast cancer risk into two groups: "our studies," dating back to 1957 (Segi, Fukushima, and Kurihara 1957) and showing a link, and "the abortion industry's studies," dating back to 1982 (Cates 1982) and failing to support a link. This tactic is currently used by the Coalition on Abortion/Breast Cancer, which lists 29 studies, dating back to 1957, that show evidence of an increased risk of breast cancer following abortion and 8 studies, dating back to a 1979 Serbo-Croatian medical journal article, that show no such evidence (2001a). (Cates' 1982 article is not cited by the Coalition on Abortion/Breast Cancer, revealing that the coalition's tally sheet is not comprehensive.) For antiabortion advocates, that the data on their side extends farther back in time is used to imply an important historical depth to their abortion-BCR claim. The implication is that those on the "other side" are challenged to disprove the original finding.

Further, Sommerville's instruction to antiabortion advocates to categorize each study as either supporting its side or the side of its opponents overlooks the complexity of epidemiological studies as well as the process of the production and interpretation of scientific knowledge and "facts" (see Gifford 1986; Longino 1990; Haraway 1991, 1996; Krimsky 1992). Antiabortion advocates are urged to view *any* evidence of an association between abortion and breast cancer as an objective fact and to view as biased those studies that reject this link or state that the data is inadequate to support a definitive conclusion. In this way, the antiabortion analysis of "good" and "bad" studies depends on the political implications of a study's findings. Medical researchers differentiate between good and bad (or strong and weak) research, yet their judgments are based (at least ostensibly) on protocols and standards set by a community of scientists and not mainly on the potential political effect of the research.[3]

But antiabortion advocates do not simply seek more data or better studies to back the truth value of their claims. It is clear that they seek also to build a constituency of "at-risk victims" who could raise others' awareness of the alleged post-abortion risk of breast cancer. Sommerville's (1993) pamphlet directly addresses the problem of how best to reach out to at-risk women: "Women who have had a miscarriage or an abortion before their first live birth may find this [Sommerville's] report to be very alarming. Women who have had miscarriages will need professional guidance from a doctor on how they should *cope with this risk*. Women who have had abortions may need additional professional assistance from lawyers and counselors" (1993:10, emphasis added). More to the point, Sommerville is offering women advice about how to cope with their *fears* about their newly discovered at-risk status; this purported risk cannot be managed, but women's feelings and desire to do something about being put at risk by abortion can.

A contradiction is contained in the message that women should see their doctors if they are worried about their heightened risk of being diagnosed with breast cancer: antiabortion activists repeatedly berate physicians for not taking seriously the abortion-BCR link. Indeed, neither of the two models widely used by clinicians to estimate a woman's breast cancer risk, the Gail and the Claus model, includes a reference to abortion (see Press, Fishman, and Koenig 2000). (The Claus model does not even include childbirth as a factor; the Gail model takes into consideration age at first live birth). Further, Sommerville points out that a doctor's advice would likely include, for most women, regular self breast exams and for others, routine mammograms (1993:10). His "see your doctor" message, therefore, supports the recommendations of medical organizations such as the American Cancer Society and National Cancer Institute, which from the antiabortion point of view have acted irresponsibly in failing to support the message that abortion increases a woman's risk of breast cancer.

At the same time, however, the "see your doctor" strategy may be designed to send anxious women to their doctors with questions about the abortion-BCR connection in an attempt to pressure medical professionals to pay greater attention to this issue. Equally, if not more important, antiabortion advocates' political interests are served by raising women's fears about breast cancer, because such fears could mobilize voters to lobby legislators to implement anti-abortion policies.

The suggestion that women seek medical advice about their fear of breast cancer risk enhances the construction of the at-risk reproductive body. Women potentially benefit from breast cancer screening because a diagnosis made early in the disease progression may be more easily and successfully treatable. But, as feminist critics argue, the screening message has the consequence of labeling women as embodying a vulnerable, at-risk status, which both renders them potential disease victims and places responsibility on them to follow experts' advice (Gifford 1986; Lock 1998; Kaufert 1999; Hunt and de Voogd, this volume). This process has implications psychologically for individual women, who must cope with the feeling that they are at risk of a serious disease. Of further potential consequence, evidence of a "nocebo phenomenon"—in which individuals who have expectations of sickness have a greater likelihood of experiencing sickness—suggests that women's feelings of being at risk may have not only psychological but also physical effects (Hahn 1999).

The recommendations that Sommerville's pamphlet offers to women promote the greater visibility of the abortion-BCR issue not only as a medical problem but also as a legal problem. His recommendation that women who have had an abortion should see a lawyer due to their newfound fear of contracting breast cancer buttresses the movement's broader efforts to bring malpractice suits against abortion providers (Russo and Denious 1998; Coalition on Abortion/Breast Cancer 2001b). Sommerville asserts that because "clear evidence" on the connection was available in 1981 (Pike et al. 1981), all women since this time should have been informed of this risk by a medical professional before making an abortion decision. The chance of winning a malpractice case is good, Sommerville-the-lawyer argues, as "juries may find it hard to believe that the average woman would knowingly choose to raise her risk of breast cancer to Russian roulette's one in six odds" (1993:10). Here, he assigns a specific measure of risk to abortion and portrays a woman's decision to have an abortion as playing a high-stakes game of chance that might result in death.

Although Sommerville's name is not connected with the most recent anti-abortion campaigns to raise awareness about the abortion-BCR connection, other advocates have mobilized many of the strategies outlined in Sommerville's pamphlet. The most broad-based organization focusing on this issue is the Coalition on Abortion/Breast Cancer, a Chicago-area group founded in May 1999. The Coalition defines its purpose as "to protect the health and save the lives of women by educating and providing information on abortion as a risk factor for breast cancer" (2001c).[4] The organization's logo features a pink ribbon, the symbol of the breast cancer advocacy movement, and its Web site offers extensive information about the "ABC" link, political and legal actions related to it, and advocacy recommendations (2001b). The Coalition models anti-abortion advocates' multidimensional efforts to convince legislators, health officials, and the public that breast cancer is a serious risk to women who have had or will have abortions.

The tactics recommended by Sommerville (1993) and taken up by other antiabortion activists illustrate how the risk concept can be used in the United States as a way to raise an individual's fears about her health status and as a tool for legislation and litigation. In these advocates' logic, abortion is harmful to women because it both causes fear of breast cancer and increases the likelihood that a woman will subsequently contract breast cancer. Antiabortion advocates urge women to blame abortion for their suffering as "at risk" or as victims of breast cancer. Further, scientific evidence suggesting a link between abortion and breast cancer risk provides the grounds for activists' work to lobby state legislatures and public health officials to institute warnings of this danger to women who are considering abortion. This evidence underlies the legal actions antiabortion advocates have taken against abortion providers for failing to inform women of the ostensible abortion-BCR connection. However, public health officials and women's health advocates have resisted the antiabortion effort to frame abortion as dangerous. The first abortion–breast cancer warning campaign inspired a counter-campaign to contest antiabortion advocates' use of science, risk, and risk communication.

ANTIABORTION ADVOCATES' "PUBLIC SERVICE WARNINGS" AND WOMEN'S HEALTH ADVOCATES' COUNTER-CAMPAIGN

In 1996, antiabortion advocates launched what one activist called a "public-health risk disclosure service" to raise awareness about the "scientific fact" that abortion raises a woman's breast cancer risk coincident with the annual March for Life and rally in Washington, D.C., to protest the anniversary of the 1973 U.S. Supreme Court's *Roe v. Wade* ruling that legalized abortion (Brad Thomas, quoted in Guiden 1996). In January 1996, Christ's Bride Ministries, a one-man operation run by Brad Thomas and based in Virginia, sponsored more than 1,000 ads in the Washington metro system and on buses.[5] The Ministries reportedly received free ad space to support their "public service" campaign (see Loose 1996:A9). Warning campaigns spread in 1996 to Baltimore, Philadelphia, and other cities in the northeast, Oregon, and Alabama, and later reemerged in 2000 in Philadelphia and North Dakota.[6] The Ministries' stark black, white, and red billboards and posters announced: "Women who choose abortion suffer more and deadlier breast cancer" and included a toll-free phone number that viewers could call "for more information."

Although this warning served to publicize the abortion-BCR link, it actually goes beyond the data that most antiabortion advocates rely on to ground their arguments. The contention that abortion is associated with a "deadlier" form of breast cancer has not been routinely included in antiabortion literature, nor was it backed by Brind et al.'s study (published one year later, in 1996). The language of the warning plays on the concept of choice, implying that a woman who opts for abortion "chooses" to put herself at increased risk of "suffering" from breast cancer. This reference to choice invokes a connection between the pro-choice movement and its failure to warn women of this alleged and alarming risk.

Advocates' use of billboards and other media outlets to promote antiabortion views, of course, is not new. Billboards, placards, and pamphlets featuring images of fetuses and messages such as "Stop Abortion. They're forgetting someone" (Condit 1990:84) support the antiabortion arguments that the fetus is a person who deserves the right to life and that it is a "scientific fact" that personhood begins at conception (see Luker 1978, 1984; Petchesky [1984] 1985, 1987; Ginsburg [1989] 1998; Morgan and Michaels 1999). Importantly, however, although many messages using fetal imagery are quite easily identified as sponsored by the antiabortion movement, the abortion–breast cancer billboard warnings and the Tennessee-based American Rights Coalition that sponsored the 1-800 information line featured in the ads are not (Loose 1996). Controversy over the ad campaign was generated from the announcement of "facts" that were not supported adequately by scientific evidence and the lack of clear antiabortion sponsorship of the ads. Callers to the 1-800 number featured on the ads were told that one in every two women who has an abortion will suffer breast cancer (Cox 1996; Guiden 1996) and given statistical information implying that the National Cancer Institute, an agency of the U.S. government's Department of Health and Human Services, supported the ad's warning (Lee 1996). Further, callers were asked to participate in a survey on women's abortion experiences and told that the purpose of the campaign was to collect enough information to file a class-action suit against abortion providers (Cox 1996; Lee 1996). The campaign clearly enacted recommendations offered in Sommerville's 1993 pamphlet.

In response, a coalition of health organizations sponsored a counter-campaign and lobbied transit authorities in several cities to remove the Ministries' posters on the grounds that abortion-BCR messages were "deceptive, false, and misleading" and "spread misinformation" (Cox 1996).[7] A sample protest letter to transit authority directors designed by one member of the coalition, the National Women's Health Network (NWHN), outlines the coalition's main arguments against the antiabortion ad campaign. The letter contends that the Ministries' claim that abortion causes breast cancer is not backed by scientific studies ("there is no evidence conclusively linking abortion to breast cancer at present") and states that public transit systems have a responsibility to provide accurate information to the public (Cox 1996). Summarizing the status of research on abortion and breast cancer and emphasizing its inconclusiveness, the letter explains, "Although there are approximately two dozen studies examining the relationship between breast cancer and abortion, the studies show no proven link. Some studies do report a strong association between abortion and subsequent diagnosis of breast cancer; other studies find no association at all" (Cox 1996). The letter closes by strongly urging the transit director to 1) remove the ads and publish a retraction and 2) "grant equal time and space for public service messages that would give women *accurate information* about abortion and breast cancer" (Cox 1996, emphasis added). Thus, the counter-campaign framed its mission as one of ensuring the public would receive scientifically backed messages about whether abortion is linked to breast cancer risk. Brind and other antiabortion advocates, however, pointed to the counter-campaign and demand that ads be removed as proof of a "cover-up" of abortion-BCR data (Brind 1997:13). In this way, antiabortion advocates could simultaneously dismiss protests against the Ministries' campaign and underscore one of their main arguments.

The coalition's protest campaign produced varied results. In Washington, D.C., the First Amendment guarantee to free speech was cited to uphold the campaign, and a Metro official actively defended the ad (Loose 1996). But transit authorities in other cities ruled differently in response to protests. In Philadelphia, the mass transit system SEPTA removed the ads and were sued for doing so by the Ministries' Brad Thomas (Guiden 1996).[8] Baltimore's Mass Transit Authority (MTA) determined that it could not violate First Amendment rights by banning the Ministries' ad; however, transit officials felt a responsibility to aid the provision of accurate information to the public (Gray 1996).

As a result, the Baltimore MTA provided a coalition of women's health advocacy organizations with free ad space to sponsor kiosk posters next to the Ministries' ads in metro stations and on both ends of the Ministries' ads on bus side boards in June 1996. The counter-message read: "Get the facts: Abortion does NOT cause breast cancer" and listed a Washington-area telephone number (Gray 1996). Speaking about the aim of the coalition's counter-campaign, one National Women's Health Network (NWHN) spokesperson stated that the coalition "wanted to provide accurate information about the relationship" between abortion and breast cancer (quoted in Guiden 1996). Voicing a different yet not incompatible aim, the executive director of NWHN contended that the purpose was to "make people doubtful about the [Ministries' risk warning] statement" by presenting side-by-side conflicting messages (Gray 1996). The juxtaposition intended to make clear the political—as opposed to scientific—nature of the claim, which would lead people to see it as a debatable statement.

Three main implications are embedded in the coalition's one-line counter advertising message. First, it discredits the Christ's Bride Ministries' statement as fiction by asserting that the "facts" indicate that abortion does not cause breast cancer. Second, it encourages people to question and investigate the issue themselves. The posters listed an NWHN phone number; callers received information on the phone and, if requested, by mail on the lack of scientific support for a link (NWHN staff member, personal communication, 2001). Third, the coalition took a stronger stand than others by claiming that abortion is not a cause of breast cancer. There is a difference between stating that abortion does not cause breast cancer and stating that scientific evidence is inconclusive about the abortion–breast cancer link.

This last point is particularly significant, because it reveals that the politicization of information about the abortion-BCR link led to claims by both antiabortion and women's health advocates that do not adequately reflect the state of medical knowledge about a possible link. Using scientific standards, the most accurate representation of the data in 1996 when the antiabortion advocates' "public service" campaign and the protest counter-campaigns were run, as well as at the time of writing, is that it is inconsistent and inconclusive: the hypotheses that abortion causes breast cancer or that it increases a woman's risk of later contracting breast cancer have been neither proven nor disproven definitively. In part, it is this ambiguous status that allows for wide-ranging interpretations and claims about the "facts" of breast cancer risk related to abortion.

Antiabortion and women's health advocates can both rightly claim that some data back their campaign positions. In the antiabortion case, some studies show a link, and in the women's health advocacy case, inconsistent evidence fails to confirm a link. The ads, however, operate on terms that are greatly reduced in complexity. The Ministries' ad implied causality (and to a "more deadly" form of the disease), and the coalitions' counterpoint explicitly denied it. The women's health advocates' message counters, "Abortion does not cause breast cancer." In the one view, abortion is dangerous, and in the other it is safe. In short, antiabortion advocates urged women to take breast cancer risk into account when making an abortion decision. The NWHN countered with the logic that "there is currently no scientifically acceptable reason for women to factor an increased risk of breast cancer into their decision whether or not to continue a pregnancy" (NWHN [1994] 1996:3). This assertion also serves to weaken the scientific legitimacy of legislative and judicial attempts to include breast cancer risk information in informed-consent materials about abortion. As more scientific data become available, advocates on both sides of the controversy will seek to bolster their arguments about whether abortion should be considered a risk factor for breast cancer.

In fact, in 1997, the year following the Ministries' campaign and the publication of Brind et al.'s (1996) meta-analysis, the publication of a new study by Danish researchers Melbye et al. (1997) provided women's health and abortion rights advocates with more data "on their side." Contradicting Brind et al.'s findings, which showed a 30-percent increase in breast cancer risk for women who had had an abortion (based on data from 11 countries), Melbye et al.'s cohort study of health data on Danish women concluded that abortion had "no overall effect on the risk of breast cancer" (1997:81). The article appeared in the New England Journal of Medicine and was accompanied by an editorial by a National Cancer Institute epidemiologist, Hartge, who asserted that Melbye's data proved that "a woman need not worry about the risk of breast cancer" in relation to abortion (1997). Other reports also labeled Melbye's study as ending the abortion-BCR controversy. Newsweek's coverage of

Melbye's research reports that Brind et al.'s (1996) meta-analysis showed abortion increases the risk of breast cancer, yet it privileges Melbye's as "the largest, most thorough study ever conducted on the issue" (Cowley 1997:48). Melbye's results, the report continues, should bring a worldwide sigh of relief because the "case is closed" until future studies prove otherwise (Cowley 1997:49).

But such assertions about the definitive nature of the scientific conclusion on the abortion-BCR link appear overstated. More correctly, the case remains open. In part, the interpretation of whether scientific data support or disprove the abortion-BCR link reflects differing values placed on types of data. Melbye et al.'s (1997) is a population-based cohort study, whereas Brind et al.'s (1996) is a meta-analysis, a study of the body of studies conducted on the topic. Although Melbye et al.'s data did not support a link, Brind et al.'s did. Not all meta-analyses, however, come to the same conclusion as Brind et al. (1996). Wingo et al.'s (1997) review of 32 epidemiological studies on breast cancer and spontaneous or induced abortion states, "Definitive conclusions about an association between breast cancer risk and spontaneous or induced abortion are not possible at present because of inconsistent findings across studies" (1997:93). What seems most prudent and accurate, then, in summarizing the data on the abortion-BCR link, is the message offered by the National Cancer Institute (NCI) that states, "There is no convincing evidence of a direct relationship between breast cancer and either induced or spontaneous abortion. Available data are inconsistent and inconclusive" (National Cancer Institute 1997). This message is more hesitant than NCI's Hartge's (1997) statement that a woman need not worry; more to the point, the current data do not support such a worry. A woman indeed could be concerned about the inconsistent and inconclusive nature of the data, as there is no definitive answer to the question of whether abortion and breast cancer are linked.

There is further indication that assurances that abortion is not linked to breast cancer may be overstated: journalists, National Cancer Institute officials, and women's health advocates (Boston Women's Health Book Collective 1998:412) rarely mention that Melbye et al.'s (1997) study reported a statistically significant increased breast cancer risk among women who had second-trimester abortions. The vast majority of abortions in the United States, 88 percent, occur during the first trimester (Centers for Disease Control and Prevention 2000); therefore, it can be argued that although the study's finding about second-trimester abortion in relation to breast cancer was of statistical significance, the conclusion that Melbye et al. (1997) and others drew from the study emphasized the finding's practical significance. The wording of a June 2000 World Health Organization fact sheet on abortion and breast cancer risk precisely reflects this main conclusion: "Results from epidemiological studies are reassuring in that they show no consistent effect of first trimester induced abortion upon a woman's risk of breast cancer later in life" (World Health Organization 2000). While women's health and abortion rights advocates seek to reassure women through such statements, antiabortion advocates have continued their efforts to represent the ABC link as scientifically proven and cause for serious concern. In the concluding section of this paper, I consider opposing views on how women should be made aware of information about the possible link between abortion and increased breast cancer risk.

CONCLUSION: "RIGHT TO KNOW" POLICY IMPLICATIONS FOR WOMEN'S "RIGHT TO CHOOSE" ABORTION

Clearly, for antiabortion advocates, risk has become what anthropologist Douglas terms a "forensic resource" (1992). Arguments about the abortion-BCR link underpin campaigns to include breast cancer risk warnings in informed-consent procedures and abortion clinic information. This enhances the legitimacy of antiabortion claims: when such risk warnings become part of medical procedures, they are divorced from the antiabortion movement and the political process that resulted in right-to-know legislation. The state's role as protector of the public's health may mislead citizens to believe that such laws are backed by an objective review of scientific data.

This is exactly the sort of association that antiabortion advocates direct people to make. In his 1998 *Wisconsin Law Review* article, Kindley argues that due to the failure of federal and state legislatures as well as health agencies to inform women about what he, too, refers to as the ABC link, the judicial/adversarial system is likely the best route (2000:251). Malpractice suits, he contends, have the ability to raise public awareness about this health risk and to demonstrate to the public that health practitioners and public health officials have irresponsibly been shirking their duties. Although an analysis of his legal arguments is beyond the scope of this paper, his article provides a range of legal strategies for malpractice suits against doctors and clinics that do not inform women of a possible breast cancer link. His position rests on the assertion that uncertainty about the potential risk of breast cancer posed by abortion should not hinder attempts to make public this possible risk: "Although the *scientific evidence may not yet prove* beyond the shadow of a doubt that induced abortion causes breast cancer, there is no doubt that abortion providers have a duty to inform women considering the procedure about this significant health risk before an abortion is performed" (2000:289, emphasis added). Kindley writes with confidence (revealed in the assertion that evidence does not yet prove the link) that future research will vindicate the antiabortion position. Women's health and abortion rights advocates also call for more research on the abortion-BCR link. Their arguments are based on the position that despite current inconclusive data, policy action to warn women about breast cancer risk is unwarranted. Each side draws an opposite conclusion about how to interpret and respond to scientific data on breast cancer in a way that supports their opposing political positions on abortion rights.

The question of medical professionals' responsibility to inform women about the possibility of an abortion-BCR link was taken up in *JAMA*, the journal of the American Medical Association, the same year the Ministries' campaign was run in response to antiabortion advocates' legislative proposals that right-to-know laws mandate informing women seeking abortion about the risks of breast cancer. Gammon, Bertin, and Terry (1996) argue that full disclosure would require what sounds close to a course in epidemiology and medical research methods. To be accurate, they contend, what would be needed is an "explanation of the inconsistent state of the research, the methodological limitations that cloud interpretation of the research, the possibility that positive findings could be real or artifactual, and the fact that most positive studies identify only a slight risk—less than or equivalent to the increased breast cancer risk associated with marital status, place of residence, or religion" (Gammon, Bertin, and Terry 1996:322). From the perspective of these medical professionals, the ethical communication of information about abortion-BCR goes far beyond a simple statement of the sort that antiabortion advocates are lobbying to have included in state-mandated informed-consent legislation. Risk communication that urges women to believe they are at risk must be backed by scientific, practical, and ethical considerations.

Taking a different approach to the issue of what type of information could be distributed to women in reaction to the abortion-BCR campaign, the National Breast Cancer Coalition (2001) argues that women should be informed both of the *controversy* over the antiabortion advocates' campaign and of the scientific evidence that has explored the abortion-BCR link. The organization, however, does not specify the mechanism for communicating this information. Nonetheless, the National Breast Cancer Coalition's emphasis on educating the public about both the abortion-BCR debate and the available scientific evidence offers a strategy to reply to the antiabortion advocates' contention that abortion rights advocates who oppose informed-consent laws are denying women access to information.

However, antiabortion advocates have attacked this sort of dual information-delivery strategy. The 1999 antiabortion lawsuit against the Fargo, North Dakota, Red River Women's clinic charged that the clinic provided false advertising and cited a clinic brochure that refuted the claim that breast cancer and abortion are linked. The brochure read, "Some antiabortion activists claim that having an abortion increases the risk of developing breast cancer. A substantial body of medical research indicates that there is no established link between abortion and breast cancer. In fact, the National Cancer Institute has stated, "There is no evidence of a direct relationship between breast cancer and either induced or spontaneous abortion" (quoted in Farmer 2000:5). The lawyer for the plaintiffs, Kindley, is a Coalition on Abortion/Breast Cancer board member and the author of the 1998 *Wisconsin Law Review* article discussed earlier that provides legal support for such litigious approaches. The success of this tactic is in jeopardy following a North Dakota judge's March 2002 ruling that the clinic need not offer a breast cancer warning (*Los Angeles Times* 2002) and the rejection the same month of a similar case by a California judge (Simon 2002). Kindley intends to appeal the case to the North Dakota Supreme Court (*Los Angeles Times* 2002).

Court challenges have as their aim not merely winning the case but "educating" the public. Coincident with the lawsuit, the Coalition worked in conjunction with a campaign organized by the director of the Pro-Life Office for the Catholic Diocese of Fargo to increase the visibility of the issue by sponsoring a college newspaper ad series, parish bulletin board notices, and billboard messages (Coalition on Abortion/Breast Cancer 2001d). The billboard ad reads simply, "Q: What increases your risk of breast cancer? A: Abortion," while the newspaper and bulletin ads urge women to visit the Coalition's Web site for "the current facts" about the increased risk of breast cancer associated with abortion and to call the Coalition to gain information about "how to protect yourself in the future ... if you have had an abortion or are considering an abortion" (Coalition on Abortion/Breast Cancer 2001d). Through this multi-faceted campaign, antiabortion advocates capitalized on the lawsuit to attempt to reach the public and build a constituency of supporters from which it could draw future litigants.

In short, the breast cancer controversy has been framed by antiabortion advocates in such a way that it puts medical professionals, public health officials, and women's health advocates in the reactive position of refuting antiabortion advocates' claims about the status of scientific evidence on the link and dispelling women's potential fears about being at risk for breast cancer if they opt for abortion. Not only science is at issue, of course, but politics—abortion politics and the politics of how health-risk data should be communicated to the public (see Balshem 1993; Lupton 1995; Parrott and Condit 1996; Petersen and Lupton 1996; Bennett and Calman 1999; Oaks 2001). One news report on the controversy states that antiabortion advocates "say that science, not politics, requires them to warn about the potential 'tragedy' of failing to alert women of the dangers they face when they have an abortion" but that critics "claim that politics—not science—is behind the study" (Lagnado 1996). This observation oversimplifies the case: Advocates on both sides of the debate have grounded their arguments in science and politics, revealing that science and politics are not mutually exclusive. Indeed, as theorists who stress the social construction of risk argue, science—like risk communication—is not value-free (see Lupton 1999a, 1999b). Social, cultural, and political processes shape the meaning of risk and the labeling of only some dangers as risks (Petersen and Lupton 1996:18).

Writing in *The Nation* in opposition to antiabortion advocates' attempts to institute mandatory abortion informed-consent regulations about breast cancer risk, feminist journalist and cultural critic Pollitt (2001) emphasizes that women and men constantly make health risk assessments and health choices without state intervention. In her analysis, abortion-BCR warnings result in "burdening the patient's choice with unsubstantiated fears" (Pollitt 2001:10).

To point out how the imposition of laws that require the delivery of breast cancer and other warnings and a waiting period before a woman is allowed to consent to abortion oversteps the bounds of a woman's individual decision-making about the possible risks of abortion, Pollitt poses a hypothetical, comparative case involving men's health. She predicts that lawmakers would never impose a waiting period on Viagra prescriptions so men can "really consider whether an erection is worth a heart attack" despite the fact that medical studies show that one of the risks of Viagra in some men is heart attack (Pollitt 2001:10). This comparison may sound trite, but it identifies as the center of the abortion-breast cancer risk debate the issue of respect for women's decision-making about their bodies and their health. The logical extension of her argument is that even if abortion were to be scientifically proven to be a risk factor for breast cancer, women must maintain the right to make for themselves the judgment about whether abortion is their best option. It should not be the case that this purported, or even future proven, risk should result in restrictions on abortion laws that erode women's decision-making and agency.

NOTES

1. Scientists hypothesize a biological link between abortion and breast cancer based on two observations: Women who give birth have a lower risk of breast cancer, and a rise in hormone production early in pregnancy causes breast cells to proliferate. These "immature" cells could be sites of cancer (see *Economist* 1996; Melbye et al. 1997).

2. Brind's research was funded by the Department of Education of the Commonwealth of Pennsylvania and Baruch College of the City University of New York.

3. I do not mean to imply that scientific research is objective and neutral; critical scholarship on science, medicine, and technology reveals how knowledge is shaped by the historical, political, and social-cultural context within which it is produced (Martin 1991, 1994, [1987, 1992] 2001; Traweek 1988; Longino 1990; Haraway 1991, 1996; Krimsky 1992; Downey and Dumit 1997; Clarke 1998; Murphy-Lawless 1999; Jacobson 2000).

4. The Coalition is based in the Chicago area and headed by its president, Karen Malec, and an advisory board composed of Joel Brind, Chris Kahlenborn (a doctor and author of *Breast Cancer: Its Link to Abortion and the Birth Control Pill*, 1999), John Kindley (a lawyer), Babette Francis (an Australian advocate), Penny Pullen (former Illinois state representative), and Jim Finnegan (no description provided) (Coalition for Abortion/Breast Cancer 2001d). That four of the six board members are men suggests that this "women's organization" is designated as such because of its work on behalf of women and not because it is composed of or run by women.

5. Although Christ's Bride Ministries' health warning tactic could be seen as the work of a single individual and not the antiabortion movement, it is a recommended strategy in *Firestorm: A Guerilla Strategy for a Pro-Life America* (1992). The book's author, Mark Crutcher, runs Life Dynamics; in 1995 the Texas-based organization report-

edly had a network of 600 lawyers trained to file suits against abortion providers on behalf of "abortion-injured" women (Russo and Denious 1998:27; see also Life Dynamics, Inc. 2001).

6. There is evidence of substantial monetary backing of this campaign. For example, the billboard that appeared in June 2000 on I-95 near Philadelphia announcing "abortion increases breast cancer risk" was sponsored by the antiabortion group Family Life Educational Foundation and cost $20,000 for a five-month period (McCullough 2000). The North Dakota campaign was backed by the Pro-Life Office of the Catholic Diocese of Fargo and the Chicago area Coalition on Abortion/Breast Cancer (2001d).

7. The counter-campaign was composed of the National Women's Health Network, the National Breast Cancer Coalition, the American Cancer Society, and the National Abortion Federation. The Public Health Services' then-Assistant Secretary of Health and Director for Public Health Service and the Congressional Caucus for Women also voiced opposition to the ad and its claims.

8. The case was appealed to the U.S. Supreme Court, which in 1999 let stand a ruling that the Ministries' First Amendment rights had been violated when SEPTA removed the ads (NARAL 2001:2).

REFERENCES

Balshem, Martha. 1993. *Cancer in the Community: Class and Medical Authority.* Washington, DC: Smithsonian Institute Press.

Bartholomew, Lynne L., and David A. Grimes. 1998. "The Alleged Association between Induced Abortion and Risk of Breast Cancer: Biology or Bias?" *Obstetrical and Gynecological Survey* 53(11):708–714.

Bennett, Peter, and Sir Kenneth Calman, eds. 1999. *Risk Communication and Public Health.* Oxford: Oxford University Press.

Best, Joel. 2001. *Damned Lies and Statistics: Untangling Numbers from the Media, Politicians, and Activists.* Berkeley and Los Angeles: University of California Press.

Boston Women's Health Book Collective. 1998. *Our Bodies, Ourselves for the New Century.* New York: Simon and Schuster.

Brind, Joel. 1997. "Abortion, Breast Cancer, and Ideology." *First Things: A Monthly Journal of Religion and Public Life* 73(May): 2–15.

———. 1998. "Abortion and Breast Cancer: Additional Evidence of Link Somehow Not Appearing in Published Studies." *National Right-to-Life News*, November. Available from www.prolifeinfo.org/risk001.html.

Brind, Joel, Vernon M. Chinchilli, Walter B. Severs, and Joan Summy-Long. 1996. "Induced Abortion as an Independent Risk Factor for Breast Cancer: A Comprehensive Meta-Analysis." *Journal of Epidemiology and Community Health* 50(5): 481–496.

Cates, Willard, Jr. 1982. "Legal Abortion: The Public Health Record." *Science* 215(4540): 1586–1590.

Centers for Disease Control and Prevention. 2000. "Abortion Surveillance—United States, 1997." *Morbidity and Mortality Weekly Report* 49 (SS-11, Dec.8): 1–43.

Clarke, Adele. 1998. *Disciplining Reproduction: Modernity, American Life Sciences, and "The Problems of Sex."* Berkeley and Los Angeles: University of California Press.

Coalition on Abortion/Breast Cancer. 2001a. *The ABC Link.* Available from www.abortion breastcancer.com.

———. 2001b. *What You Can Do.* Available from www.abortionbreastcancer.com.

———. 2001c. *About Us.* Available from www.abortionbreastconcer.com.

———. 2001d. *Catholic Diocese of Fargo, North Dakota Embarks on Ad Campaign to Educate Women about the Abortion-Breast Cancer Link.* Available from www.abortionbreastcancer.com.

Condit, Celeste Michelle. 1990. *Decoding Abortion Rhetoric: Communicating Social Change.* Urbana, IL: University of Chicago Press.

Cowley, Geoffrey. 1997. "Abortion and Cancer: No Connection." *Newsweek,* January 20, 48–49.

Cowley, Geoffrey, and Mary Hager. 1996. "Breast Cancer: Is Abortion a Factor?" *Newsweek,* October 21, 73.

Cox, Lisa. 1996. "Get the Facts and Take Action—Abortion Does NOT Cause Breast Cancer." *NWHN Policy Report* 1(1): 1–2.

Crawford, Robert. 1980. "Healthism and the Medicalization of Everyday Life." *International Journal of Health Services* 10(3): 365–388.

Crutcher, Mark. 1992. *Firestorm: A Guerilla Strategy for a Pro-Life America.* Denton, TX: Life Dynamics, Inc.

Douglas, Mary. 1992. *Risk and Blame: Essays in Cultural Theory.* London: Routledge.

Downey, Gary Lee, and Joseph Dumit, eds. 1997. *Cyborgs and Citadels: Anthropological Interventions in Emerging Sciences and Technologies.* Santa Fe, NM: School of American Research Press.

Economist. 1996. "Abortion, Breast Cancer, and the Misuse of Epidemiology." *Economist* 338(7955): 73–74.

Elliot Institute. 2001. *A List of Major Physical Sequelae Related to Abortion.* Available from www.afterabortion.org/physica.html.

Farmer, Ann. 2000. "Protestors Press Breast Cancer Ploy." *Center for Reproductive Law and Policy Reproductive Freedom News* 9(10): 5.

Gammon, Marilie D., Joan E. Bertin, and Mary Beth Terry. 1996. "Abortion and the Risk of Breast Cancer: Is There a Believable Association?" *JAMA* 275(4): 321–322.

Gifford, Sandra M. 1986. "The Meanings of Lumps: A Case Study of the Ambiguities of Risk." In *Anthropology and Epidemiology: Interdisciplinary Approaches to the Study of Health and Disease,* eds. Craig R. Janes, Ron Stall, and Sandra M. Gifford, 213–249. Dordrecht, The Netherlands: Reidel Publishing Co.

Ginsburg, Faye D. [1989] 1998. *Contested Lives: The Abortion Debate in an American Community.* Berkeley and Los Angeles: University of California Press.

Goodstein, Laurie. 1993. "Breast Cancer–Abortion Link Under Attack." *Washington Post,* November 1, A1, A4.

Gray, Ashley. 1996. "Double Negative." *Baltimore Magazine,* June.

Guiden, Mary. 1996. "Truth Be Told: MTA Caught in Battle over Abortion Messages." *Baltimore City Paper,* May 29–June 5.

Hahn, Robert A. 1999. "Expectations of Sickness: Concept and Evidence of the Nocebo Phenomenon." In *How Expectancies Shape Experience,* ed. Irving Kirsch, 333–356. Washington, D.C.: American Psychological Association.

Haraway, Donna. 1991. *Simians, Cyborgs, and Women.* New York: Routledge.

———. 1996. *Modest_Witness@Second_Millennium.FemaleMan© Meets Onco-Mouse™: Feminism and Technoscience.* New York: Routledge.

Hartge, Patricia. 1997. "Abortion, Breast Cancer and Epidemiology." *New England Journal of Medicine* 336(2): 127–128.

Hughes, Mary. 2001. "Abortion Is a Serious Cause of Breast Cancer." *Labour Life Group News*, 28 (Spring), 4–8.

Jacobson, Nora. 2000. *Cleavage: Technology, Controversy, and the Ironies of the Man-Made Breast.* New Brunswick, NJ: Rutgers University Press.

Kahlenborn, Chris. 1999. *Breast Cancer: Its Link to Abortion and the Birth Control Pill.* Dayton, OH: One More Soul Press.

Kaufert, Patricia A. 1999. "Women and the Debate over Mammography: An Economic, Political, and Moral History." In *Gender and Health: An International Perspective*, eds. Carolyn F. Sargent and Caroline B. Brettell, 167–186. Upper Saddle River, NJ: Prentice-Hall.

Kindley, John. 2000. "Abortion, Breast Cancer, and Informed Consent." *Issues in Law and Medicine* 15(3): 243–290. First published in *Wisconsin Law Review*, 1998.

Krimsky, Sheldon. 1992. "The Role of Theory in Risk Studies." In *Social Theories of Risk*, eds. Sheldon Krimsky and Dominic Golding 3–22. Westport, CT: Praeger.

Lagnado, Lucette. 1996. "Study on Abortion and Cancer Spurs Fight." *Wall Street Journal*, October 11, B4.

Lee, Philip R. 1996. "Letter to Mr. Lawrence Reuter, General Manager of the Washington Metropolitan Area Transit Authority." *'Get the Facts!': National Organizing Kit.* National Women's Health Network, April 1997.

Lerner, Barron H. 2001. *The Breast Cancer Wars: Hope, Fear, and the Pursuit of a Cure in Twentieth Century America.* New York: Oxford University Press.

Life Dynamics, Inc. 2001. Homepage. Available from www.ldi.org.

Lock, Margaret. 1998. "Breast Cancer: Reading the Omens." *Anthropology Today* 14(4): 7–16.

Longino, Helen E. 1990. *Science as Social Knowledge: Values and Objectivity in Scientific Inquiry.* Princeton: Princeton University Press.

Loose, Cindy. 1996. "Antiabortion Message Gets Free Ride on Metro System." *Washington Post*, January 22, A1, A9.

Los Angeles Times. 2002. "Abortion Clinic's Brochure Needn't Mention Cancer Risk, Judge Rules." March 29, A26.

Luker, Kristin. 1978. *Taking Chances: Abortion and the Decision Not to Contracept.* Berkeley and Los Angeles: University of California Press.

———. 1984. *Abortion and the Politics of Motherhood.* Berkeley and Los Angeles: University of California Press.

Lupton, Deborah. 1995. *The Imperative of Health: Public Health and the Regulated Body.* London: Sage Publications.

———. 1999a. *Risk.* London and New York: Routledge.

Lupton, Deborah, ed. 1999b. *Risk and Sociocultural Theory: New Directions and Perspectives.* Cambridge: Cambridge University Press.

Major, Brenda, Catherine Cozzarelli, M. Lynne Cooper, Josephine Zubek, Caroline Richards, Michael Wilhite, and Richard H. Gramzow. 2000. "Psychological Responses of Women after First-Trimester Abortion." *Archives of General Psychiatry* 57(8): 777–784.

Martin, Emily. 1991. "The Egg and the Sperm: How Science Has Constructed a Romance Based on Stereotypical Male-Female Roles." *Signs: Journal of Women in Culture and Society* 16(3): 485–501.

———. 1994. *Flexible Bodies: The Role of Immunity in American Culture from the Days of Polio to the Age of AIDS*. Boston: Beacon Press.

———. [1987, 1992] 2001. *The Woman in the Body: A Cultural Analysis of Reproduction*. Rev. ed. with a new intro. Boston: Beacon Press.

McCullogh, Marie. 2000. "Billboard on Breast Cancer Criticized as Alarmist." *Philadelphia Inquirer,* March 3, B1.

Melbye, Mads, Jan Wohlfahrt, Jorgen H. Olsen, Morten Frisch, Tine Westergaard, Karin Helweg-Larsen, and Per Kragh Andersen. 1997. "Induced Abortion and the Risk of Breast Cancer." *New England Journal of Medicine* 336(2): 81–85.

Miller, Diane Helen. 1996a. "Medical and Psychological Consequences of Legal Abortion in the United States." In *Evaluating Women's Health Messages,* eds. Roxanne Louiselle Parrott and Celeste Michelle Condit, 17–32. Thousand Oaks, CA: Sage.

———. 1996b. "Medical and Psychological Consequences of Legal Abortion in the United States." In *Evaluating Women's Health Messages,* eds. Roxanne Louiselle Parrott and Celeste Michelle Condit, 33–48. Thousand Oaks, CA: Sage.

Morgan, Lynn M. and Meredith W. Michaels, eds. 1999. *Fetal Subjects, Feminist Positions.* Philadelphia: University of Pennsylvania Press.

Murphy-Lawless, Jo. 1999. *Reading Birth and Death: A History of Obstetric Thinking.* Bloomington: Indiana University Press.

NARAL Foundation (National Abortion and Reproductive Rights Action League). 2001. "Abortion, Breast Cancer, and the Misuse of Science." *NARAL Resources.* Available from www.naral.org/mediaresources/fact/misuse.html.

———. 2002. *Who Decides? A State-by-State Review of Abortion and Reproductive Rights.* 11th ed. Washington, DC: The NARAL Foundation/NARAL.

National Breast Cancer Coalition. 2001. *Position Statement on Abortion and Breast Cancer Risk.* Available from www.stopbreastcancer.org.

National Cancer Institute. 1997. "Abortion and Breast Cancer." Bethesda, MD: National Institutes of Health.

National Women's Health Network. [1994] 1996. "Abortion and Breast Cancer: The Unproven Link. An NWHN Position Paper." Washington, DC: National Women's Health Network.

Nelkin, Dorothy. 1989. "Communicating Technological Risk: The Social Construction of Risk Perception." *Annual Review of Public Health* 10: 95–113.

Oaks, Laury. 2001. *Smoking and Pregnancy: The Politics of Fetal Protection.* New Brunswick, NJ: Rutgers University Press.

Parrott, Roxanne Louiselle, and Celeste Michelle Condit, eds. 1996. *Evaluating Women's Health Messages.* Thousand Oaks, CA: Sage.

Petchesky, Rosalind Pollack. [1984] 1985. *Abortion and Woman's Choice: The State, Sexuality, and Reproductive Freedom.* New York: Longman. Reprint, Boston: Northeastern University Press.

———. 1987. "Fetal Images: The Power of Visual Culture in the Politics of Reproduction." *Feminist Studies* 13(2): 263–292.

Petersen, Alan, and Deborah Lupton. 1996. *The New Public Health: Health and Self in the Age of Risk.* Thousand Oaks, CA: Sage Publications.

Pike, Malcolm C., Brian E. Henderson, John T. Casagrande, I. Rosario, and G. E. Gray. 1981. "Oral Contraceptive Use and Early Abortion As Risk Factors for Breast Cancer in Young Women." *British Journal of Cancer* 43(1): 72–76.

Pollitt, Katha. 2001. "This Warning May Be Hazardous to Your Health." *The Nation*, April 16, 10.

Press, Nancy, Jennifer Fishman, and Barbara A. Koenig. 2000. "Collective Fear, Individualized Risk: The Social and Cultural Context of Genetic Testing for Breast Cancer." *Nursing Ethics* 7(3): 237–249.

Rubin, Rita. 1996. "Debating Abortion and Breast Cancer." *U.S. News & World Report*, October 21, 96.

Russo, Nancy Felipe, and Jean E. Denious. 1998. "Why Is Abortion Such a Controversial Issue in the United States?" In *The New Civil War: The Psychology, Culture, and Politics of Abortion*, eds. Linda J. Beckman and S. Marie Harvey, 211–234. Washington, DC: American Psychology Association.

Segi, M., I. Fukushima, and M. Kurihara. 1957. "An Epidemiological Study of Cancer in Japan." *GANN* 48(Supplement): 1–63.

Simon, Stephanie. 2002. "Foes Seize on Reports of Cancer Link in Ad Campaign." *Los Angeles Times*, March 24, A26.

Slovic, Paul. 1999. "Trust, Emotion, Sex, Politics, and Science: Surveying the Risk-Assessment Battlefield." *Risk Analysis* 19(4): 689–701.

Sommerville, Scott. 1993. "The Link between Abortion and Breast Cancer." Purcellville, VA: Sommervile/AIM (Abortion Industry Monitor), Pamphlet.

Traweek, Sharon. 1988. *Beamtimes and Lifetimes: The World of High Energy Physicists*. Cambridge: Harvard University Press.

Wilkins, Lee, and Philip Patterson, eds. 1991. *Risky Business: Communicating Issues of Science, Risk, and Public Policy*. New York: Greenwood Press.

Wilmoth, Gregory H. 1992. "Abortion, Public Health Policy, and Informed Consent Legislation." *Journal of Social Issues* 48(3): 1–17.

Wingo, Phyllis A., Kim Newsome, James S. Marks, Eugenia E. Calle, and Sheryl L. Parker. 1997. "The Risk of Breast Cancer Following Spontaneous or Induced Abortion." *Cancer Causes and Control* 8(1): 93–108.

World Health Organization. 2000. "Induced Abortion Does Not Increase the Risk of Breast Cancer." Fact sheet No. 240. Geneva, Switzerland.

Part III

Perceptions of Health, Safety, and Hazard:
Risk Makers and Risk Takers

Chapter 5

Exporting Risk: The Cultural Politics of Regulating Traditional Medicine in Northeast Brazil

Jessica Jerome

INTRODUCTION

Toward the middle of my first month of fieldwork in Pirambu, a shantytown just outside the Northeast Brazilian city of Fortaleza, I sat down to enjoy one of the few rituals that had already become familiar to me: a mid-morning cup of tea. Isabel, the woman I lived with, had made up a small pot of mint tea for us to share and then began to prepare a medicinal tea for her teenage daughter, Fatima, to treat her persistent cough. I hadn't seen Isabel make a medicinal remedy before, and I looked on with interest as she rubbed the *malvariço* leaves (a popular medicinal plant in the state) between her hands and infused them in the steaming water.

As she worked, there came a loud clapping sound at the door, signaling the arrival of a visitor. Isabel shouted to the visitor to come in, and a trim, neatly dressed man from the Department of Health walked into her tiny kitchen and announced that he needed to check her house for any open containers of water that might contain mosquito larvae carrying the dengue virus.[1] Although I was new to the field, the Health Department agents were a familiar sight. They had been making daily visits throughout our neighborhood to advise residents about how to prevent the mosquitoes from breeding in their houses. The city's wealthier neighborhoods had yet to report any cases of dengue, but health officials were nervous and hoping to prevent future outbreaks of the disease by

The author wishes to acknowledge Laury Oaks and Barbara Herr Harthorn for their kind encouragement and perceptive commentary, Daniel Holz for lending his insight and clarity, and in Brazil, Dr. Abreu Matos, Dr. Adalberto Barreto, and the Brandão family for their warm welcome to Ceará and their unfailingly patient replies to my many questions.

stepping up dengue prevention campaigns in the shantytowns that lay on the fringes of the city.

Isabel's cramped two-room house was immaculate and it didn't take long for the health agent to complete his check. However, on his way out he noticed the medicinal tea Isabel was preparing and stopped to ask her about it.

"How many leaves are you using?" he asked.

Isabel shrugged her shoulders, "About a handful, I'm only making it for my daughter" she replied, pointing in Fatima's direction.

"You know that medicinal plants can be dangerous if they're not used correctly?" the health agent inquired.

"Dangerous?" Isabel questioned, "But this is what I've always used."

"Of course," assured the health agent, "but medicinal plants are just as potent as other medications are—you should be aware of this. Are you using any other medicines to treat your daughter's cough?"

"No." Isabel answered, "My sister was going to bring by something from the pharmacy, but she hasn't come yet."

"Good," replied the health agent, "You shouldn't be mixing medications. If she takes the medicinal tea, let her wait at least 24 hours before giving her a different kind of medication. You should stop by the health post when you have time to get more information about how to use medicinal plants safely. We have lots of brochures about it, and we'd be happy to talk to you more about it."

Isabel pursed her lips and thanked the health agent for his time. She eyed him carefully through the window as she finished making Fatima's tea. Handing her daughter her tea, she snapped, "The health agents always exaggerate. This is something my grandmother taught me to make; it could hardly be dangerous."

Although I didn't know it at the time, the confrontation between the city health agent and Isabel was emblematic of the kind of control the city of Fortaleza was trying to exert over popular medicinal practices, a realm of knowledge and practice that, in the city's lower-income neighborhoods, had traditionally belonged to women (Browner 1989; Wayland 2001). As part of an ongoing attempt to modernize the poorer regions of the city, the municipal government of Fortaleza had recently embarked on a campaign to promote the use of "scientifically valid traditional medicine." This term, coined by the World Health Organization (WHO) in the late 1970s, refers to the use of particular medicinal plants that have been pretested by pharmaceutical scientists for their toxicity and purity levels and that are taken according to a set of specific guidelines established by public health and city government officials.

The cornerstone of Fortaleza's campaign to encourage the correct use of traditional medicine was the *Farmácia Viva* (live pharmacy) program, which in 1991 had established a group of medicinal plant gardens and adjoining laboratories where "official herbal remedies" could be made and had founded a small number of clinics in low-income neighborhoods where residents could learn about the "correct" use of traditional medicine from trained doctors and a colorful assortment of brochures and comic books. According to city health officials, the ultimate goal of such a program was to ensure the safe and effective use of *medicina tradicional* (traditional medicine) by residents of the city's poorer neighborhoods while they were making the transition to *medicina clínica* (clinical medicine).

Ironically, one of the primary mechanisms city health officials used to accomplish this far-reaching goal was to construct the *current* traditional medicinal knowledge and practices of residents of low-income neighborhoods as risky. In particular, city officials used educational campaigns and patient-doctor interactions to draw attention to the ways in which medicinal plants resembled pharmaceutical drugs and thus argue that their safe use necessarily required adhering to a special set of guidelines developed by public health officials.

This strategy demonstrates how government officials can use risk warnings as an adroit means of social control. By defining medicinal plants as drugs (a category over which residents of low-income neighborhoods don't have extensive experience or control) rather than as traditional medicine (a category over which low-income residents—in particular, women—do exert quite formidable control), Fortaleza's city officials effectively shifted power away from women shantytown dwellers, who often acted as their households' primary managers of illness, and toward the doctors, public health officials, and medical assistants who were recognized by local residents as authorities on clinical medicine. As I witnessed during my fieldwork, the ultimate effect of such a shift was the slow erosion of one of the few arenas over which women of low-income communities had typically managed to gain power and authority.

Although many risk theorists have addressed the ways in which discourses on risk can work as a form of social control, particularly when embedded in the broader social processes associated with medicalization (Nelkin 1989; Riessman 1989; Beck 1995; Adam 2000), there has been a lack of attention to how these discourses play out in the developing world. In this article I offer an ethnographic account of the way in which a public health program's attempt to control the use of traditional medicine through the explicit use of risk discourses worked to erode a realm of knowledge and practice over which women living in low-income neighborhoods in Fortaleza have historically held power.

In the first section of the article I describe the community of Pirambu in which I worked and discuss the kind of authority and power female community members generated from their roles as household healers as well as the cultural categories upon which that authority was, in part, based. Next I describe the municipal government of Fortaleza's public health program, *Farmácia Viva*, in greater detail and discuss how elements of the program were shaped by international risk discourses exported by the World Health Organization. I then present several examples of *Farmácia Viva*'s educational material, using a critical discourse analysis to draw attention to the ways in which traditional medicine was presented as a drug and thus constructed as a potential risk to community residents. In the following section I use ethnographic data from two observations I made of patient-doctor interactions at a local health care clinic to demonstrate how women's authority over traditional medicine was challenged by these constructions of risk. Finally, I discuss the implications of addressing risk within a cross-cultural framework and argue that when exporting health mandates that frame certain medical practices as risky, international development agencies need to be attentive to the cultural categories upon which those constructions are based.

SETTING AND CULTURAL CONTEXTS

I conducted fieldwork in the coastal city of Fortaleza from October of 1998 to September of 1999 (Jerome 2002). Fortaleza is the capital of the Northeastern state of Ceará. With just over two and half million people, the city exhibited an uneasy mixture of wealth and poverty; luxury hotels abutted dusty crowded market places, sparkling beaches quickly merged with grossly polluted shorelines, and well-paved, tree-lined boulevards were often filled with wooden carts led by donkeys.

Throughout the entire duration of my fieldwork, I lived with a family in Pirambu, a vast shantytown that sprawls out along the coast just five miles north of Fortaleza. Pirambu is one of approximately forty shantytowns (called *favelas* in Portuguese) that have grown up around the edges of the city. It started as an urban squatter community for migrants coming from the interior of the state in the early 1930s. In 1998, with its population reaching just over 25,000 residents, Pirambu was the oldest and largest *favela* in the city.

Except for the *favela*'s most recent arrivals, residents of Pirambu lived in small but well constructed homes made from cinder block and cement. They had electricity and indoor plumbing or a nearby source of potable water and could reach the city center by municipal buses that snaked through the *favela*'s narrow, winding streets at regular intervals. The *favela* was also dotted with an intricate network of schools, churches, and health posts as well as local stores that contained an astounding range of consumer goods, from specially designed birthday cakes to the latest Hollywood videos.

When I started fieldwork I was interested in the extent to which residents of low-income communities such as Pirambu, many of whom were recent migrants from the rural interior of the state, maintained their use of traditional medicine. Fortaleza has a highly developed public and private health care system, and I wondered how or even if these residents would seek to gain access to the services it offered. To address these questions, I talked with health care providers and officials in the public health care system and with doctors and community health care workers. From these meetings I learned about the municipal government's efforts to promote the use of scientifically valid traditional medicine through the creation of the *Farmácia Viva* program.

I also conducted interviews about the use of traditional medicine in one of Pirambu's neighborhoods. During interviews with family members, I began to notice the extent to which women were relied on to provide informal household medical care. In particular, traditional medicine, a category that was, importantly, quite distinct from pharmaceutical medicine, was a realm of knowledge and practice women seemed to possess control over and from which they gained an amount of power and prestige.

The role that women play as household healers in low-income communities throughout Latin America has been widely commented on by anthropologists and other scholars (Browner 1989; Crandon-Malamud 1991; Clark 1993; Wayland 2001). In Pirambu, an important aspect of this role was their use of medicinal plants and the therapeutic remedies that are made from them. To produce these cures, women relied on an elaborate store of medicinal knowledge that had been passed to them by older family members, female friends, or traditional healers. Women's authority over this body of knowledge was not often questioned, and even when formal medical help was available, women were generally consulted first to decide how to treat a particular illness. The amount of power generated from the practice and knowledge of traditional medicine is difficult to gauge, but as one mother wryly commented to me after giving her son a *lambedor* (a syrup made from medicinal plants and sugar) for his cough, "At least there is something that he still comes to me for."

One largely ignored aspect of the authority women hold over traditional medicine in communities such as Pirambu is that it seems, in part, to be generated by a culturally reinforced distinction between traditional medicine and clinical medicine. I would argue that among the residents of Pirambu, medicinal plants tend to be categorized as a kind of food, a broad social category that includes substances with medicinal powers, rather than as a kind of drug, a narrow social category, with distinctly twentieth-century, urban origins. By categorizing traditional medicine as a food rather than a drug, it is culturally reproduced as an autonomous realm of knowledge and practice over which women are able to maintain control.

In Pirambu there were many social practices that perpetuated the categorization of medicinal plants as food. For example, within the *favela*, as in many rural areas of the state, medicinal plants were planted in the same spaces where food was grown: on people's windowsills, in their gardens, and at nearby drinking wells. Furthermore, because so many fruits and vegetables served *both* as a source of nutrition and as a medicinal remedy, it was common to be shown around a garden in which medicinal plants were not explicitly identified as such but simply listed with other plants in the garden.

Isabel's mother, Marta, for example, had a small plot of land behind her house, and one day she showed me around her garden, pointing out a passion fruit tree (the fruit of which is often used to treat high blood pressure), a guava tree (the bark of which can be used to treat stomach gas), and *capim santo* (a grass that is used to make tea that is said to reduce stress). When I asked her which of these was a medicinal plant, she looked confused. "But my child," she said, "these can *all* be used as medicine." And it is not only in people's gardens that medicinal plants are grouped with food—local markets did the same, serving up a mix of common cooking herbs, bay leaves, peppers, cloves, and ground mustards alongside *mestrastro, jatoba,* and *malvarico*—all medicinal plants used to treat specific medical conditions.

The language residents of Pirambu used to talk about medicinal plants provided another clue as to the categories they used to think about them. On the most simplistic level, the words *plantas, ervas,* and *ráizes* (meaning plants, herbs, and roots) were used in conjunction with food as well as when referring to plants with medicinal properties. Traditional remedies made from plants were often described as types of food—for example, *cha de alecrim pimento* or *suco de maracujja.* Each of these social and linguistic practices worked to reproduce the category of traditional medicine as an autonomous, familiar realm of knowledge and practice over which women in Pirambu were able to exert authority.

Pharmaceutical drugs, on the other hand, were not something over which women held much authority. Unlike traditional medicine, a person often had to procure a doctor's prescription to purchase them, consult finely lettered instructions to use them correctly, and return to the doctor for follow-up treatments. The fact that in many instances people fell ill as a direct result of the misuse of pharmaceutical drugs (in Pirambu, as all over Latin America, drugs are widely available without a prescription, and people take them without consulting a doctor according to their own inclinations) only confirmed their reputation as a product that was often unpredictable and allied with an urban, technologically sophisticated world not readily transparent to the average resident of Pirambu.

As such, pharmaceutical drugs held a peculiar place in the social world of Pirambu. Despite their associations with unpredictability, risk, and danger, their connection to the urban, cosmopolitan world meant they were regarded as prestigious and highly vaunted products. The unspoken genius of the *Farmácia Viva* program was that it drew on all these cultural associations and carefully maintained categorical distinctions to promote the use of "scientifically correct traditional medicine."

In particular, the program called into question the construction of traditional medicine as a separate realm of knowledge and practice by drawing attention to the ways in which medicinal plants resembled pharmaceutical drugs. This then allowed the suggestion that medicinal plants were potentially risky and required the supervision of the medical establishment, thereby drawing power and authority away from residents—particularly women—in Pirambu. In the following section, I describe the *Farmácia Viva* program in greater detail and discuss how its strategies were largely shaped by one of the world's foremost international development agencies, the World Health Organization.

FARMÁCIA VIVA AND THE WORLD HEALTH ORGANIZATION

The *Farmácia Viva* program was started in 1991 by a group of three university scientists, Dr. Matos, Dr. Carvalho, and Dr. Pinto, from the Department of Social Medicine and Natural Products Research at the Federal University of Ceará. The program was designed to provide Fortaleza's low-income residents with an alternative to expensive health care by providing them with medicinal plants that had been scientifically analyzed for their toxicity and efficacy as well as a small variety of medicinal remedies that were to be made from the plants (Abreu Matos 1997).

In the first stage of the program, medicinal plant gardens and adjoining laboratories were established throughout the city. The gardens provided pretested medicinal plants, and the laboratories were used to conduct ethno-botanical research on the plants and to produce basic medicinal products. The remedies consisted of any number of medicinal plants mashed up into a salve such as petroleum jelly and put in a small tube, ground up into powder form and put in capsules, or boiled together with water, alcohol, and large quantities of sugar to form a thick syrup, which was then bottled. The products were given away for free to low-income residents during clinic visits and also sold at specific sites throughout the city, including several state-run pharmacies.[2]

In addition to the gardens and laboratories, a group of clinics was also set up throughout the city and staffed with health care workers who would train people, free of charge, in the scientifically correct use of traditional medicine. The entire program was financed by the municipal government, which contributed a little more than half of the necessary funds, and by two other organizations that the founders had received grants from: Kew Royal Botanical Gardens and the World Health Organization (WHO).

Although the *Farmácia Viva* program was developed by local scientists, government officials, and public health officials, its guiding principles were largely influenced by the ideology of international medical development organizations. In particular, the concept of using "scientifically correct medicinal plants" to meet the basic health care needs of low-income communities was adopted directly from the global health policy directives outlined by the World Health Organization (WHO) in the late 1970s.

In 1978 the WHO adopted the goal of "Health for All by the Year 2000" and cited the need for worldwide access to a comprehensive primary health care system (Bryant 1980:382). According to this new mandate, medical development was to be organized, directed, and regulated by a systemization of health care resources in developing countries, with the WHO as the ultimate overseer. The fundamental ideas of the "health for all" concept included 1) the emergence of primary health care, emphasizing preventive and curative services available at or very close to communities in culturally acceptable patterns and at locally affordable costs and 2) encouragement of developing nations to scientifically research and utilize medicinal plants (Bryant 1980:383).

These objectives were exported to developing countries, such as Brazil, during international public health conferences and in the form of aid given to programs that emulated the goals of the WHO. For the founders of the *Farmácia Viva* program and the public health officials with whom they were allied, the WHO mandates provided the impetus for their program as well as a detailed set of guidelines to ensure that medicinal plants were used safely and effectively. Specifically, the WHO suggested 1) critical examination of traditional materials and medical practices, 2) accurate identification of plants and other natural products, 3) identification of useful remedies and practices and suppression of those that are partly ineffective or unsafe, and 4) overall improvement of the efficacy and safety of remedies derived from medicinal plants, many of which contain pharmacologically active agents that in an overdose may have harmful effects (Akerele 1987:178).

Part of what is suggested both by these mandates and by *Farmácia Viva*'s use of them is that a conceptual shift can be made from thinking about medicinal plants within a local, cultural framework to thinking about them and acting upon them within an abstract scientific framework in which the actions of medicinal plants can be compared to those of pharmaceutical drugs. Note, for example, the use of words such as "pharmacologically active agents" and "overdose." Both of these words, normally reserved for pharmaceuticals, are now being used to describe the actions of medicinal plants. According to the WHO, then, the kind of traditional medicine that should be promoted in developing countries is the kind that can most readily be made to resemble biomedicine.

Interestingly, although this bio-medicalized approach to traditional medicine formed the core of the *Farmácia Viva* program, the health care workers associated with the program consistently described their work as being an alternative to clinical medicine rather than a less capital-intensive version of it. For example, Dr. Eufrazina, the municipal program director at the Secretary of Health and Development, stressed, "*Farmácia Viva* offers an alternative to the fancy clinical medical regimes of the rich. Learning to use our medicinal plants is better, because it's something they can then grow at home, and they won't have to rely as much on pharmaceuticals." In a similar vein, Renaldo Ceazar, an agronomist at the Horta Municipal, the program's central garden for medicinal plants, told me, "I do this work from my heart because it is a great cycle, growing the plants and then offering a natural remedy for the poor to use in place of pharmaceuticals; it gives me great pride."

This kind of rhetoric, which closely mirrors the altruistic-sounding prose of the WHO's health directives, depoliticizes the transformation of traditional medicine into a form of biomedicine and masks the broader political-development framework in which such a program can be interpreted. For only if traditional medicine is understood as a kind of "low-tech" biomedicine can the broader political end of such programs be understood as permitting the WHO and other developers to use traditional medicine as a medical resource through which to continue the expansion of Western biomedicine. In this context, the promotion of traditional medicine represents a low-cost, technologically simplified way of circumventing the economic problems associated with providing more extensive biomedical resources, while still continuing with medical development (Greene 1998).

RISK-ING TRADITIONAL MEDICINE

By the time I arrived in the field in September of 1998, the *Farmácia Viva* program had been running strong for over six years. In the course of its life as a program, it had received backing from two different mayors, representing two different political parties, and was expected to continue receiving financial and technical support from the municipal government for the foreseeable future. Of all the program's health officials' responsibilities, the most difficult one they faced was to convince residents of low-income communities, and women in particular, that the local medicinal plants and remedies they were accustomed to using should be replaced by the "scientifically valid practice of medicinal plant use."

To accomplish this formidable task, health officials created a series of educational posters, brochures, and comic books that were distributed at local health posts throughout the targeted communities and in the occasional house-to-house visits made by health agents. Some of these booklets characterized current traditional medicinal practices as "risky" and suggested alternative "scientifically correct" practices that would be safer and more effective. Other material pointed out the ways in which medicinal plants resembled pharmaceutical drugs and thus the need to follow special precautions when using them.

For example, soon after my arrival to Fortaleza, I visited several of the local health posts scattered throughout Pirambu and noticed a series of brightly colored posters listing the dangers of medicinal plants. The posters were framed by a large yellow warning: "CAREFUL!" The poster then asked: "Are you using your medicinal plants correctly?" Below these warnings, the posters presented an illustration of a generic medicinal plant, and attached to each leaf was a warning about the dangers of medicinal plants, including:

- ATTENTION: Just because they are natural doesn't mean they are safe! The incorrect use of medicinal plants can be dangerous!
- It is important to know the correct manner of preparing plants.
- Don't use medicinal plants if you are pregnant, without a doctor's direction.
- If you don't get better with medicinal plants find a doctor!

These warnings attempt to draw a distinction between the correct and incorrect use of medicinal plants, implicitly asserting that it is the authors of the poster (and the health officials, scientists, and medical doctors with whom they are allied) who have the authority to prescribe the correct traditional medicine practices, rather than the residents of Pirambu. For example, the phrase "It is important to know the correct manner of preparing plants" does the double work of warning residents that there is a particular method by which these plants should be prepared and that it is the health authorities who know what that correct manner is.

The warning that medicinal plants cannot be considered safe just because they are natural is another attempt to subvert residents' authority over traditional medicine. Here the term "natural" can be understood as signifying not just organic but also familiar, culturally acceptable, and authentic. For residents of Pirambu do view traditional medicine as natural in the sense that it is a time-worn, at-hand, and eminently local practice. What the poster implies, then, is that just because residents are accustomed to using traditional medicine, it is not necessarily safe and that to avoid risk, they need to learn to use traditional medicine according to the methods prescribed by public health authorities.

The final warning—"If you don't get better with medicinal plants find a doctor!"—is the most explicit attempt the poster makes to wrest control over traditional medicine away from residents and to put it into the hands of health authorities. The message the poster delivers is that even if residents treat themselves with traditional medicine, clinical doctors have the ultimate authority over how that medicine will interact with the human body.

Brochures that were handed out by public health agents to residents during the house-to-house visits they made throughout Pirambu also sought to regulate medicinal plant use by distinguishing between safe and risky traditional medicine practices. For example, the brochures stated that medicinal plants must be purchased in the "correct" location for the plants to be safe. The list of correct locations included the Municipal Garden, the State Secretary of Agriculture, the Secretary of Health, the Center of Health in Jardim das Oliveiras (a neighborhood in Fortaleza), and several state hospitals.

Of course, access to medicinal plants is not confined to the short list of locations sanctioned by the brochures. Residents of Pirambu can purchase them at nearly all the local grocery stores that dot the neighborhood, at the open-air markets in the center of town, and from roadside vendors, who sell a wide array of plants and herbs. What the brochures make clear, however, is that there are only certain locations from which it is safe to purchase medicinal plants and that there are definite health risks attached to purchasing medicinal plants at any other location. By creating official social spaces for the sale of medicinal plants and defining these plants as safe, health officials have challenged residents' authority to purchase plants from a wide variety of locations and warned them that they will be safe only if they rely on government authorized locations. In so doing, traditional medicine becomes less of an independent practice that residents, and in particular women, produce, maintain, and regulate and more of a formal practice that requires the sanction of city health authorities.

But residents of Pirambu not only purchase medicinal plants, they also grow them. As I explained in the previous section, nearly all the houses I visited in

Pirambu had at least a small batch of medicinal plants growing on their window-sills, in outdoor buckets, or in recycled plastic bottles. Again, the government brochures define this behavior as potentially risky. The brochures start by asserting that "You must know the origin of the medicinal plant! Don't grow plants in polluted locations!" In particular they warn that to safely grow medicinal plants, residents must avoid polluted water and soil that is near a dump or a sewer or overrun by animals.

What is striking about these seemingly simple, common-sense warnings is how difficult they would be for most residents to heed. Directions such as find water that isn't polluted or soil that doesn't have trash strewn around it are nearly impossible for residents of Pirambu to follow. Their lives are intimately bound up with polluted water, sewers, dumps, pigsties, and strewn trash. It is a struggle to find not just clean spaces in which to grow medicinal plants safely, but clean spaces in which to *live* safely. Of course these are not risks that it would have been in the government's interest to point out, for they saw their task not as one of alerting residents to the daily risks of living on the margins of a rapidly growing urban city but rather as one of extending biomedicine to the poor through the eradication of particular traditional medicine practices. I would even go further and suggest that one of the goals of this extension was specifically *to prevent low-income residents from constituting a health risk to the rest of the city.*

Another part of the strategy the educational material used to persuade residents that traditional medicine could be risky if not practiced according to state-sanctioned guidelines was to compare medicinal plants to pharmaceutical drugs. By drawing attention to the ways in which medicinal plants resembled pharmaceutical drugs, health officials could then argue for the necessity of adhering to particular directions when using traditional medications, as well as asserting that it was doctors and not residents who had the ultimate authority over popular medical practices.

One of the cartoon books most frequently distributed by the health officials in Pirambu was titled *Farmácias Vivas* (live pharmacies). This booklet began by introducing readers to a benevolent scientist, Dr. Matos, who in turn introduced readers to two animated medicinal plants and took a walk with the plants through a medicinal plant garden to tell them about themselves and how they can be used appropriately. Throughout the story, links were made between medicinal plants and drugs. For example, the comic book starts out with Dr. Matos explaining that the plants are called medicinal because they produce the same type of pharmacological action as drugs do. "Medicines made from parts of us," the little plants exclaim, "are known as *fitoterapicos*, or *plantas medicinais.*"

Once the comic strip had introduced readers to the concept of medicinal plants, it then advised readers that there were certain risks associated with them. Here the animated medicinal plants break out into sounds of alarm: "CAUTIONS???" they cry, looking horrified. "Why do we need those?" "Because," Dr. Matos warns, "just because you are natural doesn't mean you are safe. The incorrect use of medicinal plants is DANGEROUS." "DANGEROUS," the medicinal plants cry again, "how could they be dangerous?" "Don't worry," says Dr. Matos soothingly, "medicinal plants are only DRUGS, when used correctly and with adequate orientation." He then lists some of the precautions mentioned in the poster, including that you must purchase medicinal plants in particular locations, that you shouldn't pick plants in dirty rivers or polluted places, that you must know which medicinal plants are toxic, that you shouldn't mix medicinal plant remedies with one another, and that you must consult a doctor if you don't get better. He also warned that if you make the remedies yourself, you must use them within five days, and you must remember to write down the name of the plant and the date that it was used.

Here again the comic book clearly attempts to promote the use of medicinal plants according to standards generally associated with pharmaceutical drugs. For example, directions such as "use the herbal remedies within a five-day period" work to normalize the concept that medicinal plants, like pharmaceuticals, have an expiration date and that the safe use of homemade remedies depends upon adhering to that date. Similarly, the warning that you must consult a doctor if the herbal remedy doesn't work insinuates that it is a doctor who has the ultimate authority over knowledge about traditional medicine, rather than a friend or family member.

Following the list of instructions to carefully use medicinal plants, the comic strip goes on to discuss what makes the plants effective. "Do you know," Dr. Matos asks the medicinal plants, "what an active ingredient is?" One of the medicinal plants responds correctly that it is "one or more substances that exist in plants and that produces the desired effect in order to obtain a cure." "But why would this be important?" they ask. "Because," asserts Dr. Matos, "in order for people to use your leaves as medicine, you must be sure that you have an active ingredient that is safe. If you do, then you can impress your friends!" Dr. Matos then lists fourteen plants that have been tested by his lab and found safe. The scientific name and the active ingredient of each plant are provided, as well as directions for using it correctly.

Suggesting that medicinal plants have an active ingredient and that the active ingredient is in fact the very essence of the plant is perhaps the most explicit link the educational material makes between medicinal plants and drugs. By attributing the efficacy of medicinal plants to a single ingredient that can be identified only by a medical doctor, scientist, or public health authority, the comic book effectively delegitimizes local explanations of efficacy. Here again, the health officials' construct of medicinal plants as pharmaceutical drugs works to ensure that it is they who can dictate the correct use of traditional medicine, rather than residents of communities such as Pirambu.

What all these posters, brochures, and comic books have in common is their attempt to construct low-income residents' traditional medicinal practices as risky. Part of this strategy involved pointing out to residents how medicinal plants and the remedies made from them resembled pharmaceutical drugs. By drawing attention to the ways in which the components of traditional medicinal remedies are similar to those of standard pharmaceutical drugs, the *Farmácia Viva* program sought to co-opt traditional medicine as a realm of knowledge and practice over which the medical establishment had the ultimate authority.

CLINIC VISITS

In accordance with *Farmácia Viva*'s mandates, three medical clinics were created to educate residents of Pirambu and other low-income communities about the correct use of medicinal plants. Two of these clinics were combined with preexisting, state-funded clinics that were already situated in low-income neighborhoods and provided generalized health care services. The third clinic was connected to the Federal University of Ceará and was devoted entirely to the instruction of the "correct usage" of traditional medicine.

Almost all the doctors and medical assistants with whom I spoke at these three clinics commented that the majority of the patients they saw at the clinics were women. One doctor allowed that this was probably because it was women who had time to bring family members to the clinics, and that they were the ones the family relied on to deal with illness. The fact that female community members were the primary clients of the clinic meant that, unlike *Farmácia Viva*'s educational material, which was gender neutral, the three clinics largely focused on controlling and reshaping *women's* traditional medicinal practices. As I describe later, the clinic thus became a key social space in which women's authority over traditional medicine was called into question and the power of the medical establishment was extended.

The first clinic I visited was the Água Frio Clínica, situated just outside the Federal University of Ceará. The clinic served a large *favela*, with a population of about 8,000, that had grown up along the University's west side. Behind the modest block of buildings that comprised the clinic, a small medicinal garden had been planted to grow the plants that would be given for free to visiting patients. The clinic was staffed by eight medical students from the University's social medicine program, who were referred to as medical assistants and who met with patients on a first-come, first-served basis.

One of the medical assistants, Roberto, agreed to let me observe as he treated patients. We had only just made this arrangement when a young woman named Irene came into the cramped room carrying a tiny baby girl. She sat down quietly, holding the child firmly to her chest. "My baby has the flu," Irene began. "She's had it for a week now, and it's too long. She's sick—she coughs all the time and she can't sleep."

Roberto responded that it did indeed sound as though her child had the flu and that he would give her something to stop her baby from coughing, and to help the baby get better—something she could make at home. But first, he said, she had to listen to his directions very carefully; otherwise, the remedy wouldn't work. Irene cautiously nodded her head and looked curiously at the packets of plants and mimeographed instructions Roberto was pulling out of the cupboard behind him.

"Here" he said, when he had the necessary products assembled, "This is what you do: you mix the *malvarico, mentrastro* and the *alecrim pimento* in a pot, be careful to wash them first—these are from the garden—then you boil them with water and drain that off—that's very important. Then refill the pot with water and boil them again, this time with three cups of sugar. Keep it boiling until it forms a syrup and most of the water is gone. The syrup that's left is what you'll use to give to your baby."

Throughout this explanation Irene nodded her head in agreement. Now she smiled at Roberto and pointed at the plants, "That's what my aunt always makes!"

Roberto grinned widely. "Exactly," he said, "That's exactly right."

"But," continued Irene, "she doesn't make it like that."

"No?" asked Roberto, somewhat apprehensively.

"No, she doesn't make the plants boil twice and she doesn't use this one" (pointing to the *alecrim pimento*).

Roberto picked up the small clump of leaves, "*Alecrim pimento* is very important—it's what's going to help your baby's cough. It's also important to boil the plants first, before you add the sugar—that's what makes them clean and safe to use as medicine."

Irene shook her head somewhat doubtfully, but swinging her baby onto her back, she carefully picked up the plants and clutched the free medicine in her hands, thanking Roberto for his help.

"If you have a problem," Roberto added, "be sure to come back to the clinic immediately. And remember to follow all the steps we talked about—the directions are on the sheet of paper—if you can't remember something, look at the sheet. Your baby's going to get better," he finished.

Irene smiled at this. "If God wills it," she said simply, and made her way out the door.

After Irene had left, Roberto remarked, "It's important to validate their own knowledge, to use the plants they do—but they have to learn to do it correctly—it has to be true."

In this instance what was true for Roberto and the institutions with which he was allied were medical treatments that could be proven to have scientific efficacy. The knowledge that Irene brought to the clinic visit about medicinal plants and their application was useful to Roberto only to the extent that it provided a culturally acceptable vehicle for the delivery of scientific knowledge. Thus, when Irene pointed out that the remedy was familiar to her because she'd seen her aunt make something similar, she received positive validation from Roberto. However, when she began to challenge Roberto's authority by asserting that her aunt used a different combination of plants, he swiftly drew a distinction between the kind of local traditional medicine practiced by her aunt and the effective form of traditional medicine he was advocating in the clinic.

What is particularly important about the "safe" and "effective" version of traditional medicine Roberto advocated is that it derived its authority from a group of medical experts rather than from local practitioners of traditional medicine. In this way, Irene's ability to treat her baby's illness at home according to the methods she might have learned from her aunt was constructed as potentially risky, and she was encouraged to use in its place a remedy that necessarily requires her participation in the biomedical realm.

A few weeks later I visited a second clinic, Hugo da Frota Barroso Filho. This clinic was located on the edge of another low-income community in the southwest corner of the city and was established by the State Secretary of Health in 1986 to provide basic health care services to the surrounding population. In 1995 the clinic became part of the *Farmácia Viva* program and agreed to build a small medicinal plant garden behind its facility, as well as a small laboratory in which to produce medicinal products made from the plants.

I arrived at the clinic in the middle of a hot afternoon when much of the staff had already retired for lunch or an afternoon siesta. The only doctor on call was Dr. Luis Santos, a gynecologist, who kindly agreed to speak with me and later allowed me to observe him while he treated several of his patients.

One of the first patients he treated was Louisa, a woman in her late thirties who had come to the office with complaints of severe menstrual cramps. After asking her some preliminary questions (Did she have any children? Yes, four. Was she working? Yes, she worked as a housecleaner two or three times a week in Fortaleza and occasionally took in wash for a couple of families in her neighborhood), Dr. Santos explained that there might be many reasons for her menstrual cramps, including high blood pressure, stress, or a change in eating habits, or they might be an indication of something more serious—possibly she would need a hysterectomy. He wanted to make another appointment with Louisa to perform a full examination, and he asked her if she'd be willing to come back the following day. Louisa agreed and they made an appointment for three o'clock.

Just as she was about to leave, Louisa mentioned offhand that she had also been experiencing vaginal itching and that she hadn't been able to find relief from "the normal methods." Dr. Santos asked her what she was using as a treatment. "Well," replied Louisa, "I sometimes I take a bath with *confrei* (a popular medicinal plant in Ceará) and *aroeira* at night. Or if I can't find the *aroeira*, I'll just use the *confrei*."

Dr. Santos responded that there were several other things she could do that might be more effective. For example, there was a natural cream that would be effective, Crème de Aroeira. "You might have heard of it," he added.

Louisa said that she hadn't heard of it, but that if he thought it would work, she would try it. Dr. Santos pulled a package down from a nearby shelf that included a skinny tube and a packet of instructions. Holding the package, he explained to Louisa, "You must take it just like you would the creams you would buy at the drug store. It's just as potent and you must follow the directions carefully. You should apply it three times a day, placing just enough in the plastic tube to fill it. After you insert it, you must carefully wash the tube in hot water and then place it back in the box."

Louisa looked slightly skeptically at the box and asked Dr. Santos if he was sure the medication would work. "Look," he told her soothingly, "There's a picture of the *aroeira* plant you used in your bath right here on the label—you remember that, right? It's the same thing, only packaged in a tube instead. It'll be easier for you to use."

   Louisa nodded at this and reached for the package. "And remember," Dr. Santos said as he handed it to her, "Don't take the baths anymore when you're using this cream; it's not a good idea to mix medications." Again Louisa nodded and then asked Dr. Santos if they were confirmed for tomorrow's meeting. He agreed and they said goodbye.

   Dr. Santos's remark that the remedy he was about to give Louisa was like the one she made at home neatly illustrates the way the *Farmácia Viva* program has co-opted residents' versions of traditional medicine to disseminate their own form of "traditional medicine" that is rather closely allied with clinical medicine. For example, the medication that Dr. Santos offered, though made from plants, came in the kind of packaging generally associated with pharmaceuticals: a long skinny tube, accompanied by a plastic applicator and precise instructions. Louisa was also instructed that the remedy she received at the clinic shouldn't be "mixed up" up with other traditional medicinal remedies she may have used at home. By incorporating these forms and instructions into the practice of traditional medicine, the biomedical form and all that it entails (the capital-intensive medical technology, the reliance on trained medical experts, and a biochemical understanding of the body) is itself extended.

   One of the results of the extension of biomedicine is that it enlarges the scope of ailments treated by clinical rather than traditional medicine. For example, before Louisa arrived at the medical clinic to discuss her health complaints with Dr. Santos, her common sense suggested that she take a bath with a few commonly known medicinal plants to alleviate the vaginal itching she was experiencing. Louisa had decided to go to the doctor because she had severe menstrual cramps, not because of the discomfort associated with the itching. We might therefore assume that she had categorized vaginal itching as something that was not worthy of bothering a doctor with and that, unlike the more severe menstrual cramps, could be treated with a home remedy. One might go further and suggest that, in the case of Louisa, she did not experience vaginal itching as a biomedical complaint.

   However, once Louisa arrived at the doctor's office and happened to mention that she was experiencing itching, she learned that the ailment she had thought could be treated with a home remedy could be treated by a doctor with a "safer natural remedy" that in some ways resembled the one she had used at home but in some important ways also differed from it. The remedy offered by Dr. Santos had to be prescribed by a doctor, could be purchased only from a clinic or a pharmacy, and had to be taken according to specific directions. With the safety and efficacy of Louisa's home remedy called into question and the use of effective traditional medicine promoted in its stead, her status as a household healer is also diminished, and a portion of the authority she derives from this position is given over to the biomedical establishment.

EXAMINING RISK IN A CROSS-CULTURAL CONTEXT

In the city of Fortaleza, discourses on risk have become a powerful tool through which to control, discipline, regulate, and reorganize the production and consumption of traditional medicine. Sometimes particular traditional medicinal practices were simply framed as risky and new practices were suggested in their place to make them safe. At other times, the resemblance between medicinal plants and pharmaceutical drugs was stressed, and residents of communities such as Pirambu were encouraged to follow a set of standards established by public health officials to ensure their safety. Often these two strategies were used in tandem, as when the public health agent I mentioned at the start of this chapter suggested to Isabel that medicinal plants could be risky if they weren't used correctly and that she should note the way that they were like "other medications."

As I have tried to draw out in this article, one of the significant, albeit unintended, consequences of these designations was that they wrested control of traditional medicine away from women in communities such as Pirambu and transferred it to the largely male population of public health officials, medical doctors, and government administrators. Key to this shift in authority was a concomitant shift in the conceptual categories into which medicinal plants fell. No longer were medicinal plants to be thought of a kind of food-with-medicinal-properties, a category over which women in Pirambu have traditionally held power. Rather they were to be understood as a drug, a category whose authority was explicitly linked to the biomedical establishment.

Examining the cultural categories upon which designations of risk are based is particularly important when those definitions have been exported by an international organization such as the WHO, whose understandings of medical knowledge and practice may differ significantly from those of the local cultures to whom their protocols on traditional medicine are communicated. What exactly falls into the categories of drug, food, and traditional medicine, and who exercises control over them, varies dramatically from culture to culture. In the United States, for example, the federal government passed the 1996 Dietary Supplement Health and Education Act, which defined herbal medicines as a kind of food and granted manufacturers of herbal and dietary supplements the right to sell their products without providing any proof of their safety or efficacy. This designation has been a boon to a growing subsection of the food and beverage industry that has incorporated herbal additives into their products, allowing them to market them as safe for consumers and to avoid FDA oversight.

This example not only highlights that the category into which traditional medicine falls is itself a cultural construction but also that relations of power and authority are always challenged when these categories shift. When the *Farmá-cia Viva* program in Fortaleza incorporated the WHO's definitions of effective traditional medicine into their program to promote the safe use of traditional medicine, they also challenged the status of women in low-income communities as effective household healers. We might consider that what the women of Pirambu risk in this process is their loss of authority over an important realm of medical knowledge and practice.

NOTES

1. Dengue is an acute tropical disease, generally transmitted by mosquitoes. It is characterized by high fevers and severe pain in the joints and muscles, and if not promptly treated, it can be fatal.

2. The cheapest product, Xarope de Chambá, a plant-based medicinal syrup used to treat colds, sold for 2.50$ *real* (1.25$). The most expensive product, Creme de Aroeira, a vaginal crème used for yeast infections, cost 5.00$ *real* (2.50$). In 1998–1999, pharmaceutical drugs to treat the same complaints typically cost two to three times as much.

REFERENCES

Abreu Matos, Francisco. 1997. "Living Pharmacies." *Ciência e Cultura: Journal of the Brazilian Association for the Advancement of Science* 49(5/6): 409–412.

Adam, Barbara, ed. 2000. *The Risk Society and Beyond: Critical Issues for Social Theory.* London: Sage Publications.

Akerele, Olayiwola. 1987. "The Best of Both Worlds: Bringing Traditional Medicine Up to Date." *Social Science and Medicine* 24(2): 177–181.

Beck, Ulrich. 1995. *Ecological Enlightenment. Essays on the Politics of the Risk Society.* Atlantic Highlands, NJ: Humanities Press.

Browner, Carole H. 1989. "Women, Households and Health in Latin America." *Social Science and Medicine* 28(5): 461–473.

Bryant, John. 1980. "WHO's Program of Health for All by the Year 2000: A Macrosystem for Health Policy Making—A Challenge to Social Science Research." *Social Science and Medicine* 14(A): 381–386.

Clark, Lauren. 1993. "Gender and Generation in Poor Women's Household Health Production Experiences." *Medical Anthropology Quarterly* 7: 386–402.

Crandon-Malamud, Libbet. 1991. *From the Fat of Our Souls: Social Change, Political Process, and Medical Pluralism in Bolivia.* Berkeley and Los Angeles: University of California Press.

Greene, Shane. 1998. "The Shaman's Needle: Development, Shamanic Agency, and Intermedicality in Aguaruna Lands, Peru." *American Ethnologist* 25(4): 634–658.

Jerome, Jessica. 2002. "A Politics of Health: Medicine and Marginality in Northeastern Brazil." Doctoral dissertation, Department of Anthropology, University of Chicago.

Nelkin, Dorothy. 1989. "Communicating Technological Risk: The Social Construction of Risk Perception." *Annual Review of Public Health* 10: 95–113.

Riessman, Catherine. 1989. "Women and Medicalization: A New Perspective." In *Perspectives in Medical Sociology,* ed. Phil Brown, 190–220. Belmont, CA: Wadsworth.

Wayland, Coral. 2001. "Gendering Local Knowledge: Medicinal Plant Use and Primary Health Care in the Amazon." *Medical Anthropology Quarterly* 15(2): 171–188.

Brazilian Educational Material

1995. Malva-Santa Um Medicamento Para Seu Estômago. Assoçiacão Plantas do Nordeste. com Conselho Nacional de Desenvolvimento Cientifico e Technologia.

1996. Planta Medicianal Saúde Para Quem Usa Corretamente. Secretária Municipal de Desenvolvimento Social.

1995. Programa Estaudal de Fitoterapia. Estado do Ceará, Secretária da Saúde.

1997. Quadrinhos da Saúde No. 1. Farmácias Vivas. Secretária Municipal de Desenvolvimento Social.

1997. Quadrinhos da Saúde No. 3. Uso Racional de Medicamentos e Fitoterapicos. Secretaria Municipal de Desenvolvimento Social.

Chapter 6

Risk, Remediation, and the Stigma of a Technological Accident in an African American Community

Theresa A. Satterfield

INTRODUCTION

Kai Erickson (1994) has described technological hazards as "a new species of trouble" that constitutes its own kind of trauma wherein victims are haunted both bodily and psychologically. This chapter documents one such experience of chemical contamination in an African American community in rural Georgia.[1] It begins with a description of the setting and contamination events in which this study took place. This is succeeded by a brief discussion and critique of the theoretical construct—technological stigma—a construct central to emerging work on perceived risk. I argue that this new construct needs to properly explore and incorporate the social, psychological, and bodily consequences of exposure and thus recognize the relationship between technological stigma, social stigma, and the contamination experience. My approach relies on both ethnographic and qualitative findings, with the ultimate goal of speaking to and

This chapter was originally published in *Human Ecology Review*, Volume 7, Number 1, Summer 2000. Reprinted with permission, copyright 2000 by The Society for Human Ecology.

The material in this chapter is based on work supported by the National Science Foundation under grant SBR-9731533. Any opinions, findings, and conclusions or recommendations expressed in this material are those of the author and do not necessarily reflect the views of the National Science Foundation.

The author would like to thank the Annenberg School for Communication for their support of this work and to extend particular thanks to William Pannell, Anne Winther, Laurence Stathem, and Beth Mallard for their exemplary help in the field. Finally, the author would like to thank several anonymous reviewers as well as Paul Slovic, Robin Gregory, and James Flynn for their extensive reviews and comments on earlier drafts of this chapter.

of experience rather than data per se. Consistently, the chapter's discursive format is part narrative, in that it tells an image-laden story, and part expository, in that it presents some quantitative and qualitative evidence for its central points.

CONTEXT

Marshall, Georgia, situated in Pecan County in southern Georgia, hosts an historically Black college, a population of 5,000, and a very limited stock of inexpensive housing. Railroad tracks and a major thoroughfare separate the Alouette Chemical Works plant and an adjacent African American neighborhood from the town's more prosperous residential and commercial center. The Alouette Company began operating in 1910 as a lime-sulfur plant, later (1927) becoming a supplier of arsenic-based pesticides for agricultural, lawn, and garden markets (Hillsman and Krafter interviews, 1996). Locals refer to the plant as "the dust house," a designation that invokes the particulate matter that once permeated neighborhood air and life. A ditch carrying untreated waste from the plant traveled through the adjacent neighborhood until it was covered in the late 1970s. Adult residents of the neighborhood recall playing in the ditch as children, and their parents were said to have waded across the ditch to avoid the longer walk to the plank bridges at the ends of each block.

For most of its history, the plant was owned and operated by a prominent local White family; it was sold to a corporate chemical manufacturer in 1985. In 1986, the state's Department of Environmental Quality requested that the company clean contaminated areas within the commercial facility where arsenic had adhered to the soil on plant property. Nothing was said to the predominantly African American residents living nearest the plant at that time.[2] In 1990 the site was recommended to the U.S. Environmental Protection Agency (EPA) for listing on the National Priority or "Superfund" list. Three years passed before the EPA notified affected citizens and issued cleanup orders to the plant.

Beginning in 1993, residents of the plant neighborhood learned that several probable carcinogens, in particular arsenical compounds, had permeated the soil in neighborhood yards and the dust inside local homes. Testing in 1994 through 1997 on the plant property and throughout the adjacent neighborhood indicated dust- and soil-based arsenic levels of 15 to 800 parts per million despite the cessation of arsenic production during the mid-1980s. The plant grounds include hot spots of up to 30,000 parts per million (ppm). The background level for arsenic in comparable geographic regimes was judged to be about 7 ppm. Chronic arsenic exposure has been associated with skin, lung, liver, bladder, kidney, and colon cancers (ATSDR, 1990); arsenic is also believed to be a cancer progressor, as is benzene and asbestos (Steingraber 1997, 244). A 1996 study conducted in Marshall, Georgia, by the Agency for Toxic Substances and Disease Registry (ATSDR) concluded that significant dangerous exposures had occurred in the past but that current post-remediation levels of exposure were not dangerous to residents (ATSDR 1996).

THEORETICAL FRAMEWORK

Risk scholars recognize that physical harm results from exposure to chemicals, heavy metals, and radioactive isotopes and that the social and psychological experience of that harm is both fully rational and central to the risk experience (Slovic 1987, 1992; Edelstein 1988; Kasperson 1992; Erikson 1994). A prominent extension of risk work involves the study of technological stigmas as first defined by Edelstein (1987) and later spelled out by Gregory, Flynn, and Slovic (1995) in the periodical *American Scientist*. Technological stigma occurs when certain products, places, or technologies are identified by the public as dangerous and subject to avoidance, given their affiliation with health risks (Gregory, Flynn, and Slovic 1995). Stigma targets are generally affiliated with risks the public views as dreaded, potentially fatal; involuntarily imposed, or regarded as beyond individual control (Slovic 1987).

The primary evidence for technological stigmas is the coexistence of negative cognitions about a place, product, or technology—negative word associations, imagery, affective descriptors, and perceived risks—with detrimental changes in consumer behavior (Flynn et al. 1997; Flynn et al. 1998). Ultimately, the stigmatized object becomes an epicenter from which severe economic impacts emanate. The millions in lost revenues incurred by Johnson and Johnson in the wake of fear about further Tylenol poisonings, the collapse of the British beef industry in the face of reports about Creutzfeldt-Jakob or mad cow disease, the decline in land values near nuclear facilities or chemical plants, and the devaluation of real property alongside electromagnetic fields are classic cases of (respectively) product, place, and technological stigma (Mitchell 1989; Slovic, Layman, and Flynn 1990; MacGregor, Slovic, and Morgan 1994).

Defining technological stigma in terms of market impacts is logical to the extent that economic viability and public acceptance are necessary for the commercial development of modern technologies. An emphasis on economic impacts may also be driven by tort laws that permit citizens to sue for damages when real property is devalued due to its proximity to a hazardous facility. Regardless, a focus on pecuniary impacts sustains a model of stigma that implicitly narrows the definition of impact to altered purchase habits or fluctuating market values. This narrows the position of human proponents to one of consumers whose spending drops to *avoid* suspect painkillers (Tylenol) or buyers whose worries prompt them to *think negatively about* housing purchases; in so doing, something of the "complex interplay of psychological, social, and political forces" that fall within the web cast by technological stigmas is lost (Gregory, Flynn, and Slovic 1995:222).

In contrast, a model that recognizes the full social expression of stigma has the potential to accommodate the important association between the stigmatizing of a technology or place by external society and the adverse effects on the people most immediately affected. The relationship becomes more pertinent in light of recent speculation about the disproportionate presence of technological hazards in socially stigmatized, especially minority, communities (Bullard 1990; Johnston 1994, 1997; Szasz 1994; Lee 1987).[3] Those groups historically subject to social stigmas—defamation due to race, class, or economic status—might also be contemporarily subject to technological hazards and thus, in some circumstances, technological stigmas.

Hereafter, this chapter seeks to demonstrate the non-economic effects of stigma on one community subjected to the experience of contamination. Research conducted in Marshall shows that the experience of living in a contaminated and stigmatized place includes both physical and psychological invasions. Neighborhoods are structurally altered, domestic routines are profoundly disrupted, and long-time residents come to be haunted by the inversion of home as a safe haven, an inversion that insinuates itself into thoughts about health and leads to the nagging fear that one's body has been infected by toxic substances. Residents notably invoke their sociopolitical experiences of racism, of being socially marginalized, to interpret how they are viewed by the outside world and to explain why some citizens are protected from contaminants while others are not, why their concerns go unheard, or why they are blamed for the economic woes of the larger community. This study suggests that these opinions may be tied to the defeating social climate that can accompany the experience of contamination and thus warrant study as symptoms of the link between technological and social stigmas.

METHODS

In the spring and summer of 1996, 206 questionnaire-based interviews employing open- and closed-ended questions were administered to 66 past and 140 current residents of the contaminated neighborhood. Interviewees were selected from over 600 past and current residents listed as plaintiffs in litigation pending against the Alouette plant. Plaintiffs included all but a few past and present residents of the plant neighborhood who were (a) traceable, (b) had lived in the neighborhood for at least 5 years, and (c) were said by a medical doctor to have clinical signs of arsenic exposure. Interviewees (all 206) were selected not at random but because they lived or had lived in the houses closest to the plant or because their house or yard had already been tested for the presence of arsenic. Only one of the 206 interviewees currently works at the plant, and fewer than 10 have ever worked at the plant for more than three months. All but 3 of those interviewed were African American, although a larger proportion of the 600 litigants (approximately 5 percent) are White.[4]

Twenty-six of the 140 people referred to here as current residents moved or were moved in response to the news about contamination. The other 114 (of 140) still live in the neighborhood. The second group of people referred to here as past residents (66) include only those people who left the neighborhood well before (often many years before) the news of contamination broke. Most in this latter subset of interviewees live in comparable though not contaminated communities elsewhere in rural Georgia. They do not otherwise differ from current residents with regard to age, gender, or race; the mean age of past residents is 46.3 years and of present residents is 46.9 years.[5] Thirty-nine percent of all present residents are male, and 61 percent are female. Thirty-five percent of past residents are male and 64 percent are female.

Questionnaire items were developed with reference to the extant literature on social responses to technological hazards and on the basis of background ethnographic interviews conducted by the author. Questionnaire items were pretested and, when necessary, rewritten for simplicity and ease of administration. The instrument included word-association tasks, affective ratings, reported behaviors, and opinions about remediation procedures. The questionnaire was read aloud to each interviewee, and answers were recorded by the interviewer. Questionnaires were administered by nine African American school teachers, all of whom were trained as interviewers. Many of the teachers had taught in the neighborhood, but none of them lived there. After the questionnaires had been completed, approximately 15 follow-up interviews were conducted by the author. This last group of interviews was, again, open-ended.

THE STIGMATIZATION OF PLACE: RECONFIGURING HOME AND ENVIRONMENT

Community studies have documented the physical deterioration of contaminated places, including the potential for infrastructural, social, and psychological upheaval that follows a disclosure of contamination (Edelstein 1988; Fitchen 1989; Erikson 1994). In Marshall, Georgia, multiple houses on each of the blocks closest to the plant were purchased by the company and torn down and/or encircled with chain-link fences. The "Hazardous—keep out" signs that hang on the fencing inform residents that the fractured landscape they occupy is no longer, and perhaps never has been, safe. The soil on the plant-purchased lots remains too contaminated for habitation (the plant is not obligated to clean its purchased properties), negating the potential for rebuilding the neighborhood's residential infrastructure. Neighborhood gardens, fruit trees, and farm animals (e.g., chickens and some goats) were removed from properties registering 30 ppm of arsenic or greater. Remaining residents see the fences and signs appearing where neighbors once lived and conclude that perhaps their properties are also unsafe; consequently, they cease to garden or trade locally produced fruits and vegetables. The overall inability for neighbors to maintain the quotidian behaviors that typify a comfortable domestic routine—such as gardening, permitting children to play outside, completing yard work, visiting neighbors—represents a "collective trauma ... a blow to the basic tissues of social life" that "impairs [any] prevailing sense of communality" (Erikson 1994:33).

Residents also portray their immediate neighborhood as a "ghost town" of vacant lots and the aesthetic quality of the neighborhood as "concentration-camp like."[6] Houses are uneasily occupied, devoid of the intrinsic merits of home as a safe haven from the predicaments of public life. Betty Fields thus prefers to stay late at her job rather than face "going home to my *arsenic house* [where] I can't breathe." Her neighbor, Helene Johnson, finds only that her home "feels like a trap ... like there's something hiding in the shadows waiting to jump." Many feel there is little they can do to protect themselves, a defenselessness articulated by Leroy Roberts as the feeling of "living in a place I'm afraid of, like it's [the contamination] coming in the cracks." Long-term neighbors regard these insults as historically rooted, a continuation of decades of plant encroachment into residential territory given the meteoric rise of the plant's productive capacity after the Second World War.[7]

Individual expressions of feeling trapped or feeling unable to breathe should not be mistaken as idiosyncratic, indicative only of exemplars of severe impact. Word-association tasks, credited for revealing the content and thought pattern of the respondents' minds without the complication or burden of discursive language (Szalay and Deese 1978), confirmed that both past and current residents define their environs in extremely negative terms. Respondents were asked to provide image or word associations for context-specific prompts (fences, soil, dust, etc.) and subsequently rated their responses on a five-point affective rating scale: very bad (-2); bad (-1); neutral (0); good ($+1$); or very good ($+2$). The rating scores for each stimulus and a sampling of the consistently immoderate image content are displayed in Figure 6.1.

Seventy-eight percent of respondents rated their associations with the fenced-in areas in the neighborhood as highly negative ("very bad" or " -2" on the affect scale), and 81.6 percent and 84.3 percent of respondents, respectively, rated images associated with "soil" and "dust" as highly negative. Across all three stimuli, no single item generated a combined very positive, positive, and neutral response in excess of 14.0 percent. The apparent absence of neutral responses, which usually include synonyms and visual or sensory descriptors (e.g., dimension, color, sound) is distinctly revealing in that responses of this kind would be expected in circumstances perceived as benign or generally less threatening. The logical coherence of these affective scores is that the stimuli closest to home and thus closest to one's physical body (dust inside a house and soil immediately outside a house) are rated more negatively than are more distant stimuli (such as fenced-in lots).

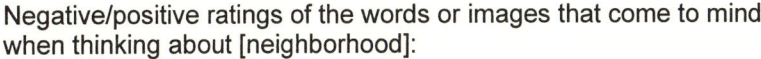

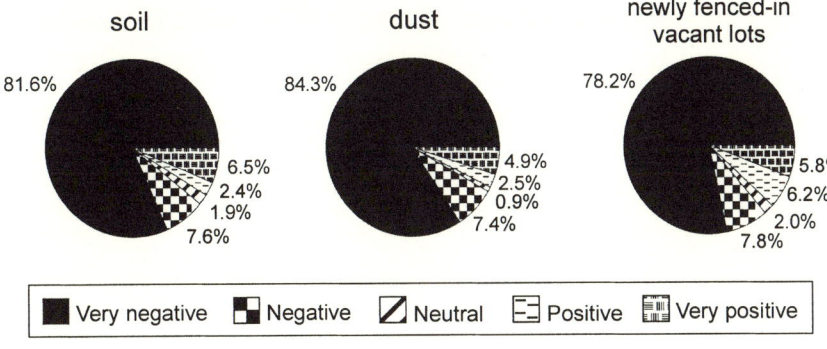

Figure 6.1 Image/word associations and affect ratings ($N = 206$)

AVOIDANCE BEHAVIORS

The decayed sense of safety within and around the homes is confirmed, equally, by parallel efforts of residents to avoid activities that normally comprise the acts of everyday life (Edelstein 1988). Current residents were asked whether they found themselves unable to do some activities, given concern about the plant. If the response was affirmative, respondents were then asked if the avoided behaviors were missed a great deal, missed slightly, or not at all missed ("I don't miss it," "I miss it slightly," or "I miss it a great deal"). The majority of residents reported changes in their domestic routines. Residents easily distinguished restrictions that were extremely bothersome from those that were less so. Table 6.1 demonstrates activity avoidance attributed to the plant and reports frequency distributions for those who missed the avoided activity "a great deal."

Residents are much more likely to avoid ordinary activities such as opening a window on a breezy day (79.8 percent) or sitting in the yard on a nice day (74.6 percent) than less frequent or necessary activities such as going under the

Table 6.1
Activity Restrictions: Residents
Percentage who do an activity "less often because of the plant," who miss
the activity "a great deal," and the percent of total respondents who agreed
to both (n = 114)

Activity	"I do it less often because of the plant"	"I miss it a great deal"	Percent of total sample
Opening the windows in your house on a breezy day	79.8%	84.6%	67.5%
Sitting in your yard on a nice day	74.6%	84.7%	63.2%
Yard work	66.7%	64.5%	43.0%
Flower gardening	65.8%	70.7%	46.5%
Allowing children in your care to play in your yard	64.0%	72.6%	46.5%
Investing money or time to improve the quality of your house or fix something that is broken	63.2%	66.7%	42.1%
Allowing children in your care to play in a friend's or relative's yard that is near the plant	62.3%	71.8%	44.7%
Walking near the open ditch	54.4%	29.0%	15.8%
Visiting someone whose house or yard is said to have high arsenic levels	50.9%	51.7%	26.3%
Going up in the attic of your house	47.4%	53.7%	25.4%
Going under the house to fix something	44.7%	47.1%	21.1%
Allowing children in your care to play in uncovered ditches	43.0%	34.7%	14.9%

house to repair something (44.7 percent), going up into the attic (47.4 percent), or allowing children to play in exposed ditches at the edge of the neighborhood (43.0 percent). When asked which activities respondents "miss a great deal," a similar pattern emerges. Commonplace activities generally associated with a pleasant sense of domestic environment are those most heartily missed. These include opening windows on a breezy day (84.6 percent), sitting in the yard on a nice day (74.6 percent), and allowing children to play in the yard (72.6 percent). Alternately, activities such as walking near the remaining, though distant, open ditches (29.0 percent) or allowing children to play in those ditches (34.7 percent) were "missed a lot" by a minority of respondents.

EMBODIED STIGMA

Alterations in household routines signify the inclination of individuals to protect their physical bodies. Worry about bodily harm is often regarded as the defining feature of toxic emergencies: the fear is that contaminants have been absorbed into one's tissues and perhaps the genetic material of survivors (Erikson 1990:121; see also Edelstein 1988; Oliver-Smith 1996; Kroll-Smith and Floyd 1997). In Marshall, Georgia, residents were forced to interpret these fears while haunted by the image of remediation workers protected from exposure to contaminants—an invading army of cleanup contractors and soil-testing technicians, each of whom benefited from the prophylactic suits used in industrial hygiene. This other-worldly attire seals face, head, body, feet, and hands from external contaminants. Workers also were protected and physically distanced from soil and dust through the use of immense backhoes and HEPA Vacs (backhoes assist the removal of contaminated topsoil, and HEPA Vacs function as powerful dust-extracting vacuum cleaners). Such acts of caution are understandable under the circumstances, yet the symbolic weight of these protected workers lingered in neighborhood residents' discourse and helped articulate poignant misgivings. Visually compelling recollections of heavy machinery and "suited knights" seemed to say that the residents ought to have been safeguarded these many years, that the residents' bodies were already "poisoned," rendering protection futile, or—more cynically—that the residents were a socially disposable population, unworthy of protection in the first place.

Congruent with this symbolically charged backdrop of protected workers versus vulnerable residents, the interview notes reveal the markings of residents' physical selves. Residents learned to regard the long-familiar patches of atypical skin color and density on different parts of their bodies as evidence that contaminants were systemically present. Hyperpigmentation, hypopigmentation, and hyperkeratoses manifest as epidermal discolorations and lesions and constitute the primary clinical sign of chronic inorganic arsenic exposure (ATSDR 1990). ATSDR physicians and clinicians examined the health records of 274 current and past residents for signs of exposure. A subset ($n = 75$) of this group showed evidence of simultaneous occurrence of hyperkeratosis, hyperpigmentation, and hypopigmentation. Though clinically associated with exposure, these signs are not expertly defined as health risks unless they progress to cancer (ATSDR 1996:3–6). Those diagnosed with skin cancers as well as those merely suspicious about the implications of their symptoms considered their skin discolorations constant reminders that their physical well-being was potentially amiss. During interviews, individuals would draw attention to their "spots," point them out, or absentmindedly press on them as though they were a kind of worry bead, a point of reference that redirected thoughts to the consequences of contamination.

Toxicologists speak of "body burdens," the sum total or physical history of exposures through all routes of entry (inhalation, ingestion, skin absorption) and through all sources (food, air, water, office building, etc.) (Steingraber 1997:236). Denizens of the plant neighborhood refer instead to the burden of worry: worry about health, childhood exposures, and especially the heightened expectation of pending disease. Eighty-eight percent and 83 percent of all respondents define themselves, respectively, as "worrying a lot" about "birth defects in children" and "the impact of the plant on my health." Every child with asthma and every virus is thought to be symptomatic of something larger and more foreboding: "Am I going to come down with something in my throat and die?" Individual bodies have become physically inscribed (marked) in the eyes of the owners; atypical pigmentation, perceived risks, and socially mediated fears about health have, together, gotten under the collective skin of neighborhood residents (Erikson 1994). Residents thus come to regard their lives as "one long lethal injection" or "feel that they are something that will slowly kill" them. These observations are corroborated by the vast majority of respondents reporting a deep sense of dread, "a quality well-documented as central to lay characterizations of toxins" (Slovic 2001), and persistent thoughts about the inhalation and ingestion of contaminants. A full 94.2 percent of past and current neighborhood residents agreed that thinking about the contaminants left them with "a creepy, frightened feeling," and 90 percent of current residents agreed with the statement "When I'm in my house, I often wonder if I'm breathing in something poisonous."

Older residents carry the additional burden of prior wounds and the unexplained deaths of loved ones. Further, the opportunity to reconsider old griefs in light of recent knowledge about contamination is, for many, unavoidable. Mary Aimes is in her late 60s. Her first child, a daughter, lived only 20 days—the result of a heart defect. Her disabled adult son died of asphyxiation in 1982, the result of a severe allergic reaction to "something" in the air. Mary's "bad nerves" began after the release of information about contamination and the concurrent threat that she might be moved from her home.

You don't worry about it if you don't know, but once you know, it makes you remember everything that happened before. . . . All these things I remember. I have nightmares about them now. Like when [as a child and teenager in the late 1940s and 1950s] men from the plant would knock on doors in the middle of the night and tell me and my family to leave the house immediately. There was a leak at the plant. They had giant gas masks, like creatures from outer space. They would tell us we had to run, and my mother would try to get all of us up; I was the youngest. When they told me I had to move [due to remediation], I woke up one night in the middle of the night, like as if my mother was trying to get me out of the house. I don't know [Mary stops herself] it's almost more than a body can stand after a certain age.

Mary's psychological and bodily peace is greatly disturbed by this recurrent nightmare and anxious ruminations about the premature deaths of both her children. Her fixation on the "middle of the night" memory has a particular capacity to crystallize and re-create a pivotal moment of horror for her and is indicative of the "intrusive" states that characterize trauma (Herman 1997:38).

Extreme distress of this kind is unusual, although most residents spoke at length about their diseased life histories and typically enumerate kinship ties and deaths-by-cancers in the same breath ("He was my uncle, he died of bladder cancer, and my sister died last year from breast cancer," and so on). The reporting of physiological expressions of stress was equally common. A majority of current and past residents reported suffering from "nausea," "feelings of hopelessness," the "feeling of being trapped," "nervous/shaky feelings," and the feeling of being "tense or keyed up." Over 60 percent of the subset of respondents who reported being "bothered a lot" by these symptoms attributed their symptoms to the plant. This did not, however, preclude a credible tendency to attribute other symptoms to noncontaminant causes. Only a minority of respondents reporting symptoms of lower back pain, crying easily, or temper outbursts subsequently attributed their sufferings to the plant (Table 6.2, column 2). Similarly, only one symptom, low energy, was reported by a slim majority of all respondents (50.5 percent) both as "bothering them a lot" *and* as "caused by the plant" (column 3). Table 6.2 depicts both the distribution of symptoms and the subset of respondents who thereafter attributed their symptoms to the plant.

SOCIOPOLITICAL STIGMA

Stigma is a discrediting judgment that in turn evokes a response from those stigmatized (Goffman 1963; Jones et al. 1984; Gregory, Flynn, and Slovic 1995). In contaminated communities, the complex interplay between technological and social stigmas constructs a tangled mass of attributional actions and reactions. That is, we can speak of those "constructing" the stigma versus those managing it, and we can speak of the racial stigmatization that is likely at play in minority communities versus the technologically derived stigma that residents simultaneously project and suffer because of the plant. Some of this complexity is clarified by acknowledging two basic points. The first is that the occupant of a stigmatized environment can suffer damage simply because of association with that place. This "suggests that beyond a direct fear of a stigmatizing condition in its own right, there is a concern that any association with the marked setting may serve to mark oneself" (Edelstein 1987). To this end, residents consciously worry that they are viewed by the outside world as socially contaminated, contagious, and therefore unfit as members of the larger human community. Consider by way of example Marvia Lou Smith's characterization of herself as chaffing under media's occasionally ghoulish eye:

People come through here now and you see them outside with TV cameras taking pictures and all that. I reckon they said: well, what kind of neighborhood is this that has fences and barbed wire? That must be a bad neighborhood. They bad folks that got fences up around here.

Table 6.2
Stress-Related Symptoms (N = 206)

Symptom	Symptom "bothers me a lot" [a]	Believe plant is the cause [b]	Percent of total sample [c]
Low energy	85.4%	59.1%	50.5%
Lower back pain	68.4%	41.8%	28.6%
Headaches	68.4%	60.3%	41.3%
Body weakness	65.5%	65.2%	42.7%
Memory trouble	64.1%	50.0%	32.0%
Nervous/shaky feeling	63.6%	62.6%	39.8%
Sore muscles	61.7%	44.9%	27.7%
Trouble getting breath	60.2%	73.4%	44.2%
Tense/keyed up	59.7%	60.2%	35.0%
Heart/chest pains	59.7%	58.5%	35.9%
Heaviness in arms/legs	57.8%	54.6%	31.6%
Depression	53.4%	62.7%	33.5%
Easily annoyed/irritated	52.4%	52.8%	27.7%
Nausea/upset stomach	51.9%	70.1%	36.4%
Trouble concentrating	51.5%	49.1%	25.2%
Heart pounding/racing	51.5%	62.3%	32.0%
Hopelessness	51.0%	74.3%	37.9%
Feeling trapped	49.0%	77.2%	37.9%
Confusion	48.5%	51.0%	24.8%
Faintness/dizziness	48.5%	58.0%	28.2%
Fear	44.2%	64.8%	28.6%
Others do not understand you	43.7%	35.6%	15.5%
Easily hurt feelings	42.7%	38.6%	16.5%
Feeling lonely/alone	41.7%	44.2%	18.4%
Avoidance due to fear	40.8%	67.9%	27.7%
Blaming yourself	37.4%	40.3%	15.0%
Crying easily	33.5%	40.6%	13.6%
Temper outbursts	26.2%	46.3%	12.1%
Critical of others	25.7%	47.2%	12.1%
Poor appetite	22.8%	55.3%	12.6%

[a]Percentage who answered "yes" to being bothered a lot by the symptom or problem.
[b]Of those who are bothered "a lot," percentage who believe the plant is the cause.
[c]Percent of total sample who are bothered "a lot" and believe the plant is the cause.

Marvia faults both the physical consequences of remediation (fencing, barbed wire) and the media's amplification of those effects (see Kasperson 1992) for the negative light they cast upon herself and her community.

Troubling reflections of this kind coexist with a second basic point—that contamination events often involve the stigmatization of the already stigmatized. Exposure to environmental hazards is not random but rather selective of social and economically vulnerable populations. Risks are not distributed equally across social groups; there is a greater-than-average likelihood that the victims of hazardous technologies will be people of color and/or those occupying the economic margins of society (Bullard 1990; Johnston 1997). At the same time, those living in environmentally degraded contexts are often subject to psychosocial debasement and dehumanizing innuendo (lazy, ignorant, backward) that destroy self-esteem and the motivation of individuals to control their destiny (Appell, quoted in Johnston 1994:10).

In Marshall, this fusion of social stigma and environmental risk engulfs local disputes about the consequences of exposure. To this end, all talk about "the plant" is somehow also talk about race. Arguments about the nature of legitimate evidence for injury, the appropriateness of different compensatory actions, or the logic of soil-testing were invariably articulated as concerns that would have been addressed or never would have happened in a White neighborhood. These articulations closely follow Capek's (1993) environmental justice frame, a set of dimensions common to the "claims-making" (Spector and Kitsuse 1987, quoted in Capek 1993) interactions that characterize most antitoxic movements. The civil rights movement is the shaping historical event with regard to these claims; community members define their struggle as one in which political access, access to information, the right to protection and compensation, and fair treatment from elected officials, agency representatives (EPA, ATSDR, etc.), and legal institutions are paramount (Capek 1993:7–9).

In Marshall, most residents of the contaminated neighborhood believed the plant and the EPA ignored pertinent local input that might have ensured a mutually agreeable plan for the testing of soils and thus cleanup. EPA engineers posited a linear model of contaminant dissemination; properties immediately adjacent to the facility were tested, as were those radiating outward from the source. When a safe property was encountered, testing would extend one or two houses further and then cease. It was assumed that all further properties were safe. Locals opposed this model by insisting that wind patterns, the ditch's history of flooding into some properties and not others, the plant's trucking routes through the neighborhood, and the historical tendency for employees to carry contaminants into their homes via soiled work clothing had each contributed to an erratic dispersal of contaminants. Widespread discontent of this kind was expressed by survey respondents: 71.8 percent disagreed with the contention that "EPA experts considered all the important ways in which chemicals traveled from the plant into the neighborhood," and 74.8 percent believed that the EPA did a poor job of "testing for contaminants in the neighborhood."

The dismissal of local concerns was eventually tempered by the hiring (on behalf of residents) of outside experts who confirmed a more extensive pattern of contaminant dissemination; the EPA subsequently verified these findings with further testing by their own technical staff.

Racist motives were also attributed to the EPA's procrastination regarding the distribution of knowledge about contaminants. The time lag between the 1990 Superfund listing and the 1993 official proclamation of exposure (a fact noted earlier in this chapter) was widely interpreted as an act dismissing Marshall's African American community as peripheral and thereby unworthy of urgent attention. Further, African American residents cite a late 1980s exodus of White residents from the plant neighborhood's periphery as evidence that knowledge of contamination was divulged well in advance to White residents. The suspicion is that White residents knew about the contamination early on and thus sold damaged residential properties at "good prices" to unsuspecting African Americans.

Representatives of Marshall's White community deny the persistent accusations of racism and instead accuse (African American) plant-neighborhood residents of acting against the plant for easy economic gain via the several pending litigation efforts. Residents of the plant neighborhood are also censured by more affluent locals (White and some African American) for denigrating the town's reputation and its commercial prospects through exaggerated and false claims of plant-derived health impacts. Other White residents are not critical per se but fear the repercussion of voicing support for those in the plant neighborhood and fear being socially isolated because of perceived disloyalty toward their White peers (including the plant's founding family) or for being "too close" to the town's poorest and racially stigmatized residents.[8]

Local African Americans' pointed critiques of testing procedures and the racist undertones of interactions between some local citizens and responsible parties can be read as healthy, proactive signs of resistance to economic and racial stigmatization (Schwab 1994; Szasz 1994). Yet the impressions from my own field observations confirm something different. Neighborhood residents often appeared to be overwhelmed by a pervasive mood of hopelessness, a few resilient activist voices aside. The neighborhood's emotional landscape was marred by despair and a resignation not unlike the psychological numbing described in Lifton's (1967) work on radiation poisoning. Similarly, Jones et al. (1984:4) defined the essence of the stigmatizing process as producing devastating consequences for emotions, thought, and behavior. The argument is that marked individuals are often unsuccessful at maintaining positive self-regard when the evaluations elicited from other people are disproportionately negative (Jones et al. 1984:111). Other scholars of power and subordination have defined this defeated disposition as a quiescence of political participation despite a relatively open political system (Scott 1990:71).

To obtain some indication of the injuries of racism as they apply to political will, Srole's (1965) political-alienation questions were modified to fit the Georgia context. The responses produced suggestive results. Compare, especially, responses of current residents with those offered by prior residents. These demographically similar groups differ from one another to the extent that current residents have lived through the full range of consequences of exposure: the parade of suited hygiene experts, exacerbated racial tensions, battles for voice in decisions about remediation, and, most dramatically, the resonating presence of a denuded landscape signified as hazardous—while prior residents have faced these events from a more removed and thus arguably protected position.

Both current residents and prior residents demonstrate an impaired sense of political efficacy. This impaired political efficacy is more prominent among current residents than prior residents on each of four questions, though only one of these differences is statistically significant at greater than .05. Figure 6.2 demonstrates that current residents are more likely (by 10.0 percent) than prior residents to disagree that "local officials really do care about what I think"; less likely (by 12.9 percent) to believe that "people like me have a say about what will be done about the plant"; and much more likely (by 34.2 percent) to disagree with the suggestion that their point of view was heard and attended to. Both respondent groups disagreed with the contention that voting was no longer worthwhile, though prior residents were more supportive of voting (by a margin of 13 percent) than were current residents. The combined findings capture something of the flat affect about political efficacy expressed by both groups. The between-group differences suggest, however, that current residents share a greater sense of defeat with regard to political processes than do prior residents. Given that the two groups are demographically similar save for current residents' greater exposure to plant and cleanup-specific events, it is likely that remediation procedures have contributed to the loss of democratic control expressed by current residents.

DISCUSSION

This chapter began with the contention that the personal trauma of toxic exposure merits a central position in theorizing about technological, product, or geographic stigma. An expanded theory of stigma requires an understanding that extends well beyond the measure of market losses or adverse behavior by consumers. Accordingly, I considered the ravaging of home, neighborhood, and individual well-being that characterize Marshall's contamination events. An overwhelming majority of residents adjacent to the chemical plant think only negatively about soil, home, and neighborhood. Individuals change their daily routines, close windows, rest uneasily both inside and outside their homes, and abhor the "concentration camp" aesthetic that has taken over their lives. Implicit and explicit definitions of home as a place that promises safety for self and family, as an affective anchor in an otherwise chaotic world (Fitchen 1989), are supplanted by the fear of dust in the attic and the feeling that "something will slowly kill me." The fear among Marshall's plant-adjacent residents is a state of mind that "gathers force slowly and insidiously, creeping around one's defenses

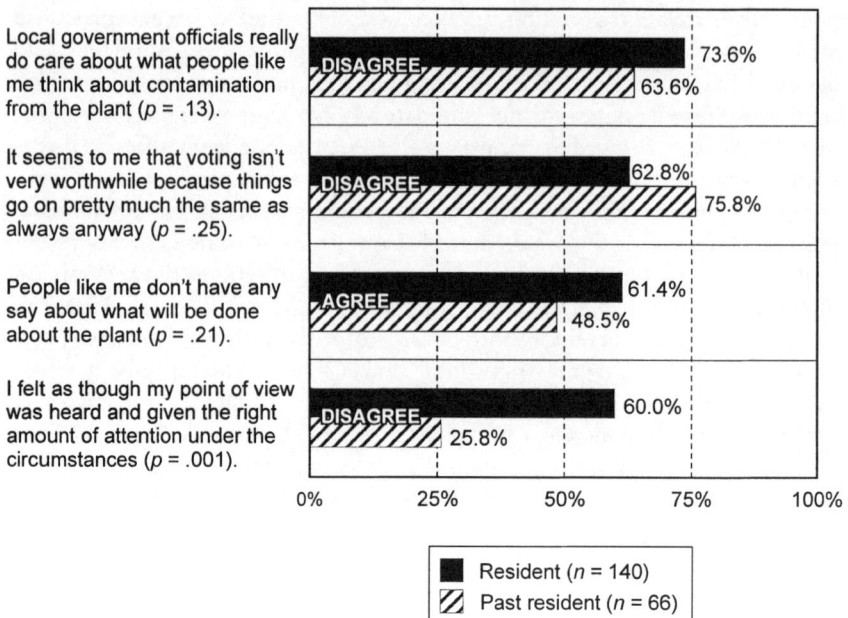

Figure 6.2 Expressions of political efficacy

rather than smashing through them" (Erikson 1994:21). This insidious "creeping" quality is evident in the psychological recoil that follows the sight of workers in hygiene suits and in individuals' graphic articulations of invasion (e.g., "My life feels like one long lethal injection").

Both body and place assist the reflective processes fundamental to human thought. The body is the means by which we experience and apprehend the world (Merleau-Ponty 1962), and place (as in home, neighborhood, environment) is a basis for direction and self-reflection, for who one is in the larger social world (Basso 1996). In Marshall, Georgia, the physical experience of a contaminated neighborhood and body intersect with disturbing reflections about the self. In this sense, the hazard signs, the emergence of vacant lots, and the browning of the neighborhood can be understood as discrete injuries and as vehicles that repeatedly summon, indeed trap residents in a vacuum of negative reflections. Dramatic changes in the landscape become insistent reminders of the presence of contaminants, forcing those who live there to cognitively register and re-register the possibility of "poison in [their] systems."

These reflections interact with larger sociopolitical realities. In the contaminated neighborhood studied here, worry about one's health or the safety of one's home merged with racial discrimination from some sectors of the town's White community, with anguished musings about denigrating the portrait of one's neighborhood and its residents on television, with implications about the worthiness of protecting remediation workers but not residents, and with experts' rejection of local complaints about remediation or the testing of soil. This combination of affronts encourages resignation among residents who define themselves as *not* cared for, listened to, or able to have a say in what will be done about the plant.

Ultimately, the Marshall, Georgia, experience can enhance our understanding of the contamination experience and of stigmas. Much of what is documented here refers to the contamination experience, that is, the physical, psychological, and social consequences of exposure. These are direct reactions to hazardous environmental stimuli. Stigmatizing influences consist instead of signals that exacerbate the experience of contamination. The origin of stigmatizing impacts is in part media-fueled, as suggested by Kasperson et al. (1988) and as evidenced by one woman's response to the presence of camera crews in her neighborhood. More important, the Marshall, Georgia, context demonstrates unremittingly that public agency (EPA, ATSDR) efforts to remedy hazards often contribute to the experience of stigmas locally. So-called remedies for protecting exposed communities (e.g., the stripping of vegetation, the removal of contaminated properties, the invasion of "suited knights," and the relabelling of pigmentation patterns as exposure symptoms) can foster the very fears they ought ideally to alleviate.

Finally, in this context one must come to some understanding of the combination of racial and technological stigmatization. We know from Goffman's (1963) early work that some visible minorities are fully cognizant of and need to actively manage their "spoiled" identities.[9] In minority communities faced with the ramifications of extant hazards, preexisting experiences of racial stigmatization can constitute a dominant lens through which the new experience of contamination and technological stigma passes. Technological and social stigmas can thus form an ugly loop, where each follows and thus intensifies the impact of the other. A more comprehensive, interactive, and socially astute model of technological stigma would acknowledge this interplay and thereby seek to define the links and relationships between social stigmas, technological stigmas, and the local experience of vulnerability and contamination.

NOTES

1. All person, place, and company names cited have been altered to respect the privacy of those involved.

2. A significant White population lived in the neighborhood until the late 1970s or early 1980s. As well, middle-class Whites and African Americans work and live in the proximate and residential areas across the railroad tracks. It is probable that both groups were exposed to contaminants over the years. Few came forward in the period covered by this research, and almost all avoided litigation efforts (see Methods section). Recently, a small handful of this group have become active in a remediation task force led by the mayor.

3. I use the term "speculation" here because the validity of claims of widespread environmental justice is still being examined (see, for example, Zimmerman 1993).

4. Relying on a litigant sample is admittedly problematic. On the one hand, the legal team did not exclude anyone who fit the above criteria and reported to me that only a very few (fewer than 10) of all traceable past and present residents declined participation. At the same time, current residents refer to an earlier period during which more Whites resided on the periphery of the plant neighborhood. This seems to suggest that more Whites should have been included in the litigant list. Regardless, the litigants who make up the sample for this chapter are drawn from the areas closest to the plant and include those whose properties were regarded by EPA and litigant experts as appropriate for contaminant testing. This subset represents neighborhood areas that are currently, and were historically, primarily African American.

5. Thirty-four percent of the resident group are between 18 and 39 years of age, 43.6% are between 40 and 59, and 20.7% are 60 or older (remaining unknown). Thirty-three percent of nonresidents are between 18 and 39 years of age, 39.4% are between 40 and 59, 19.7% are over 60 (remaining unknown).

6. All quoted unreferenced speech is derived from word-association tasks and open-ended interview notes.

7. In the United States, the post-1945 production of synthetic organic chemicals accelerated exponentially and by 1955 had captured 90% of the agricultural pesticide market. By the early 1990s, 860 active pesticidal ingredients were registered with the federal government (as compared to 32 ingredients in 1939). They are disbursed into more than 20,000 products (Steingraber 1997:95).

8. Though I think this paragraph accurately represents the tenor of racial tensions in the period covered by this chapter, I do not mean to deny the presence of White residents working actively toward a better end for those in the plant neighborhood. Two recent events bode well: the replacement of an EPA site coordinator regarded by many in the plant neighborhood as ill-disposed toward the community and the election of a new mayor who is White but is actively supported by residents of the plant neighborhood, has close ties to the community's African American churches, and recognizes the continued cleanup as a first-order priority.

9. I do not mean to ignore subsequent work that argues that minorities do not have spoiled identities or low self-images (for example, Porter and Washington 1982). I simply mean to state that the evidence here suggests a strong interaction between experiences of discrimination and injustices specific to contamination events (Capek 1993 makes this point as well).

REFERENCES

Agency for Toxic Substances and Disease Registry (ATSDR). 1990. *Case Studies in Environmental Medicine: Arsenic Toxicity, June.* Washington, D.C.: U.S. Department of Health and Human Services.
―――. 1996. *Exposure Investigation: CR#40W1, March 6.* Washington, D.C.: U.S. Dept. of Health and Human Services.

Basso, Keith H. 1996. *Wisdom Sits in Places: Landscape and Language among the Western Apache*. Albuquerque: University of New Mexico Press.

Bullard, Robert D. 1990. *Dumping in Dixie: Race, Class and Environmental Quality*. Boulder, CO: Westview.

Capek, Stella H. 1993. "The 'Environmental Justice' Frame: A Conceptual Discussion and an Application." *Social Problems* 40(1): 5–24.

Edelstein, Michael R. [1986] 1987. "Disabling Communities: The Impact of Regulatory Proceedings." *Journal of Environmental Systems* 16(2): 87–110.

———. 1987. "Toward a Theory of Environmental Stigma." In *Public Environments*, eds. Joan Harvey and Don Henning, 21–25. Ottawa, Canada: Environmental Design Research Association.

———. 1988. *Contaminated Communities: The Social and Psychological Impacts of Residential Toxic Exposure*. Boulder, CO: Westview.

Erikson, Kai. 1990. "Toxic Reckoning: Business Faces a New Kind of Fear." *Harvard Business Review* 68(1): 118–126.

———. 1994. *A New Species of Trouble: The Human Experience of Modern Disasters*. New York: W.W. Norton.

Fitchen, Janet M. 1989. "When Toxic Chemicals Pollute Residential Environments: The Cultural Meanings of Home and Home Ownership." *Human Organization* 48(4): 313–324.

Flynn, James, Roger E. Kasperson, Howard Kunreuther, and Paul Slovic. 1997. "Overcoming Tunnel Vision: Redirecting the U.S. High-level Nuclear Waste Program. *Environment* 39(3): 6–11, 25–30.

Flynn, James, E. Peters, C.K. Mertz, and P. Slovic. 1998. "Risk, Media, and Stigma at Rocky Flats." *Risk Analysis* 18(6): 715–727.

Goffman, Erving. 1963. *Stigma*. Englewood Cliffs, NJ: Prentice-Hall.

Gregory, Robin, James Flynn, and Paul Slovic. 1995. "Technological Stigma." *American Scientist* 83(3): 220–223.

Herman, Judith. 1997. *Trauma and Recovery: The Aftermath of Violence from Domestic Abuse to Political Terror*. Rev. ed. New York: Basic Books.

Hillsman, Reverend Morris, and Marvin Krafter. 1996. Interview by author at the Shiloh Baptist Church, Marshall, Georgia, July 29.

Johnston, Barbara R., ed. 1994. *Who Pays the Price?: The Sociocultural Context of Environmental Crisis*. Washington, DC: Island Press.

———. 1997. *Life and Death Matters: Human Rights and the Environment at the End of the Millennium*. Walnut Creek, CA: AltaMira Press.

Jones, Edward E., Amerigo Farina, Albert H. Hastorf, Hazel Markus, Dale T. Miller, Robert A. Scott, and Rita de French. 1984. *Social Stigma: The Psychology of Marked Relationships*. New York: W.H. Freeman.

Kasperson, Roger E. 1992. "The Social Amplification of Risk: Progress in Developing an Integrative Framework of Risk." In *Social Theories of Risk*, eds. Sheldon Krimsky and Dominic Golding, 153–178. New York: Praeger.

Kasperson, Roger E., Ortwin Renn, Paul Slovic, Halina Szejnwald Brown, Jacque L. Emel, Robert L. Goble, Jeanne X. Kasperson, and Sam Ratick. 1988. "The Social Amplification of Risk: A Conceptual Framework." *Risk Analysis* 8(2): 177–187.

Kroll-Smith, J. Stephen, and H. Hugh Floyd. 1997. *Bodies in Protest: Environmental Illness and the Struggle over Medical Knowledge*. New York: New York University Press.

Lee, Charles. 1987. *Toxic Waste and Race in the United States.* New York: United Church of Christ Commission for Racial Justice.

Lifton, Robert J. 1967. *Death in Life: Survivors of Hiroshima.* New York: Random House.

MacGregor, Donald, Paul Slovic, and M. Granger Morgan. 1994. "Perception of Risks from Electromagnetic Fields: A Psychometric Evaluation of a Risk-Communication Approach." *Risk Analysis* 14(5): 815–828.

Merleau-Ponty, Maurice. 1962. *The Phenomenology of Perception.* London: Routledge and Kegan Paul.

Mitchell, Mark L. 1989. "The Impact of External Parties on Brand-Name Capital: The 1982 Tylenol Poisonings and Subsequent Cases." *Economic Inquiry* 27(4): 601–618.

Oliver-Smith, Anthony. 1996. "Anthropological Research on Hazards and Disasters." *Annual Review of Anthropology* 25: 303–328.

Porter, Judith R., and Robert E. Washington. 1982. "Black Identity and Self-Esteem: A Review of Studies of Black Self-Concept 1968–1978." In *Social Psychology of the Self-Concept,* eds. Morris Rosenberg and Howard B. Kaplan, 224–234. Arlington Heights, IL: Harlan Davidson, Inc.

Schwab, James. 1994. *Deeper Shades of Green: The Rise of Blue Collar and Minority Environmentalism in America.* San Francisco: Sierra Club Books.

Scott, James C. 1990. *Domination and the Arts of Resistance.* New York: Yale University Press.

Slovic, Paul. 1987. "Perception of Risk." *Science* 236(4799): 280–285.

———. 1992. "Perception of Risk: Reflections on the Psychometric Paradigm." In *Social Theories of Risk,* eds. Sheldon Krimsky and Dominic Golding, 117–152. New York: Praeger.

———. 2001. *The Perception of Risk.* London: Earthscan.

Slovic, Paul, Mark Layman, and James H. Flynn. 1990. *What Comes to Mind When You Hear the Words "Nuclear Waste Repository"? A Study of 10,000 Images.* Report No. NWPO-SE-028-90. Carson City, NV: Nevada Agency for Nuclear Projects.

Srole, Leo. 1965. "Social Integration and Certain Corollaries." *American Sociological Review* 21(6): 709–716.

Steingraber, Sandra. 1997. *Living Downstream.* New York: Addison-Wesley.

Szalay, Lorand B., and James Deese. 1978. *Subjective Meaning and Culture: An Assessment through Word Associations.* Hillsdale, NJ: Lawrence Erlbaum.

Szasz, Andrew. 1994. *Ecopopulism: Toxic Waste and the Movement for Environmental Justice.* Minneapolis: University of Minnesota Press.

Zimmerman, Rae. 1993. "Social Equity and Environmental Risk." *Risk Analysis* 13(6): 649–666.

Chapter 7

Safe Exposure? Perceptions of Health Risks from Agricultural Chemicals among California Farmworkers

Barbara Herr Harthorn

Farmwork is arguably the most hazardous and lowest paying occupation in the country, largely performed by approximately four million migratory and seasonal workers, of whom over a quarter reside and work in California (Villarejo et al. 2000). It has a death rate five times the average for all industries, attributed to the long work hours, direct work with heavy machinery, and chemical exposures (National Safety Council 1999). In spite of increasing public concern in the United States about the hazards and safety of agricultural chemicals, the production and application of chemicals has increased exponentially in the past decade, directly exposing agricultural workers to a known health hazard. A recent report by the U.S. Government and General Accounting Office, *Pesticides: Improvements Needed to Ensure the Safety of Farmworkers and Their Children* (2000), points to the failures of the Worker Protection Standard to limit pesticide exposure by agricultural workers and their families (Taylor 2000).

In this chapter I examine the occupational "risk subjectivities" (Lupton 1999:104) of Mexican-origin farmworker women and men in central coastal California in relation to their exposure to agricultural chemicals. This analysis demonstrates how these Latina/-o immigrant agricultural workers construct

I am most grateful to the farmworkers who gave their time and thoughtful responses for this research. The UCSB Center for Chicano Studies and the UC MEXUS program provided multiple grants of support. Susan Stonich was a key collaborator in the first farmworker study referenced here. Sarah Rodriguez has contributed in numerous ways to this project; her dedication and capability have helped make it a success. Jessica Jerome, Leo Chavez, and Thomas Arcury provided valuable comments on an earlier version of this chapter. Laury Oaks deserves my special thanks for her insightful comments and patient attention to this and all the other contributions to the volume.

risk knowledge in the context of their everyday lives, and how this knowledge is linked to behavior (e.g., taking self-protective measures).

Perception of risk has been shown by many scholars to vary widely by social position and stakeholder status. Some of the key actors in the U.S. debate over agricultural chemicals include the federal government (e.g., the EPA, USDA, CDC), state government, agribusiness, corporate manufacturers of agricultural chemicals and seeds, university researchers from toxicologists to sociologists, other industry experts, state and local public health officials, community and environmental health advocates and nonprofits, workers' advocates, educators, and "the public." In this chapter the social and cultural definition of "risk" is a critical point of struggle between key stakeholders in the battle over farmworkers' health and broader environmental health and justice issues. Slovic (2000) has repeatedly shown that defining risk is at its essence an exercise of power, regardless of how it is cloaked in the language of science. This analysis focuses on farmworkers' views of hazardous exposure and work because their perceptions and experiences have been conspicuously ignored in the public debates over exposure.

More specifically, I argue that the particular exposures to environmental health hazards by immigrant, often undocumented, working poor women and men are linked to health inequality. My analysis follows Sobo (1995) and Lopez (1997) in showing how difficult and risky choices, in this case "choosing" high-risk work, can be both oppressive and empowering. I ask how risk is embodied and explore how the embodiment of risk, perceiving risk, and becoming perceived as "at risk" can be tools for individual and community agency.

RISK MAKERS

This approach to the study of risk is influenced by an interdisciplinary dialog about the global systematic production of health inequality through processes labeled by some as structural violence (Farmer 1992, 1996, 1999). Farmer's and others' analyses at the level of the nation-state trace the differential exposure of groups to health risk factors (especially by class and ethnicity) and the differential provision of care to them. They have convincingly demonstrated links between accelerating social and economic inequality and increasing health inequality (Wilkinson 1996). The factors most often identified as producing health inequality are excessive workplace and environmental exposures, increased susceptibility, and inferior health care (Frumkin, Walker, and Friedman-Jiménez 1999). Socially inflicted trauma and targeted marketing of harmful substances and commodities should also be included (Krieger 1999).

In this analysis, I use these approaches as a frame to critically analyze the way "risk" that is constructed by "risk makers" is experienced, revised, or resisted by "risk takers" (cf. Taylor 1999), in this case, immigrant Latinas/-os working in agriculture in central coastal California. Indeed, farmworkers are an almost paradigmatic case of risk takers whose exposures to risk are largely determined by those other than themselves, a set of more powerful actors who are risk makers (Grieshop 1997; Bennett and Calman 1999).

The features of structural violence that I believe are particularly relevant to farmworkers include differential allocation of health risks to a particular segment of society, the system of stratified health care evident in multiple limitations to access to care by the working poor, and ethnic discrimination, normalized through processes of racialization. Others have demonstrated how present racial practices in California mirror past practices in allocating workers to disparate economic sectors that fill the demand for cheap labor (Morales and Bonilla 1993). This analysis asserts a direct link between these practices and emergent health inequality.

FARMWORKERS AS RISK TAKERS

There is a growing, although still inadequate, body of literature about the health consequences for farmworkers of their living and working conditions. A recent health survey of more than 900 farmworkers in California, resulting in the report *Suffering in Silence* (Villarejo et al. 2000), found high rates of chronic degenerative diseases, nutritional deficiencies, dental problems, median income of less than $10,000/year, and greatly impaired access to health care. These findings mirror results of a number of other studies showing rampant health problems and dire difficulties with access to care among farmworkers (e.g., Von Essen and McCurdy 1998; Bade 1999).

Often cited as their most serious health issue, farmworkers and their children are at high risk of pesticide exposure (Bradman et al. 1997; Arcury and Quandt 1998; Eskenazi, Bradman, and Castorina 1999). Pesticide exposure has been linked to many forms of cancer, reproductive health problems, noninfectious respiratory conditions, impaired child health, and a number of other medical problems (e.g., Zahm, Ward, and Blair 1997; Arcury and Quandt 1998; Goldman 1998; Gorell et al. 1998; Ji et al. 2001). In the United States, farmworkers can legally include children age 12 and above, and the detrimental effects on children of most agricultural chemicals are generally assumed to be greater than for adults (Zahm and Ward 1998; Lu et al. 2000). Pesticides are immunosuppressive and pose a most serious risk in populations with high exposures to infectious and parasitic disease, malnutrition, and poor health care (Repetto and Baliga 1997).

Directly measuring effects of pesticide exposure is problematic. Clinical differential diagnosis of pesticide exposure is difficult (Wagner 1997), and chronic as opposed to acute exposure often manifests in the short term with subclinical symptoms (Arcury and Quandt 1998; Gomes et al. 1998). There is a longtime lag between exposure events and many of the most severe health consequences, so looking only at health outcome data is not a fully satisfactory approach. Additionally, epidemiological data provide important indices of population-wide health problems, but they cannot answer questions about how individual people make sense of their lived experience, which problems seem more severe to them, and how they confront the tasks of living and working and, in many cases today, raising a family in the context of risk-taking. This is important because failure to understand and take into account determinants of people's views on risks has been identified as the key impediment to successful risk communication and intervention (Bennett and Calman 1999). The breakdown of trust, a key theme in Giddens' (1990) and Beck's (1992) analyses of the escalating prominence of risk concerns in late capitalist global societies, is also of great interest in this analysis, where employers and governmental regulators declare workers' exposures to be "safe," but workers' views diverge significantly.

FARMWORKERS AND RISK PERCEPTION

The limited work that exists on perceptions of environmental health risk among farmworkers has been based primarily on men. This emphasis is understandable, given the far greater participation in farmwork by men. For example, 82 percent of California farmworkers in 1997 were men (Rosenberg et al. 1998). However, since the early 1990s, more women and families with children have migrated to the United States, and farmworkers' living conditions have changed accordingly (Vaupel 1992; Palerm and Urquiola 1993; Chavez 1998). This analysis in particular has sought to investigate women farmworkers' perceptions of risk, along with those of their male partners and co-residents, because so little is known about women's views.

Vaughan (1990, 1993, 1995), in her studies of California farmworker men's perception of risk, found that farmworkers in more limited economic circumstances perceived a greater risk of future adverse health effects from their work and a lower likelihood of benefits from safety precautions. The perception was negatively correlated in her analysis to workers' degree of willingness to use protective safety measures. Her finding emphasizes that poverty is connected to perceptions of workplace vulnerability.

Two recent studies have compared farmer and farmworker perceptions of risk. Grieshop, Stiles, and Villanueva (1996) surveyed two large samples of central valley California farmworkers ($n = 302$) and farmers ($n = 399$), exploring their beliefs about locus of injury control. They found that farmworkers believed accidents to be beyond their control (and often viewed accidents to be in the control of farmers). In contrast, farmers believed in personal control of safety and took more personal safety measures. More recently, Quandt and Arcury (Quandt et al. 1998) have compared farmworker and farmer perceptions of exposure to agricultural chemicals in the North Carolina tobacco industry. This analysis found that farmers were uniform in their beliefs and differed profoundly from farmworkers in judgments of risk. In fact, farmers assessed there to be *no* risk to farmworkers, because farmers do not believe that pesticide exposure of workers occurs; farmworkers had varying perceptions of risk that the researchers speculate may be linked to differences in age, experiences in agriculture, and national origins.

Based on work in Chiapas, Mexico, Hunt et al. (1999) provide a particularly useful analysis of the cultural, practical, and perceptual factors underlying pesticide-use behavior among 119 *campesinos* (peasant farmers). They found that *campesinos* had a clear understanding that pesticides were toxic and perceived that weak or old people could get sick from contact with them. They also were aware of self-protective behaviors to mitigate exposure, yet they rarely took protective measures for themselves. The authors argue that the findings support Vaughan's (Vaughan and Nordenstam 1991; Vaughan 1993, 1995) argument that the immediacy of negative health outcomes as well as the frequency of exposure affect perception of risk, because in Mexico even direct contact with chemicals through spills was seen as not very risky if there were no immediately perceptible negative effects. Personal and observed experience, thus, are seen to be powerful determinants of perception of risk. It is noteworthy that in another study these *campesinos* showed high levels of pesticide blood toxicity (Tinoco-Ojanguren and Halperin 1998).

PARTICIPANTS, LOCALE, AND METHODS

This analysis examines perceptions of risk from workplace chemical exposures among three samples of farmworkers in rural central coastal California. The findings are drawn from detailed ethnographic interviews on perception of chemical exposures conducted in 1998–99 among a small number (10) of Mexican-origin women farmworkers who were new mothers living in northern Santa Barbara County, California.[1] Additional supporting materials are drawn from interviews in 1996–97 with another 32 women and 11 men farmworkers.[2] All but one interview took place in the participants' homes, and all were conducted in Spanish and audio-recorded with permission of the participants, subsequently transcribed, and translated into English. For this analysis, blocks of pertinent narrative were extracted and sorted into a matrix, along with categorical and other variables of interest and a qualitative content analysis performed to identify main themes and concerns (Bernard 1994).

The study sites were the two adjacent farming communities of Guadalupe and Santa Maria, California. Guadalupe is a small coastal-proximate town surrounded by agricultural fields. It has a population of approximately 5,500, and over 98 percent of residents are Latina/-o, almost all working in agriculture. Santa Maria is located 9 miles inland and is a rapidly growing rural agricultural town of about 80,000 residents. A Mexican-origin farmworker population of several thousand residents is clustered in the northwestern quarter of the city.

Santa Barbara County agriculture, like much in California, demonstrates a marked shift away from mechanization and toward hand labor (Palerm 1991; Palerm and Urquiola 1993; Wells 1996). California coastal agriculture is notable for the diversity of fruit and vegetable crops grown (the top five crops in dollar revenue planted in 2000 were broccoli, strawberries, grapes, lettuce, and cauliflower), moderate climate, and year-round cultivation patterns. Because fields are in continuous production throughout the year, opportunities for chemical exposure are likewise nearly continuous, although there are seasonal patterns of use of numerous fungicides, pesticides, herbicides, and chemical fertilizers. The area is known to be windy, so pesticide drift is a constant risk and evaporation rates (which increase exposure) are high.

Although all farmworkers in this research were born in Mexico and almost half hope to return to live there one day, migration patterns include the maintenance of permanent home bases in central coastal California, from which workers may migrate to other work in off seasons or when local work is unavailable. Workers all lived in private residences, primarily rental apartments or homes. The range of people per household was two to fifteen and the number of rooms per household was one to four. Impermanence of living and working arrangements is almost universal throughout the farmworker households I have studied, and discourses of near continual flux permeate personal accounts. Social and economic exclusion operates on many levels for these farmworkers as well (Harthorn 2002).

The farmworkers in this research were a heterogeneous group. They ranged in age from 19 to mid-40s, in education from 6 to 12+ years, had been in the United States from less than 1 year to more than 15 years, had from 0–4 children, and came from 5 different Mexican states. Most were undocumented.[3] All participants were either currently or recently engaged themselves in farmwork, dependent partners or adult children of farmworkers, or co-residents with farmworkers. Most had partners; about half were married, a little less than half were living in consensual relationships, and two were divorced.

Poverty underlies every aspect of farmworker health and living conditions (cf. Bade 1999). Most had barely enough money to cover expenses at the end of the month, and the rest did not have enough to cover expenses. Poverty, lack of health insurance, and high worker co-payments for those who do have health insurance profoundly limit access to medical and dental care (see Harthorn 2002). Poverty also places harsh limits on access to desired food, transportation and communication, clothing, and other necessities.

RISKS IN AGRICULTURAL WORK

All the farmworkers we have talked with categorize their work first in terms of the crop(s) in which they work. Women in our studies have consistently expressed preference for work with smaller, "lighter," and "drier" crops such as strawberries, lettuce, and grapes as opposed to crops such as broccoli and celery that they typify as "heavy" and "wet" and more appropriate for men. They report that farmworker men prefer working in the heavier crops, many of which are grown year-round and also have more mechanized components (and thus involve the use of heavy machinery). Industry analyses show that each crop industry may have distinctly different patterns of production (see Wells 1996), so the complexity of exposure patterns even in a relatively small geographic area can be great.

These patterns are producing a complex gendered process of occupational exposures. For example, combination with water heightens many pesticides' effects, which may make the "heavy/wet" crops higher risk, but the "light" crops of strawberries, grapes, and lettuce and their associated higher-heat summer work periods are considered among the highest risk for pesticide exposures (Moses 1993). Growers here exclusively use men for direct pesticide application activities, which should increase the men's risk, but these workers (usually) are provided with and wear protective gear. Women, who most often do not have protective gear (an exception is in strawberry fields after soil fumigation with methyl bromide), may end up with higher exposures. Clearly these effects should be examined much more closely in the future.

PERCEPTIONS OF PATHWAYS OF CHEMICAL EXPOSURE

Following Quandt and Arcury (Quandt et al. 1998), interviews in the most recent research started by exploring the perceptual basis for knowledge of chemical exposures before discussing perceived health consequences of exposure. Women in this study displayed varying degrees of knowledge about pesticide exposure pathways. Eight said they know when they have been exposed to pesticides because they can smell them; two said they know because they can see people spraying the crops; one said she can taste the chemicals on food (from the fields); and one said she knows when she is exposed because she can see the residue on the plants. Five women named the lungs or respiratory system as the bodily point of entry for pesticides; five mentioned the skin as a point of entry; two mentioned the mouth as an entry point, via food; and one said she did not know how the chemicals get into the body. Half (five) assessed pesticides to be "very dangerous," three assessed them to be "moderately dangerous," and one said they were "somewhat dangerous."

The significance of this response pattern is twofold. First, most workers already feel confident, based on personal experience, that they know how pesticide exposure takes place. However, the belief of half of the women that their primary exposure is by breathing pesticides is contradicted by scientific studies that show farmworker pesticide exposure is primarily transdermal, particularly from the hands (and, in the case of men, the genitals) (Arcury et al. 2000; Hakkert 2001). Hence, there may be worker education implications from this finding, showing the need to enhance worker understanding of pathways of exposure and alert them to the most likely points of entry.

As further evidence of their knowledge, some of the women had received training by growers and free-listed possible symptoms of pesticide exposure, and two-thirds of them knew of, cited, and practiced (if imperfectly) preventive measures such as laundering work clothes separately, bathing after work before touching children, keeping away from posted areas at work, not eating unwashed produce in the fields, and wearing protective clothing when provided. An interesting empirical question (that this research cannot answer) is whether farmworker women have more or less knowledge than men about these practices and particularly whether there are gender differences in putting knowledge into practice (e.g., in protecting their children from known points of contact).

PERCEIVED HEALTH EFFECTS OF PESTICIDE EXPOSURE

Health problems from pesticides were often the first health hazard volunteered when women and men talked about their health in relation to the workplace in all three samples during open-ended interviews. When we probed women's perceptions about the relationship between chemical exposure and health, we elicited both normative statements and actual symptoms from almost all of them that either they themselves (or their partners) had experienced. Of the nine women interviewed most extensively, eight affirmed health problems resulting from chemical exposure and one claimed no ill health effects. The types of their own or their partners' health problems attributed to chemical exposures included rashes, allergies, skin problems (4); eye problems or diseases (3); flu-like symptoms (2); dizziness and/or nausea (1); excessive colds (1); headache (1); and sore throat (1). This list looks strikingly like the list of "subclinical morbidity patterns" reported recently in a controlled comparison of morbidity profiles of long-term farmworkers and recently employed ones. Long-term workers in this study had statistically significant higher morbidity in terms of irritated conjunctiva, watery eyes, blurred vision, dizziness, headache, muscular pain, and weakness (Gomes et al. 1998).

Many workers perceived that agricultural work caused upper and lower respiratory problems and in particular "weakened their lungs" (cf. Nichter 1994). This was particularly evident among those in the tuberculosis (TB) study, virtually all of whom attributed their vulnerability to TB infection to chemical exposures at work. For example, fieldnotes recorded the following:

A 25-year-old woman says her 30-year-old husband, a lettuce field supervisor, thinks the people who work in the fields are more susceptible to TB because the ground in which they are working and planting contains a lot of fertilizer and insecticides that get into the throat and into the lungs and infect them and make them weak. Also, she says planes fly very low, spraying insecticides, and even though the planes are not overhead, the winds bring the smell to their noses when they are working. It must get into the lungs.

This perception was not limited to those with acute lung disease.

A woman of 28 who used to work in cauliflower reports that her 28-year-old husband, a field hand in broccoli, is in contact with pesticides at work, where he inhales them from the air, causing allergies and problems with his sinuses every day in the morning. He takes drops and pills, but the problem has not kept him from work.

Dermatological problems, particularly rashes, were another widely reported illness attributed to agricultural chemical exposure. These symptoms develop even though all workers wear clothing in the fields that provide full body coverage, although their hands are often not well protected.

One woman who works in lettuce reports that workers in the field have skin rashes caused by fertilizers. She says there is contact with the fertilizers at work. Sometimes it is a lot, sometimes not very much. After they fertilize, the people at work get rashes on their legs from walking through the lettuce. Because her job was to cut the lettuce, she also got rashes on her arms up to her elbows. She says she did not receive any training or information about how to protect herself. She is concerned about this and particularly about her kids. She explained that when they arrive home from work they have some of the spray on their clothes. Her husband, also a farmworker, came home from work and their daughter ran out to hug him and she kissed him and she got a rash on her face from touching his shirt.

That workers are not always well informed by growers about the chemical exposures they experience seems clear from many accounts.

There is a distinction between workers who seem concerned about the possible effects of residue exposures (contact with the residues remaining on plants and soil after the "safe entry" period has been reached) and those with little or no expressed knowledge about these possible effects. The latter position is consistent with what we know about farmers' understandings and communicated knowledge to farmworkers that residues pose no hazard to workers (Quandt et al. 1998). Other workers know they are being exposed to chemicals but express little concern about their own personal vulnerability. These accounts, which are frequent, have a distinct "it couldn't happen to me" quality that does not dismiss hazards but discounts personal likelihood of experiencing their effects. This parallels Hunt's finding (Hunt et al. 1999) in Mexico of personal invulnerability to the negative consequences of pesticide exposure among young, healthy peasant farmers. One example from my research:

A woman in her late 20s who has a child with serious neurological problems says her husband has had quite a lot of contact with pesticides at work, but he has been given some training for dealing with them, and therefore she is not worried about her children or herself because they have no direct contact.

In fact, in addition to the chemical residues with which farmworkers experience direct contact daily in their hand labor, residues have been found to occur at high (and probably toxic) levels on farmworkers' clothing, on food brought home from the fields, in the dust in workers' homes, on their children's hands in the home, and in the cars used to transport them to and from the workplace (Bradman et al. 1997; Lu et al. 2000).

Still other workers have not personally experienced serious health problems that they attribute to pesticides, but they have directly observed such effects in others, and this has affected their perceptions of the risks, which may be non-specific or may include fear of cancer or other life-threatening illness.

One couple, ages 27 and 30, work in lettuce and have contact with pesticides in their work. They explained that when they're working, helicopters are spraying in the field right next to them. They can smell it, and it makes them feel sick to the stomach. They personally haven't experienced serious bad effects, but people they work with have. One day when the helicopter was too close and the winds were blowing, many of the people in the crew began to vomit. They had to send a bunch of people to the hospital immediately. The woman adds that there was even a pregnant woman in the group. After that accident, everyone was a bit scared at work for a while, but then they slowly forgot and things got back to normal. The husband says he gets rashes on his hands sometimes, which he thinks are from the pesticides on the lettuce he cuts.[4]

More specifically about reproduction and farmwork, there is a clear sense among women that pregnancy is a time of vulnerability to pesticides (cf. Hunt et al. 1999). One Oaxacan woman with TB was three months pregnant and not working, because of her pregnancy rather than the TB, although this caused financial hardship. Another woman on preventive TB treatment (INH) because of another family member with active TB reported working in strawberries while pregnant and on INH. She said she was taking the INH pills "to protect the baby," but she lost this pregnancy later. Others among the new mothers who had worked in the fields during their pregnancies revealed their anxiety about the risks to fetal health after the fact, expressing relief at the delivery of a healthy baby.

In response to a series of questions about working conditions and chemical exposures, the new mothers in general showed optimistic bias regarding relationships between exposures and the consequences for their own and their children's health, but made generic, nonspecific negative judgments about the community's exposures—they tended not to personalize risk. Many responded "no" initially when asked if they thought they had been exposed to pesticides, but then in the course of the interview they cited health problems in their families that they attributed to chemical exposures. As noted, the list of health problems tended to be mild subclinical symptoms, and only skin and eye problems had resulted in their seeking treatment. This may partially account for the initial negative response. However, this response pattern seems to reflect a tendency to denial, more pronounced among those working in the fields than those working in the home, supportable as long as the health effects are subclinical with little associated dysfunction.

Their stories about health problems of others outside the immediate family were more complex, detailed, and associated with attributions of blame. For example, one woman recounted a story about three of her coworkers who were assured by their employer that it was safe to enter a field to work adjacent to another being fumigated. All three fell ill. Her assessment clearly points to the discrepancy between farmers' judgments about a "safe" field and coworkers' lived experiences of exposure and subsequent illness in the "safe" field.

The issue of residues, which farmworker men and women are warned to wash from their bodies and clothes and to keep separate at all times from their children, is another murky area in which risk takers clearly question the truthfulness of risk makers, in this case growers and the state that regulates them. How can chemicals be dangerous and safe at the same time, farmworkers' accounts ask? The whole concept of safe exposure is problematized in these accounts. Women and men in this research attribute blame for their risk exposure to growers, who make the decisions to apply pesticides, but especially to the government for allowing this to happen. However, retrospective accounts of exposures in Mexico by research participants seemed uniformly to assess the situation in Mexico to be worse: more pesticides are used, both quantities and types, they are administered with far fewer controls, and more direct contact is experienced by workers (cf. Hunt et al. 1999). This past experience must serve as a key lens for viewing risks (and the balance of choices) here in the United States by Mexican immigrants.

DISCUSSION

These data readily support an argument about how race, class, and gender figure in the production of health inequality. Themes of mobility and impermanence in their accounts show how this immigrant workforce is forced by economic constraints to continually move, shifting residence and workplace along the way—even those who are living continuously in one community for many years (Chavez 1998; Harthorn 2002). The isolation produced by flux in living and working contexts mirrors, though more harshly, the criterion of worker isolation described by Nelkin and Brown (1984) as an effective tool of industries for reducing the ability of their exposed workers to organize and voice their concerns.

The processes of social differentiation that enable recruitment and allocation of Mexican farmworkers to low-quality work are consistent with those evident in California for most of the past century, but arguably are accelerating now, along with economic and health inequality. There is more hand labor (as opposed to mechanized processes) in local agriculture today than in the past 50 years (Palerm and Urquiola 1993; Wells 1996), and growers' profits continue to increase, while farmworkers' income in real dollars has actually declined in the past 15 years. This system depends completely on the continued exploitation of poor, immigrant workers, preferably docile ones who will "suffer in silence" (cf. Gutierrez 1995; Villarejo et al. 2000).

The racialization of Mexican immigrants in California is a process that traces back to the mid nineteenth century (Almaguer 1994). The marginalization of present immigrants, of whom farmworkers are a particularly instructive example, takes place in the workplace, where risk makers perform the "forensic" judgments of acceptability of risk that Douglas has written about so persuasively (Douglas 1992). It also unfolds in communities, in housing, in schools, and in contexts of medical care, where processes of structural violence are amply evident both in farmworkers' limited access to care and in the quality of care they receive. The resilience of workers in the face of such obstacles is a testimony to other factors and processes at work, not the safeguards in place either to fulfill the social contract in a more general sense or to protect workers, including children, in a dangerous workplace in particular (see Chavez 1998).

I argue that the patterns of risk perception in relation to workplace exposures among coastal California farmworkers seem more complicated than most previous studies would lead us to predict. Previous studies on perception of risk and exposure to occupational hazards suggest that high perception of workplace health risk is predicted by relative poverty (Vaughan 1995), doing work that one doesn't like and where one has little autonomy (being powerless) (Nelkin and Brown 1984), directly observing or experiencing the negative consequences of exposure (Hunt et al. 1999), involuntary rather than voluntary risk-taking (Slovic 2000), ethnicity (Hahn, Vesely, and Chang 2000), and a host of other factors. Lack of trust, particularly lack of trust in an employer's or risk maker's likelihood of protecting from or adequately communicating about the risks, is a particularly important associated factor to assess (MacGregor, Slovic, and Malmfors 1999).

Most farmworkers, particularly women, expressed nonspecific concerns about their children's likelihood of suffering unspecified future health consequences from their daily exposures. Almost all were aware of, and treated as commonplace, general knowledge about wearing protective clothing in the fields, washing clothes separately from household clothing, washing hands and skin immediately upon return from the fields, and not eating unwashed food from the fields. But from both observations and accounts of behavior, we know, too, that these practices are often only imperfectly followed. For example, parents want to hold their children when returning from work. How is a farmworker parent to pick up her child safely from a childcare provider after work? However, in specificities of knowledge about risks, farmworkers showed only partial awareness of transdermal exposure risks, and the dangers of residues, which are skirted but not directly addressed in safe-exposure guidelines, seem nonspecific to most workers.

Privatization and individualization of risk-factor knowledge is a well-identified trend in the United States that seeks to shift responsibility for risk avoidance to the individual (Rockhill 2001). Exemplifying this trend, much current intervention work is aimed at enhancing farmworker knowledge about self-protective behavior. In the light of abysmal pesticide regulation, worker education for self-protection has for the past decade seemed to many the most fruitful approach to farmworker health and safety (Pease et al. 1993). However, my analysis, like Hunt's (Hunt et al. 1999), suggests that other forces than knowledge deficits about risks may better account for failure of workers to take self-protective measures.

Age and its related variables of years of work experience in agriculture seem to be important in understanding differences in perceptions of choices about work, risk-taking, and the future among farmworkers. Age and education appear to be negatively correlated in these samples. Those in their mid-30s and above had the lowest education, had worked in agriculture and in the United States for longer periods of time, and tended to be least hopeful about the future, their ability to change their living or working conditions, and their children's likely future economic security. They saw little choice about the work they felt compelled to do and the risks associated with it and, with increasing age and number of years in farmwork, also seemed more likely to begin experiencing adverse health effects. The deleterious effects of social and economic discrimination seemed to be taking a significant toll.

By contrast, the accounts by younger workers and those with fewer years of work experience in agriculture in the United States were interwoven with numerous threads of autonomy, dignity, and hopefulness. In spite of fairly dire financial circumstances and realistically negative assessments about changing this in the short term, almost all the younger workers believed that an improvement in their situations is possible, and virtually all identified adult education as the achievable route to that end. They expressed the belief that their children's future would be better than theirs—they thought their children would become productive professionals either here in California or in Mexico. Virtually all mentioned a need for language training in English in their plan-making, as well as the need for computer training. None of them envision their children working as farm laborers.

Economic necessity was mentioned over and over as the impetus driving farmworkers to work, particularly farmworker women—often with conflicted feelings. Women display a range of preferences about working and not working. Most would prefer to take care of their young children themselves; some have husbands who feel shame at the need for their wives to work. All would prefer other work than farmwork, but they see no prospect of obtaining such work, and it is hard enough just to find agricultural employment and especially to keep it. In this sense, farmworkers are clear about making the choice to work in the present, even with the risk of long-term health consequences for themselves and possibly their children. Women choose this unsafe work because they and their families need to eat and have a place to live; they make the work more tolerable through camaraderie with other women workers and the support of family (including having childcare for their small children provided at home by other women or girls who are kin if at all possible) and by considering the future with hope.

Another important way that farmworkers make unsafe work palatable is to minimize the risks whenever possible. In general, I found lower stated perceptions of risk from chemical exposures among those experiencing the highest workplace exposures, which seems evidence of self-protective denial in the service of personal agency (cf. Lopez 1997). Those who do not produce these kinds of responses seemed at far greater risk for depression and other stress effects. Workplace events that seem to inhibit resort to denial include personally experienced or closely observed adverse health consequences, either when the illness is relatively severe or when it immediately follows exposure. Except for those with TB, most of the workers in my research have been in relatively good health and thus far have experienced only mild symptoms from their exposures, although with age, people's judgments about risk seem to increase, along with reduced trust in workplace safety. Those directly involved in agricultural field work tend not to assess personal risk as high—they might be argued to follow Luker's (1975) distinction of making a judgment of uncertainty rather than risk—but they do nonetheless express more nonspecific worry about risks, particularly regarding their children's health and safety and the community at large. Thus, personalized risk and generalized risk seem to be two quite distinct judgments for farmworkers, perhaps more emphatic among women than men.

This research provides evidence that risk perceptions are socially and culturally constructed through multiple lenses of personal and community experience, cultural beliefs, and socioeconomic conditions. The "risk subjectivities" of farmworkers show that particular workplace experiences shape and reflect personal agencies and that this may be the overriding factor in determining risk judgments, with knowledge of exposure pathways, possible health consequences, and preventive and treatment possibilities of secondary importance at most. In choosing hazardous work to produce "the healthy family" (i.e., one that is economically viable), farmworkers embody risk. Farmworkers are demonstrably doing the best they can with what they've been given by a ruthless transnational system of industrial agricultural production (Griffith, Camposeco, and Kissam 1995) and a xenophobic society. The resilience and stamina of these immigrant, working poor women and men in the face of these conditions is truly remarkable (cf. Grieshop, Stiles, and Villanueva 1996; Chavez 1998).

These findings present a number of implications for policy makers and activists. As others have shown, temporary seasonal workers, who are immigrants and often undocumented, have limited power to change the policies and practices of the agricultural workplace (Valdes 1998), and farmworkers we have talked with show little inclination to jeopardize their already precarious employment by complaining or overtly resisting workplace exposures (cf. Nelkin and Brown 1984). Lack of trust of growers and the government (the same government that is often pursuing them for deportation) is widespread but carefully articulated in private. With lack of trust comes fear and feelings of vulnerability for most farmworkers, at least some of the time. These feelings seem to increase over years of work in agriculture, and because inequality is accelerating in this industry, additional forces are acting on workers' perceptions. Thus risk is a particularly illuminating lens for examining the ways that farmworkers make sense of issues of employment, personal and family health, denigrating processes of racialization, and the future.

In one direction, these data are consistent with second-generation studies of the immigration process, particularly those by Portes (1996), Vega (Vega and Amaro 1994; Vega et al. 1997), and others that point to declining expectations and health of the second generation of Latino immigrants. In this vein, optimistic accounts of the first generation's expectations are predicted to be unfulfilled in the second generation as realities of migration and ethnicity and forces of "downward assimilation" impact immigrants (e.g., see Fernandez-Kelly and Schauffler 1996). Health inequality is a predictable result of the multiple discriminatory forces at work in farmworkers' lives: excessive workplace exposures to harmful substances; poverty associated with poor nutrition; difficult, exhausting work hours; numerous barriers to health care; lower quality health care; and the corrosive effects of progressive racial denigration that is experienced as an overwhelming force by these immigrants. Embodied risk is one powerful idiom through which these multiple effects are seen by workers to converge. If current assessments about accelerating economic inequality are realistic, these predictions about the next generation seem almost certain to be realized. However, an account of processes of immigration in California offered by Palerm (1999) in his analysis of the revitalization of rural California communities by Mexican immigrants provides an alternative vision of personal agency, resisting oppression, and restructuring community. In his account, vibrant new rural enclaves are emerging with young immigrant families, and he sees grounds for hope that the second generation now under their care will be successful on their own terms. The study of the second generation will need this more complex approach to the diverse immigrant population in California and its changing needs, urban and rural residence, gendered experiences, and more.

NOTES

1. These farmworkers were participants in three studies conducted in Santa Barbara County between 1996 and 1999. The latest study (1998–99) explored issues of pesticide exposure in interviews with ten Mexican-origin farmworker women who were new mothers. Women were recruited through a diverse set of educational, social service, legal aid, and health care organizations and interviewed in their homes; sampling was opportunistic within contact points. Interviews focused on reproductive health and access to care, family life and migration histories, plans for the future, and perceptions of health risk from farmwork, including agricultural chemical exposures. An approved

verbal consent procedure was followed for study participation to protect participants' identities. This study was conducted with grants from the UC MEXUS program and the UCSB Center for Chicano Studies. An earlier focus-group component of the research was conducted in collaboration with Dr. Sylvia Guendelman, UC Berkeley Department of Public Health. Sarah Rodriguez has assisted in all aspects of this research.

2. These data are drawn from two studies conducted in 1996–97. In one study, individual and small-group interviews were conducted with a heterogeneous sample of 18 women and 4 men farmworkers drawn from a migrant housing project, a grower who had accepted migrant outreach mobile clinic visits, community-run Healthy Start programs, and a migrant health clinic. Participants were interviewed in their homes or, in one case, workplace, at their preference, about their own and their dependents' living and working conditions, health histories, health concerns, and health care experiences, using a loosely structured interview protocol. In a second study, treatment interventions were followed and interviews conducted with all current Mexican-origin participants in a Santa Barbara County-run program for treating active tuberculosis (6 women, 5 men). Interviews focused on participants' experiences with tuberculosis and health care but also included discussion of work, health, and living experiences comparable to the other study. These studies were funded by a grant to the author and Susan Stonich and another to the author alone from UC MEXUS. Dana Petersen assisted in all aspects of the field research for the project. Patricia Ospina assisted in one interview.

3. We did not directly ask participants about their immigration status, in order to protect them as human subjects. However, in virtually all cases we either learned directly or could make inferences about their status (cf. Wells 1996). The great majority of the workers were undocumented.

4. In my experience, most growers provide emergency access to health care for workers injured on site, usually at a private urgent-care facility with which they have a contractual arrangement. However, those who do provide this care often withhold a part of each worker's paycheck against such expenses, and there is no provision for continued care or replacement of lost wages. For most workers, the only way to get employer-provided medical care for workplace-induced injuries or illness is to continue to work, regardless of the amount of dysfunction they are experiencing.

REFERENCES

Almaguer, Tomas. 1994. *Racial Fault Lines: The Historical Origins of White Supremacy in California.* Berkeley and Los Angeles: University of California Press.

Arcury, Thomas A., and Sara A. Quandt. 1998. "Chronic Agricultural Chemical Exposure among Migrant and Seasonal Farmworkers." *Society and Natural Resources* 11(8): 829–843.

Arcury, Thomas A., Sara A. Quandt, Colin K. Austin, Rosa Saavedra, Pamela Rao, and Luis F. Cabrera. 2000. *Preventing Agricultural Chemical Exposure: A Safety Program Manual—Participatory Education with Farmworkers in Pesticide Safety.* Winston-Salem, NC: Department of Family and Community Medicine.

Bade, Bonnie L. 1999. *Is There a Doctor in the Field?: Underlying Conditions Affecting Access to Health Care for California Farmworkers and Their Families.* Berkeley and Los Angeles: University of California, California Policy Research Center.

Beck, Ulrich. 1992. *Risk Society: Towards a New Modernity.* Translated by Mark Ritter. Newbury Park, CA: Sage.

Bennett, Peter, and Sir Kenneth Calman, eds. 1999. *Risk Communication and Public Health, Oxford Medical Publications.* New York: Oxford University Press.

Bernard, H. Russell. 1994. *Research Methods in Anthropology: Qualitative and Quantitative Approaches.* 2nd ed. Thousand Oaks, CA: Sage.

Bradman, M. Asa, Martha E. Harnly, William Draper, Sharon Seidel, Suzanne Teran, Diane Wakeham, and Raymond Neutra. 1997. "Pesticide Exposures to Children from California's Central Valley: Results of a Pilot Study." *Journal of Exposure Analysis and Environmental Epidemiology* 7(2): 217–234.

Chavez, Leo R. 1998. *Shadowed Lives: Undocumented Immigrants in American Society.* 2nd ed. Fort Worth, TX: Harcourt Brace College Publishers.

Douglas, Mary. 1992. *Risk and Blame: Essays in Cultural Theory.* New York: Routledge.

Eskenazi Brenda, Asa Bradman, and Rosemary Castorina. 1999. "Exposures of children to organophosphate pesticides and their potential adverse health effects." *Environmental Health Perspectives* June, 107 (Supplement 3): 09–19.

Farmer, Paul. 1992. *AIDS and Accusation: Haiti and the Geography of Blame.* Berkeley and Los Angeles: University of California Press.

———. 1996. "Structural Violence, Suffering, and Social Justice: Five Questions and Five Challenges for Medical Anthropology." *Series in Health and Social Justice* 3(2):8.

———. 1999. *Infections and Inequalities: The Modern Plagues.* Berkeley and Los Angeles: University of California Press.

Fernandez-Kelly, M. Patricia, and Richard Schauffler. 1996. "Divided Fates: Immigrant Children and the New Assimilation." In *The New Second Generation*, ed. Alejandro Portes, 30–53. New York: Russell Sage Foundation.

Frumkin, Howard, E. Darryl Walker, and George Friedman-Jiménez. 1999. Minority Workers and Communities. *Occupational Medicine* 14(3): 495–517.

Giddens, Anthony. 1990. *The Consequences of Modernity.* Stanford: Stanford University Press.

Goldman, Lynn R. 1998. "Chemicals and Children's Environment: What We Don't Know about Risks." *Environmental Health Perspectives* 106 (Supplement 3): 875–880.

Gomes, James, Owen Lloyd, Mike D. Revitt, and Mansour Basha. 1998. "Morbidity among Farmworkers in a Desert Country in Relation to Long-Term Exposure to Pesticides." *Scandinavian Journal of Work, Environment and Health* 24(3): 213–219.

Gorell, Jay M., Christine Cole Johnson, Benjamin A. Rybicki, Edward L. Peterson, and R. J. Richardson. 1998. "The Risk of Parkinson's Disease with Exposure to Pesticides, Farming, Well Water, and Rural Living." *American Academy of Neurology* 50(5): 1346–1350.

Grieshop, James I. 1997. "Transnational and Transformational: Mixtec Immigration and Health Benefits." *Human Organization* 56(4): 400–407.

Grieshop, James I., Martha C. Stiles, and Ninfa Villanueva. 1996. "Prevention and Resiliency: A Cross Cultural View of Farmworkers' and Farmers' Beliefs about Work Safety." *Human Organization* 55(1): 25–32.

Griffith, David Craig, Jerónimo Camposeco, and Edward Kissam. 1995. *Working Poor: Farmworkers in the United States.* Philadelphia: Temple University Press.

Gutierrez, David G. 1995. *Walls and Mirrors: Mexican Americans, Mexican Immigrants, and the Politics of Ethnicity.* Berkeley and Los Angeles: University of California Press.

Hahn, Robert, Sara Vesely, and Man-Huei Chang. 2000. "Health Risk Aversion, Health Risk Affinity, and Socio-Economic Position in the U.S.A: The Demographics of Multiple Risk." *Health Risk and Society* 2(3): 295–314.

Hakkert, B. C. 2001. "Refinement of Risk Assessment of Dermally and Intermittently Exposed Pesticide Workers: A Critique." *Annals of Occupational Hygiene* 45 (Supplement 1): S23-S28.

Harthorn, Barbara Herr. 2002. "Choosing Unsafe Work: California Farmworkers' Living and Working Conditions and Perceptions of Health Risk." Paper presented at the Society for Applied Anthropology/Society for Medical Anthropology, Atlanta, March 6–10.

Hunt, Linda M., Rolando Tinoco Ojanguren, Norah Schwartz, and David Halperin. 1999. "Balancing Risks and Resources: Applying Pesticides without Using Protective Equipment in Southern Mexico." In *Anthropology in Public Health: Bridging Differences in Culture and Society,* ed. Robert A. Hahn, 235–254. New York: Oxford University Press.

Ji, Bu-Tian, Debra T. Silverman, Patricia A. Stewart, Aaron Blair, G. Marie Swanson, Dalsu Baris, Raymond S. Greenberg, Richard B. Hayes, Linda M. Brown, Keith D. Lillemoe, Janet B. Schoenberg, Linda M. Pottern, Ann G. Schwartz, and Robert N. Hoover. 2001. "Occupational Exposure to Pesticides and Pancreatic Cancer." *American Journal of Industrial Medicine* 39(1): 92–99.

Krieger, Nancy. 1999. "Embodying Inequality: A Review of Concepts, Measures, and Methods for Studying Health Consequences of Discrimination." *International Journal of Health Services* 29(2): 295–352.

Lopez, Iris. 1997. "Agency and Constraint: Sterilization and Reproductive Freedom among Puerto Rican Women in New York City." In *Situated Lives: Gender and Culture in Everyday Life,* eds. Louise Lamphere, Helena Ragoné and Patricia Zavella, 151–171. New York: Routledge.

Lu, Chensheng, Richard A. Fenske, Nancy J. Simcox, and David Kalman. 2000. "Pesticide Exposure of Children in an Agricultural Community: Evidence of Household Proximity to Farmland and Take Home Exposure Pathways." *Environmental Research* 84(3): 290–302.

Luker, Kristin. 1975. *Taking Chances: Abortion and the Decision Not to Contracept.* Berkeley and Los Angeles: University of California Press.

Lupton, Deborah. 1999. *Risk.* London: Routledge.

MacGregor, Donald G., Paul Slovic, and Torbjorn Malmfors. 1999. "'How Exposed Is Exposed Enough?' Lay Inferences about Chemical Exposure." *Risk Analysis* 19(4): 649–659.

Morales, Rebecca, and Frank Bonilla, eds. 1993. *Latinos in a Changing U.S. Economy: Comparative Perspectives on Growing Inequality.* Newbury Park, CA: Sage.

Moses, Marion. 1993. "Farmworkers and Pesticides." In *Confronting Environmental Racism: Voices from the Grassroots,* ed. Robert Bullard, 161–178. Boston: South End Press.

National Safety Council. 1999. *Deaths and Injuries in the Workplace.* Available at www.nsc.org/lrs/statinfo/99report.htm#WORK.

Nelkin, Dorothy, and Michael Stuart Brown. 1984. *Workers at Risk: Voices from the Workplace.* Chicago: University of Chicago Press.

Nichter, Mark. 1994. "Illness Semantics and International Health: The Weak Lungs/TB Complex in the Philippines." *Social Science and Medicine* 38(5): 649–663.

Palerm, Juan Vicente. 1991. *Farm Labor Needs and Farmworkers in California 1970 to 1989.* Sacramento, CA: Employment Development Department.

———. 1999. "Current Research." Talk presented in the Department of Anthropology, University of California, Santa Barbara. Fall quarter.

Palerm, Juan Vicente, and Jose Ignacio Urquiola. 1993. "A Binational System of Agricultural Production: The Case of the Mexican Bajio and California." In *Mexico and the United States: Neighbors in Crisis,* eds. Daniel G. Aldrich and Lorenzo Meyer, 311–367. San Bernardino, CA: The Borgo Press (for UC MEXUS).

Pease, William, Rachel A. Morello-Frosch, David S. Albright, Amy D. Kyle, and James C. Robinson. 1993. *Preventing Pesticide-Related Illness in California Agriculture: Strategies and Priorities.* Berkeley and Los Angeles: University of California, California Policy Seminar.

Portes, Alejandro, ed. 1996. *The New Second Generation.* New York: Russell Sage Foundation.

Quandt, Sara A., Thomas A. Arcury, Colin Austin, and Rosa M. Saavedra. 1998. "Farmworker and Farmer Perceptions of Farmworker Agricultural Chemical Exposure in North Carolina." *Human Organization* 57(3): 359–368.

Repetto, Robert, and Sanjay Baliga. 1997. "Pesticides and Immunosuppression: The Risks of Public Health." *Health Policy and Planning* 12(2): 97–106.

Rockhill, Beverly. 2001. "The Privatization of Risk." *American Journal of Public Health* 91(3): 365–368.

Rosenberg, Howard R., Anne Steirman, Susan M. Gabbard, and Richard Mines. 1998. *Who Works on California Farms?: Demographic and Employment Findings from the National Agricultural Workers Survey.* Washington, DC: Office of the Assistant Secretary for Policy Office of Program Economics, U.S. Department of Labor and the Agricultural Personnel Management Program. Oakland: University of California Agricultural and Natural Resources.

Slovic, Paul. 2000. *The Perception of Risk.* London and Sterling, VA: Earthscan Publications.

Sobo, Elisa J. 1995. *Choosing UnSafe Sex: AIDS-Risk Denial among Disadvantaged Women.* Philadelphia: University of Pennsylvania Press.

Taylor, David A. 2000. "A New Crop of Concerns: Congress Investigates Pesticide Safety." *Environmental Health Perspectives* 108(9):A408-A411.

Taylor, Ian E. 1999. "Political Risk Culture: Not Just a Communication Failure." In *Risk Communication and Public Health,* eds. Paul Bennett and Sir Kenneth Calman, 152–169. New York: Oxford University Press.

Tinoco-Ojanguren, Rolando, and David C. Halperin. 1998. "Poverty, Production, and Health: Inhibition of Erythrocyte Cholinesterase via Occupational Exposure to Organophosphate Insecticides in Chiapas, Mexico." *Archives of Environmental Health* 53(1): 29–35.

U.S. Government and General Accounting Office. 2000. *Pesticides: Improvements Needed to Ensure the Safety of Farmworkers and Their Children.* Washington, DC: General Accounting Office.

Valdes, Dennis N. 1998. "Activism and Farm Labor Unionism: A Brief History." Paper presented at Society of Applied Anthropology, San Juan, Puerto Rico, April 25.

Vaughan, Elaine. 1990. *Some Factors Influencing the Nonexpert's Perception and Evaluation of Environmental Risks.* New York: Garland Publishing, Inc.

———. 1993. "Chronic Exposure to an Environmental Hazard: Risk Perceptions and Self-Protective Behavior." *Health Psychology* 12(1): 74–85.

———. 1995. "The Socioeconomic Context of Exposure and Response to Environmental Risk." *Environment and Behavior* 27(4): 454–489.

Vaughan, Elaine, and Brenda Nordenstam. 1991. "The Perception of Environmental Risks among Ethnically Diverse Groups." *Journal of Cross-Cultural Psychology* 22(1): 29–60.

Vaupel, Suzanne. 1992. *A Study of Agricultural Workers in Ventura County, California.* Ventura, CA: Committee on Women in Agriculture, Cabrillo Economic Development Corporation.

Vega, William A., and Hortensia Amaro. 1994. "Latino Outlook: Good Health, Uncertain Prognosis." *Annual Review of Public Health* 15(12): 39–67.

Vega, William A., Rick Zimmerman, Andres Gil, George J. Warheit, and Eleni Apospori. 1997. "Acculturation Strain Theory: Its Application in Explaining Drug Use Behavior among Cuban and Other Hispanic Youth." *Substance Use and Misuse* 32(12–13): 1943–948.

Villarejo, Don, David Lighthall, Daniel Williams, Ann Souter, Richard Mines, Bonnie Bade, Steve Samuels, and Stephen A. McCurdy. 2000. *Suffering in Silence: A Report on the Health of California's Agricultural Workers.* Davis, CA: California Institute for Rural Studies.

Von Essen, Susanna G., and Stephen A McCurdy. 1998. "Health and Safety Risks in Production Agriculture." *Western Journal of Medicine* 169(4): 214–220.

Wagner, Sheldon L. 1997. "Diagnosis and Treatment of Organophosphate and Carbamate Intoxication." *Occupational Medicine* 12(2): 239–249.

Wells, Miriam J. 1996. *Strawberry Fields: Politics, Class, and Work in California Agriculture.* Ithaca: Cornell University Press.

Wilkinson, Richard G. 1996. *Unhealthy Societies: The Afflictions of Inequality.* London: Routledge.

Zahm, Shelia Hoar and Mary H. Ward. 1998. "Pesticides and Childhood Cancer." *Environmental Health Perspectives* 106(Supplement 3): 893–908.

Zahm, Shelia Hoar, Mary H. Ward, and Aaron Blair. 1997. "Pesticides and Cancer." *Occupational Medicine* 12(2): 269–289.

Part IV

Regulating Risk and the Public's Health

Chapter 8

Governing Migrants' Sexual Behavior: Work, HIV/AIDS, and Condom Use Campaigns in Southeast Asia

Peter Chua

In the media and in political debate, the epidemiological category of risk group has been used to stereotype and stigmatize people already seen as outside the moral and economic parameters of "the general population." [United States Senator] Jesse Helms's success in October 1987 in getting the Senate to prevent federal dollars from being spent on safe sex information for gay men—the hardest hit "risk group" in the U.S., and the only group in which reported transmission of the virus has declined due to safe sex education by gay men themselves—makes clear the social and political as opposed to epidemiological functions of the risk group concept: to isolate and condemn people rather than to contact and protect them. (Grover 1988:27–28)

Nearly 20 years since AIDS first emerged, the medical concept of risk group remains in use without sufficient civic accountability. As cultural critic Grover recounts in the opening quote, the concept of risk group resulted in the stigmatization of group members during the early years of the AIDS epidemic in the United States (see Schiller, Crystal, and Lewellen 1994). She emphasizes the ways dominant institutions construct groups that are already marginalized socially by saddling them with the added classification of being "at risk" for HIV/AIDS.

This chapter examines two of these risk group constructions, the "woman sex worker" and the "male truck driver," through an historical analysis of pub-

I presented earlier versions of this research at the 2000 American Sociological Association Annual Meeting in Washington, DC, and at the 2000 Women, Culture, Development Graduate Conference at the University of California, Santa Barbara. I am thankful to the panel organizers and participants for their thoughtful suggestions. Barbara Herr Harthorn's and Laury Oaks's editorial comments improved my argument in many ways. The University of California Pacific Rim Research Grant provided financial support for data collection.

lic health monitoring and intervention along the border regions in mainland Southeast Asia. These regions include northern Thailand, eastern Myanmar (formerly Burma), Cambodia, southern Vietnam, and Lao People's Democratic Republic (PDR) and extend into Yunnan in China and Manipur in India. Epidemiological data suggest that AIDS remains on the verge of being an uncontrollable epidemic in Asia and pinpoint the prevalence of "at risk" categories such as injecting drug use and risky heterosexual behavior in mainland Southeast Asia (MAP 1997:5). In response, governmental and nongovernmental programs have been expanded to curtail further HIV transmission in the border regions.

My analysis compares the practices of social inclusion and exclusion in this Southeast Asian case. Focusing on the strategies employed by AIDS prevention and condom promotion programs, I maintain that national and transnational health agencies such as the U.S. Agency for International Development strive to regulate the sexual practices of women sex workers through inclusion and male truck drivers through exclusion. These programs stigmatize truck drivers for their reported "promiscuous" sexual practices as well. The programs assume that their geographical mobility facilitates HIV transmission across large distances rapidly. Paradoxically, these programs also normalize and increase social tolerance for the work of already stigmatized sex workers by seeking to educate them about condom use and by encouraging their active participation in the expansion of the programs. This normalization of sex-work activities in Southeast Asia—by U.S.-funded programs—differs from strategies that led to the exclusion of U.S. gay men in HIV/AID programs during the same period. Consequently, this chapter focuses on (1) the expansion of scientific and governmental monitoring in the Thai border regions, constructing certain groups as at risk, (2) the expert use of logics about borders and poverty to sustain constructions of HIV risk categories, and (3) the implementation of both inclusion and exclusion strategies through prevention programs designed for sex workers and truck drivers.

The theoretical issue here involves the construction of epidemiological risk and social regulation through the practice of inclusion and exclusion, that is, *why and how does the regulation of certain sexual practices rely on the use of risk construction?* Current understandings wrestle with the perception and communication of risk in various sociocultural contexts (Douglas and Wildavsky 1982; Southwell 2000). The issue that remains unexplored is that of the *materiality* of social regulation and risk construction, the non-symbolic processes and practices that shape the perception and communication of risk, and how they in turn imbue materials and objects with meanings. In the context of sexual regulation, this materiality involves corporeal bodies and their social identities (Foucault [1978] 1990; Fout 1992; Weeks 1996). Yet other material objects have been part of sexual regulation—for example, in the context of governmental programs, modern contraceptives—in the effort to restrict population growth (Hartmann 1995; also see Appadurai 1986). Here, male condoms serve as the commodified object under investigation. The condom as a social object facilitates particular relations of power and inequalities, because a social inquiry into condoms and condom social relations offers a distinct answer to the main theoretical question, different from the focus on corporeal bodies, in which answers focus on individual risk perception.

Shifting our attention to condoms and the materiality of risk construction also turns our focus to the activities and logics of medical and public health experts in their construction of epidemiological risk categories. In the AIDS context, experts use the logic of cultural practices and logic of antipoverty strategies (Parker, Barbosa, and Aggleton 2000; Farmer 2001). The logic of cultural practices suggests that HIV transmission results from hypersexualized cultural practices and that condom use would increase if such practices were reduced (Caldwell, Caldwell, and Quiggin 1989). One of the problems with this logic is that it reinforces racist tropes—in particular, colonial and orientalist tropes of sexual promiscuity initiated under conquest and empire rule and prior to the advent of HIV (Said [1978] 1990; Hall 1996). The logic of antipoverty strategies suggests that HIV transmission results from dire economic conditions and that condoms provide a partial resource to prevent transmission. This underlying logic is found in many epidemiological studies on HIV/AIDS (World Bank 1997). It insists that certain groups, particularly in the Third World, are susceptible to HIV/AIDS and that risk construction, however problematic at times, is necessary to prevent further poverty and any further decline in the health and well-being of the groups. Accordingly, what sorts of social and sexual regulation strategies do health promotion agencies use that arise from these expert logics and practices of risk construction? Historically, in the Southeast Asian context, social and sexual regulation strategies relied on state violence—through military and police actions—and on restrictive legislative measures (Leinbach and Ulack 2000). This reliance has been particularly salient to the state regulation of sexual behavior related to prostitution, homosexuality, and sexual assault. In view of this history, we might ask whether state violence and legislative strategies of sexual regulation lend support for social inclusion and exclusion via condom use campaigns. Or are there newer strategies of local, national, and transnational governance in use?

Disputing explanations that predominantly focus on state violence and repressive legislation, I argue for a *managerialistic* explanation to understand the development of condom use campaigns directed at sex workers and truck drivers in mainland Southeast Asia. First I suggest, unlike Grover's quote that opens this chapter, that the medical and epidemiological construction of risk is also and already social and political due to the expert practice of monitoring and data collection, resulting in unreliable conclusions. Second, I suggest that there is a need to reevaluate the poverty assumptions in epidemiological research and monitoring programs, especially the flawed assumption that poverty causes unhealthy sexual practices and HIV transmission. Third, I suggest that expert risk construction and monitoring programs lead to increased reliance on managerialism as a governance and social regulation strategy. Managerialism is best defined as the institutional growth and restructuring of welfare policies and programs with an increasing use of market, bureaucratic, and social science solutions.

By focusing on the materiality of risk and social regulation through condoms, this chapter provides an ethnographic analysis of the capitalist world-system (Marcus 1998; Enloe 2001) and contributes to a sustained political-economic analysis of global public health that goes beyond a mere sociopsychological understanding of risk (Bunton, Nettleton, and Burrow 1995; Labonte 1998). Extending existing theories on managerialism as a governance and social regulation strategy, I argue for greater civic consultation and accountability of health programs that aim to control risk-group members' sexual practices.

MONITORING ACTIVITIES: EVOLVING CONTEXTS, UNCHANGING RISK CATEGORIES

Although AIDS cases were reported as early as 1984 in Thailand, constructions of AIDS risk categories by medical and policy officials began to emerge only in 1988, and these group categories continue to be used today (UNAIDS 1998:5). Medical researchers in 1988 reported an "alarming" increase in HIV seroprevalence transmitted through injecting drug users and female sex workers. Their findings were drawn from ad hoc HIV antibody testing (Sittitrai and Brown 1994:S143). In the following year, the Thai Ministry of Public Health began to develop and implement national AIDS-related activities with World Health Organization assistance. These activities included "educational efforts in perceived 'high-risk' groups, [and the] strengthening of blood screening, testing, and surveillance efforts" (Ungphakorn and Sittitrai 1994:S156). Targeted groups included sex workers, injecting drug users, men visiting sexually transmitted infections clinics, women visiting antenatal clinics, and blood donors. This surveillance effort, known as the HIV sentinel system, involved the anonymous monitoring of a given cohort group's blood or other bodily fluids; this early detection system tested the same groups annually. This testing procedure was designed to track and monitor the changing levels of prevalence for particular groups.

Government monitoring also extended beyond HIV surveillance testing; it involved gathering information about specific risk groups, many of whom the experts considered poor, such as male truck drivers and female sex workers. From 1989 to 1992, the U.S. Agency for International Development provided technical and financial assistance to Thailand's AIDS prevention efforts as part of its global initiative directed at 35 countries (FHI 1992a; 1992b). Of the 20 U.S. AIDS programs in Thailand, 2 focused on injecting drug users, 2 on male truck drivers, 10 on female sex workers, and 7 on populations in northern Thailand (FHI 1992b:162–81). Many of these programs focused on educating specific populations about the need for increased condom use. The United States contracted Family Health International, a nonprofit U.S.-based organization, to oversee other governmental and nongovernmental entities implementing the programs. It also subcontracted out the necessary quantitative and rapid-assessment qualitative studies, which were conducted by research groups at Columbia University (U.S.) and Mahidol University (Thailand) (see Morris et al. 1995; Morris et al. 1996; Podhisita et al. 1996; Wawer et al. 1996).

For instance, the United States supported a program researching the "multiple partner networks" of urban sex workers and their clients to "determine the exponential spread of HIV into groups with identifiable characteristics" (FHI 1992b:164). Another program conducted a study on the "lifestyle, norms, and the conflicting pressures" of 200,000 long-haul truck drivers to understand their "risk of contracting and transporting HIV because of their extended periods away from home, their reported use of amphetamines with alcohol, and their multiple sexual partners" (FHI 1992b:166). A third program developed and distributed HIV-prevention flip charts for use by health educators working with Burmese female sex workers to increase condom use in the Mai Sai district along the Lao-Myanmar border, which has one of the highest HIV prevalence rates in northern Thailand (FHI 1992b:173).

In 1992, the United States extended its assistance to the region, with new prevention activities in Cambodia and Lao PDR (FHI 1997a:111–14). These new activities nevertheless continued to focus on sex workers and truck drivers as identified risk groups. Through its Cambodia program, the United States implemented an "HIV sentinel surveillance" program in 1995 to track HIV transmission across international borders with Laos, Thailand, and Vietnam. The program monitored HIV prevalence among women sex workers and other sentinel groups. In addition to the annual HIV antibody testing, the United States also implemented an "HIV risk behavioral surveillance" system, relying on self-reported condom use surveys. These behavioral surveys contained questions involving "behaviors related to high-risk behaviors," such as using drugs and alcohol, knowing someone with HIV/AIDS, not using condoms, and "other items often preceding high-risk sexual behavior" (FHI 1997b:29). U.S.-survey training materials highlighted the need to include samples of "highest-risk (core-transmission) groups," "'bridge' population groups" who connect the core and the public, and general population groups (FHI 1997b:19). This behavioral surveillance allowed governmental and nongovernmental AIDS organizations to infer HIV prevalence from self-reported condom use rather than relying solely on more intrusive blood testing. In this way, these organizations were able to continuously monitor and scrutinize the behavior of sex workers and acquire an analytical map of their social networks.

Moreover, the U.S. program in Cambodia funded a study on "sexual networks [that] connect Thai men with female Cambodian and Vietnamese commercial sex workers, who in turn have extensive contact with local Cambodian men" (FHI 1997a:110). The study provided an example of its "areas of affinity" principle, explaining "how domestic epidemics are ignited and perpetuated" through "high-risk ... border crossing" (110). The United States, through the Lao PDR program, also initiated an HIV sentinel surveillance program along the Lao-Thai border. A summary of the program stated:

Despite the low levels of detected infection, the proximity of northern Lao PDR to one of the highest prevalence areas of the region (northern Thailand and Burma) creates an environment conducive to the transmission of HIV into Lao sexual networks. Every Lao province borders on another country, and travel is easy and frequent between Thailand, China, Vietnam, and Lao PDR. (112)

Despite such increased surveillance of sexual activities in the regions along Thai borders, information about risk remains incomplete. For instance, in February 1998, researchers at Bangkok's Chulalongkorn University released a U.S.-funded report on the population movements across borders between mainland Southeast Asian countries; the report mentions "concern about the spread of HIV/AIDS across the border, based mainly on perceptions about the risk behaviors of migrants" (Stern and Crissman 1998). Although the report aims to provide a spatial and social description of the sexual and health behavior of migrant groups, it nonetheless repeats the description throughout the report for all the border crossings. In the case of migrant labor activities along the Thai-Cambodian border, the report states the following:

In Klong Yai, there are apparently no Thai commercial sex workers, only Cambodian and Vietnamese. According to one estimate, there are roughly 100 Vietnamese and 20 Cambodian commercial sex workers in Klong Yai. In Klong Son and Kan Kang, two villages near Klong Yai, there are estimated 120 commercial sex workers, about 80 percent Cambodian and 15 percent Vietnamese. There are many fishermen in the Klong Yai and many people believe they frequently visit brothels. (1998:22)

This quote typifies the slippage of experts from unconfirmed reports of risky behaviors to risk-group construction and the blending of information sources (from local anecdotes, mass media, and official estimates). Moreover, it reveals a reliance on the assumed importance of focusing on the sexual networks of migrant workers, particularly in "areas of affinity."

Historical records of risk-group monitoring for AIDS in mainland Southeast Asia reveal evidence of extensive surveillance, but it is clear that the quality of these monitoring activities has been uneven. National governments, transnational quasi-governmental organizations (such as Family Health International), nongovernmental organizations, and university research centers participated in these monitoring activities. Monitoring ranged from sentinel surveillance (blood testing) to behavioral surveillance surveys and rapid assessment ethnographies. The surveys and ethnographies focused on pre-identified at-risk behavioral factors for HIV, including unprotected sexual activity (the lack of condom use) and sex with a sex worker. Such monitoring activities easily conflated at-risk behaviors and risk-group membership. One of the documents, for instance, states

Risk behaviors are not evenly distributed in population groups. . . . Findings from Thailand, for example, suggested that risk behavior is greater among adult men than adolescents. . . . In a very young or slow-growing epidemic, it is important to include male and female groups who are at highest risk or members of core-transmission groups, i.e., those who have the highest numbers of multiple partners. . . . Typically, these groups include female sex workers and men who regularly pay for sex. (FHI 1997b:19)

The danger posed by such (epidemiological and policy) expert construction of risk categories is that it lends a sense of fixity and naturalness to such categories. These experts rely on limited understanding and the idea of risk construction to generate new information about risk through intensive monitoring of the identified at risk group. One expert, for instance, would find increased HIV prevalence for sex workers as compared to other groups; another expert would study condom use by sex workers or their sexual and social networks; still others would conduct a behavioral surveillance study of this group. Methodologically, the very practice of risk construction is questionable. The adoption of risk-behavioral categories across experts and studies fosters the persistent identification of certain groups as at risk. Increased availability of funding for monitoring and technical expert assistance further encourages this metaphoric borrowing or traveling of ideas. In turn, epidemiological theories about HIV risk become accepted as facts among these medical and policy experts without any reevaluation of the initial epidemiological aspects of risk.

THE LOGIC OF REPEATED MONITORING: SUB-SAHARAN AFRICA, SOUTHEAST ASIA, AND CAPITALIST VECTORS OF TRANSMISSION

Although cases of HIV and AIDS were described among Asians in the early to mid-1980s, HIV only became visible as a problem for Asia when it appeared among sex workers, transforming sex workers from the sexual/tropical home-away-from-home for Westerners into a vector within Asia. . . . Once "Asian AIDS" was launched, blame concerning the diasporal relations of migrant Western homosexuals was subordinated to hysteria about heterosexual vectorial transmission. Asia's plight was compared to "African AIDS," not to the unmarked, but unmistakable queer AIDS which the media suggested formed the centre of the epidemic in white America. (Patton 1997:249)

Increased monitoring of AIDS risk groups by public health officials, non-governmental organizations, and academic researchers took a distinct form of implementation in the Southeast Asia region and since then has relied on a particular logic of risk-group construction and monitoring that did not originate in the region. This logic traveled from Sub-Saharan Africa in the same way that experts explain HIV's transnational migration. In this section, I first highlight the development of this logic in Africa involving heterosexual transmission in general and sex workers and their clients in particular. Second, I show how experts transferred this logic from Sub-Saharan Africa to Southeast Asian sex workers and truck drivers. Third, I analyze the Sub-Saharan African and Southeast Asian logics as extensions of the corresponding rise in waged work and capitalist relations in these areas. The trajectories of this economic argument on Third World heterosexual risk groups differ from those that shaped the sexualized risky logic of Western gay behavior, as Patton hinted in the section's opening quote, such that "Southeast Asian AIDS" has become quintessentially about sex and work.

As we have seen, the expert construction of AIDS risk groups and behaviors has been built on politically and epidemiologically questionable claims. Since the initial mass media hysteria about the "gay cancer" in 1981–82, AIDS stigmatization in the United States and other First World countries seemed to spread even more insidiously than HIV itself. By 1983–84, medical researchers and media coverage began to draw attention to the possible origins of HIV in Sub-Saharan African countries such as Zaire and Rwanda (Cohn 1983; Vandepitte, Verwilghen, and Zachee 1983).[1] Published research and medical journal commentaries in 1984–85 raised the possibility of male-to-female and female-to-male sexual transmissions of HIV in AIDS cases of African-origin in contrast to male-to-male sexual transmission (and infected-blood transmission) in cases in the First World (Clumeck et al. 1984, Clumeck et al. 1985; Piot et al. 1984; Van de Perre et al. 1984). Moreover, while highlighting the importance of heterosexual HIV transmission, Piot et al. (1984) presented a rare early speculation that being *middle class* in urban Zaire was a risk factor for AIDS, based on 38 cases: "While rates of disease by socioeconomic status cannot yet be calculated, these figures do suggest that a disproportionate number of cases may be occurring in the higher income population" (Piot et al. 1984:67). In the same July issue of the *Lancet,* Van de Perre et al. (1984) presented empirical findings about the financially stable status of 26 AIDS patients, supporting the speculation of Piot and his colleagues that "Almost all patients were middle or upper class. They worked in the private or public sector in urban centres [of Rwanda]" (63). Importantly, Van de Perre and his coauthors also mentioned that some of their female patients were sex workers.

By the following July, some of the same authors of the earlier Van de Perre et al. study published another article, "Heterosexual Promiscuity among African Patients with AIDS," discussing most of the same patients (Clumeck et al. 1985). Here they highlighted extramarital sex with prostitutes as a significant risk factor for HIV based on their findings about 10 Rwandan prostitutes (who were living in Kigali, Rwanda, or in Brussels as immigrants) out of a total of 42 patients. Their conclusion was that "In Central Africa, infection with HTLV-III or lymphadenopathy-associated virus is linked with heterosexual promiscuity and female prostitution" (Clumeck et al. 1985:182). This brief and significant research note received global mass-media attention (Haney 1986) and inspired further academic inquiry into AIDS, promiscuity, and prostitution (Mann et al. 1988; Wilson et al. 1989). Later it also resulted in sex workers being seen as a core transmission group for HIV/AIDS in Africa. This 1985 "Heterosexual Promiscuity" article also initiated greater focus on the sexual attitudes and practices of African men who can pay for sex. In other words, although the earlier research speculated that being middle class in Africa was an HIV risk factor, experts began to reconstruct, momentarily, this socioeconomic risk factor into sexual risky behavior with prostitutes. They also speculated about the significant social impact of male migrant workers, who travel from rural towns to find work in busy urban centers and who sometimes become clients of female sex workers (Hunt 1989). In particular, they focused on long-haul truck drivers as a potential vector for HIV transmission because these drivers also moved people across Africa (Bolin 1987; Bwayo et al. 1991; Orubuloye, Caldwell, and Caldwell 1993).

Hence, by 1989, as governments in Africa, Asia, Latin America, and the Middle East began to develop their national AIDS "control" programs with assistance such as from the United States and the World Health Organization, heterosexual transmission of AIDS became a central focus, and female sex workers and their clients began to be regarded as important risk groups based on the Sub-Sahara African model. Governments consequently monitored the sexual activities of members of these and other groups in the hope of preventing the rapid spread of HIV. The U.S. government, in particular, sponsored projects and research on women sex workers and their male migratory clients in many Third World countries.

The expert logic of "African AIDS" was specifically transferred to AIDS-prevention activities in South Asia (particularly in India) and Southeast Asia, places that were known for their sex industries (see Singh et al. 1993). Having a risk logic that focused on heterosexual transmission—mainly on female sex workers and their male clients—allowed governments to focus on AIDS transmission at the social margins and borders of their countries. Geographic borders also are metaphoric and denote politico-geographic locations.

A growing number of research studies have been published on AIDS and female sex workers across Thailand (such as Swaddiwudhipong et al. 1990; Sawanpanyalert et al. 1994; Hanenberg and Rojanapithayakorn 1998). Several studies have focused primarily on AIDS and the male clients of Thai female sex workers, such as truck drivers (Havanon, Bennett, and Knodel 1993; Maticka-Tyndale et al. 1997). Htoon et al. (1994) explored AIDS and sex work in Myanmar; Thuy et al. (1998) examined these issues in Vietnam. In this way, these disparate experts have helped to solidify the HIV-risk construction around a particular form of heterosexual transmission, providing Southeast Asian governments with information to track and monitor continuously the behavior and attitudes of these sex workers and their clients. It is important to ask why, beyond their concern about the well-being of these groups, governments have chosen to patrol their borders in this manner.

To answer this question, I want to turn to a 1997 United States—and United Nations—funded report that briefly addresses the clustering of the HIV epidemic in Asia. Here we see how monitoring and surveillance shape managerialistic strategies:

Populations in Asia are moving across land and sea borders in increasing numbers. International trade and commerce support this growth in population mobility, which is also facilitated by the growing number of international highways and construction of new bridges. ... As in Africa, truckers on international land routes move vast quantities of goods between mainland countries. ... The fact of being away from home, family, and community, and the anonymity and loneliness of traveling are factors that increase vulnerability to HIV acquisition. ... Crossing land or sea borders often required overnight stays, leaving the individual with idle time and opportunities to visit drinking and gambling establishments and brothels. HIV surveillance data for female sex workers, male STD clinic patients, and young men in the countries in the region—Thailand, Myanmar, Cambodia, and Vietnam—show a clustering of high prevalence sites around international borders and ports. (MAP 1997:18–9)

This quote summarizes the prevailing logic used by academic and policy experts to describe one aspect of AIDS risk in parts of Asia. It shows the African origin of the logic and the idea that international borders are "areas of affinity" for the rapid transmission of HIV/AIDS. In addition, the movement of workers in the quote is distinctively gendered. This logic connotes that truck drivers move goods from new factories to ports and distribution centers, such truck drivers cross national borders, they are men, they are away from home and family and are lonely, they have idle time, and therefore they visit brothels.

This expert logic interweaves AIDS, money, and migrants. The logic traces and connects different kinds of movement—movement of trade and commerce, movement of workers, and movement of diseases such as AIDS, either in Africa or Asia. Because commerce, workers, and diseases cross national borders, governments focus on the workers involved in transnational commerce to control the spread of AIDS. That is, the governments take the exponential spread of cross-border economic activities as a given and consequently focus on the movements of workers. As a result, this logic linked AIDS transmission and the new and emerging free-market activities in economies of Third World borders, particularly in 1980–90s Southeast Asia. With the global expansion of large-scale manufacturing activities throughout many border regions, governments have had to address the alarming growth of AIDS in these newly industrializing zones. In other words, for-profit economic activities have brought both waged work and HIV/AIDS to these regions. Although these Southeastern Asian governments have sought to increase trade and economic activities in the border regions, they have also aimed to limit HIV transmission by focusing on risk groups such as male truck drivers, who have been classified as "bridge" groups because they serve to link one of the "core" transmission groups, women sex workers at truck stops, to the general public, including truckers' female partners at home.

Theoretically, there is a peculiarity in the economic logic of risk applied to women sex workers and their clients that links poverty (or economic activities), promiscuity, and the lack of condom use with HIV transmission. This peculiarity is a key component of an understanding of the materiality of risk construction (Giffin 1998). In this case, truck drivers and sex workers have money irrespective of their individual economic origins or the amount of money earned. As speculated in the early research by Piot et al. (1984) and presented by Van De Perre et al. (1984)—whose work is now considered erroneous—sex workers were described economically as middle- or upper-class. In a similar fashion, the economic logic that truck drivers are a risk group frames poverty in a distinct manner. As previously quoted: "international trade and commerce support this growth in population mobility ... [and increase the] vulnerability to HIV acquisition" (MAP 1997:18–9). Public health entities in the region viewed risky behavior under conditions of poverty as not simply unprotected sex but, more broadly, as unprotected sex in unhealthy expanding market economies. Through this logic, I argue—by providing a partial material understanding of risk construction and social regulation—that the meaning of poverty has not been simply the lack of income or access to affordable healthcare.

Poverty has also meant the lack of social alternatives to the local sex industry that is situated in the unhealthy context of capitalist activities and waged relations. Accordingly, expert and government monitoring and tracking of female sex workers and their male truck-driver clients generate particular notions of risk, poverty (uncontrolled capitalism), and heterosexual promiscuity: poverty (however vaguely defined) and promiscuity foster risk. This epidemiological construction of risk, one that is also already political, remains flawed because it simply focuses on the individualized health perception of HIV risk and fails to account fully for the development of commercial activities, whether based on sexual practices or not. In other words, a material theory of risk construction necessitates placing greater attention on particular sites of capitalism as a route for HIV transmission to reframe the perception of risk beyond mere interpersonal relationships.

INTERVENING THROUGH MANAGERIALISM

So far I have discussed how various institutional entities construct and monitor HIV/AIDS risk at the national borders in mainland Southeast Asia. In this section I analyze these constructing and monitoring activities within a model of state managerialism by focusing on how they normalize the status of sex workers and stigmatize that of truck drivers. "Managerialism" is defined as a public governance strategy with the goal of instituting organizational reform that increases programmatic efficiency, restructuring welfare policies and programs and increasingly relying on market, bureaucratic, and social science solutions (see Lewis, Gewirtz, and Clarke 2000). I argue that managerialism as a governance strategy attempts to regulate the sexual practices and agency of risk groups through communication-based "behavioral change" programs.

Although First World countries have produced welfare-state institutions to manage social and economic crises and balance democratically competing interest groups, Third World countries have had a more limited history in the modern development of welfare-state management practices (Leinbach and Ulack 2000). With increased internal and external pressures for more open, transparent, and democratic governmental practices to end elite control and bureaucratic corruption and provide for legal reforms, many Southeast Asian governments are opting into the managerial model of state governance and providing greater social welfare services (Chua 2001). Turning away from prior governance strategies of state violence and restrictive legislative measures, this managerialism offers a technocratic solution lacking civic accountability to address the "social problems" of AIDS.

For example, with managerialism comes a new form of social regulation through HIV/AIDS monitoring and prevention activities. At the borders of mainland Southeast Asian countries, this managerialism means that a central national government has a new way to interact with people who are living as labor migrants and war refugees, many of whom are ethnic minorities. Ethnic groups living along the Thai borders, for instance, include Laotians, Hmong, Mon (from Myanmar), and Khmer (from Cambodia) as well as "hill-tribe dwellers" such as Karen, Lawa, and Sewang. Through managerialism, governmental activities along the Thai border become less punitive toward ethnic minorities, whereas in the past they relied on formal repressive means of social control. AIDS prevention programs have become more publicly legitimated due to the greater reliance on policy, scientific, and social welfare experts and nongovernmental organizations (FHI 1997a; World Bank 1997).

For women sex workers along the border regions, managerialism has meant the normalization of their sexual practices. Conventionally, government authorities control prostitution and sex work by making them illegal and often use antierotic morality-based arguments to permit the continual legal and police harassment of sex workers. Authorities also argue that these women are driven into the sex industry because they are victims of economic poverty and male domination. However, with the advent of HIV surveillance and AIDS education programs, government authorities have turned away from simply relying on legal restrictions and police repression to regulate the work, sexual identity, and sexual behavior of these women. Instead, health authorities have had to include and "empower" these women for HIV prevention programs to be successful (MAP 1997). In this way, new forms of state regulation through managerialism normalize and legitimate these ethnic women sex workers, even if provisionally. The Thai government proclaims success of condom-use prevention programs directed at female sex workers who have a near 100-percent condom use rate (UNAIDS 1998).

This sexual and ethnic normalization of the women workers and their sexual identities occurs in several ways. Women become clients in health programs sponsored by governments and other health organizations. They are actively sought after to take part in behavioral and epidemiological research, and they are invited to receive social services and modern medical treatment. They receive counseling about negotiation and communication skills to use with male clients and with their employers to increase condom use and similar health-seeking activities. Moreover, women are recruited to be peer educators and to teach HIV/AIDS prevention strategies to other sex workers. Some have also received counseling on how to leave the sex industry and seek other forms of income-generating activities.

As a result, women sex workers along the national borders of mainland Southeast Asia face a multifaceted form of sexual regulation that integrates repressive and legislative restrictions with normalizing managerialism. Authorities have come to accept sex workers as a legitimate group for social welfare provision and have come to view them as a "normal" group. For these women, work is no longer (or minimally) stigmatized, because experts classify them as engaging in one of the "core" risk behaviors for HIV transmission.

By contrast, for male truck drivers in the region, managerialism has not meant normalization. Instead, for them, managerialism introduces a new form of stigmatization that associates their form of employment with a propensity to engage in sexual promiscuity and "risky" sexual behavior. Male truck drivers working along the national borders of mainland Southeast Asia and traversing the long-haul highways have become increasingly monitored. State authorities and health-related organizations promote harm-reduction behavior to counteract the possible effects of combined risky behaviors such as intoxication, injecting drug use, and engaging in commercial sex without using condoms.

Such programs encourage truck drivers to engage in health-seeking behavior as the result of learning about HIV prevention. However, these managerialism programs also stigmatize the truck drivers as a group by associating their occupation with risky behaviors. That is, experts and officials believe that both the occupation and the associated truck-driver lifestyle foster HIV transmission. This includes assumptions that link being away from one's family (and wife), sexual promiscuity, and being working class and an ethnic minority. Stigmatization is fostered through a specific form of heterosexual morality that promotes the stability of a Western monogamous nuclear family arrangement. If this morality was not there before, it was generated through the health programs. Further, the assumed tendency of truck drivers to engage in sexual promiscuity was linked to the idea that they had multiple sexual networks, such as female sex workers, which then led to the idea that the drivers "bridged" HIV transmission between sex workers and their wives and other sexual partners in urban areas. In this way, programs consider sexual promiscuity as not just a problem of morality but also as a public health risk that could give rise to a major medical epidemic.

In particular, governments and health promotion organizations work to change individual behavior through communication-based programs. In these programs, communication refers to activities ranging from interpersonal exchange to mass-media marketing. The programs, which have extended the parameters of traditional public health promotion, include condom distribution, outreach activities, and promotion strategies. Such intervention programs aim to "meet the needs of populations unaccustomed to sharing concerns about sexuality and of societies whose customs and structures inadvertently encourage risky behavior" (FHI 1997b:8). The programs attempt to "influence individual behaviors and the social contexts in which they occur" (FHI 1997b:8). Program messages are crafted to motivate and appeal to the needs, beliefs, concerns, and readiness of specific target audiences such as women sex workers and male truck drivers (FHI 1996:9). That is, these coded messages encourage the audience to change their "attitudes" and to learn "skills" to protect themselves from HIV infection. They also present certain behaviors as "undesired" and present the advantages and disadvantages of adopting "desired" behaviors (FHI 1996:12–14). The U.S. and Lao PDR governments, for example, developed an HIV-prevention campaign that aimed to encourage sexual behavior change among vulnerable border and urban populations—populations that include traders, businesspeople, truckers, migrant workers, and ethnic minorities who cross the Thai-Lao border (FHI 1997c:28).

Therefore, the HIV/AIDS prevention programs directed at women sex workers and male truck drivers attempt explicitly to change their sexual practices—viewed as significant HIV risk factors—and, thus, regulate their behavior by promoting condom use and other health-seeking activities. The programs also strive to reduce the number of sexual partners and decrease the extent of the at-risk sexual networks. In this way, these programs allow managerialism to become part of the lives of these women and men. The result of these risk-intervention programs targeted at women sex workers and male truck drivers is that if these groups do not change their sexual practices, they will be blamed for the further spread of the epidemic.

Managerialism consequently provides for the containment of AIDS risk and epidemic along the border regions. Through the social regulation of women sex workers and male truck drivers through HIV-prevention programs, I argue, that this border containment is also designed to provide for the "de-risking" and deregulation of the country's metropoles—urban areas situated far from rural landscapes that combine long stretches of highway, border checkpoints, and brothels. In this way, among the nonmigratory elite and middle-class people of Bangkok, AIDS can be conceptualized as a health-risk issue isolated at the Thai border among ethnic migrants and one that threatens the new urban localities.

Nevertheless, the rise of managerialism also provides new avenues for women sex workers and male truck drivers to negotiate any attempt by health authorities and organizations to regulate their sexual practices. This negotiation process highlights the constraints introduced by social regulation. I suspect that some workers choose to be complicit with health authorities and conform to the authorities' desire to see them engage in more health-seeking behaviors. Workers may opt to change their ways of life and adopt new ideas of health; these values may then be passed on to the next generations of sex workers, truck drivers, and people in surrounding communities. Alternatively, workers might also reinterpret the "influential" (value-laden) messages involving AIDS prevention, sexual promiscuity, and condom use to create new and unexpected meanings and practices different from those desired by health authorities. The experts might consider such reinterpretations as evidence of the difficulty of certain populations "learning" to get the proper message and might suggest that migrant workers remain uneducable. But it may also be that such reinterpretations provide workers with new ways to *resist* and grapple with competing desires and pressures in their lives and to actively create new meanings for sexual practices without wholly accepting expert constructions of medical and social risk.

REORIENTING RISK

In sum, governmental and affiliated social-welfare entities strive to regulate and control marginalized groups at the same time as they attempt to improve the health conditions of these groups through managerialism. Coalescing around public health activities and this managerial process, power, as social theorist Michel Foucault (1980) argues, creates knowledge, subjects, domination, and resistance. This managerialism produces—as a generative act of this power—a whole host of risk-group categories at the national borders of mainland Southeast Asia. It also produces often inadequate information through monitoring and surveillance of risk activities involving women sex workers and male truck drivers, social regulation (through a combination of normalization and stigmatization), and resistance to the social regulation. I would argue that to conduct further studies on their condom use, risk perception, and prior experience with epidemiological experts, however well meaning, would merely perpetuate the faulty construction of their risk. It would also disempower research subjects through the use of patronizing inclusion and exclusion strategies. As Foucault suggests, transforming power relations necessitates changing the social relations that produce knowledge claims.

Moreover, the peculiar features of this managerialism involve the medical, policy, and social-service expert construction of the economic logic of HIV/AIDS risk. Health authorities and organizations have constructed a particular logic that isolates poverty as the primary cause of risk, all the while working hard to mitigate the negative health consequences of capitalist economic activities. That is, authorities have judiciously worked to change the individual behavior of ethnic and migrant women sex workers and male truck drivers and have simply accepted that new capitalist economic activities might be a more salient risk factor for HIV transmission. Governments have not wanted to limit economic activities; instead, they have limited the scope of their agenda to the apparent inability of certain migrant groups to behave in sexually "proper" ways by using condoms.

My analysis, therefore, raises questions about the conventional wisdom that says these health authorities and organizations merely want to curtail the rapid growth of HIV transmission in the border regions. Instead, in this situation and historical context, authorities accept capitalist economic growth as a given, and rather than identify and challenge some of the negative health consequences it has produced, they merely aim to minimize the negative effects of such rapid growth. Further, the authorities draw on managerial techniques simultaneously to legitimize, control, and monitor groups of people whom they assume to be the fundamental cause of the rise in HIV/AIDS. Thus, by maintaining their focus on changing the sexual behavior of border area migrants, health authorities and associated organizations have directed public attention away from the health risks associated with capitalist development. Consequently, this case theoretically provides a richer understanding of the material links associated with the social practices of risk construction and social regulation, moving beyond mere sociopsychological perceptions of harm caused by individual "risk takers" and "risk makers."

To reorient the expert risk construction of sexual behavior, I would argue for greater scrutiny through epidemiological studies and individual behavior-change projects of a different class of people, the transnational middle and upper classes, as being able to rapidly transmit HIV/AIDS. As medical geographer Peter Gould has suggested, this elite group has not yet been targeted:

Do not misunderstand me: the truck routes with their drivers and migrant passengers are still the same force in the geographic spread of the pandemic, but superimposed on those ... [routes are air travel networks used] by the modern elite, a group rich from business or government sponsorship, generally well-educated; in brief, the engineers, doctors, military officers, and particularly and especially, the politicians. (1993:82–3)

If even one comprehensive epidemiological study on AIDS and transnational elites in mainland Southeast Asia existed, the historical scrutiny and promotion of condom use among marginalized people to reduce risk of HIV/AIDS might be more convincingly regarded as unbiased and well intentioned.

More concretely, this chapter identifies four preliminary ways to reorient risk construction and its related social regulation to provide greater feedback and accountability from various civic constituencies. First, medical and epidemiological researchers need to curtail the use of risk categories in statistical and ethnographic studies and policy formulations, at least until experts and policy makers are able fully to disentangle and reexamine political and epidemiological construction of risk. Second, experts need to articulate the meanings of poverty in relation to HIV risk without simply using the poverty logic as a convenient rationale to justify research studies and prevention programs.

Third, experts and policy makers need to make explicit (if they aim to uphold democratic ideals) their attempts to change the behavior, through their reliance on managerial governance, of particular groups who are already often socially marginalized. And finally, experts and policy makers need to change their mode of operation and allow marginalized groups greater ability to define what they themselves consider good health and social well-being, thereby seeking their own alternate means of promoting and sustaining good health.

NOTE

1. I relied on condom-use journal articles involving mainland Southeast Asia groups published in English up to 1998 as primary evidence for this chapter and supplemented them with precursory epidemiological studies on AIDS.

REFERENCES

Appadurai, Arjun. 1986. "Introduction: Commodities and the Politics of Value." In *The Social Life of Things: Commodities in Cultural Perspectives,* ed. Arjun Appadurai, 1–63. New York: Cambridge University Press.

Bolin, H. 1987. "AIDS in Africa." *Jordemodern* 100: 402–403.

Bunton, Robin, Sarah Nettleton, and Roger Burrow, eds. 1995. *The Sociology of Health Promotion: Critical Analyses of Consumption, Lifestyle, and Risk.* London: Routledge.

Bwayo, Job J., Mohammed A. Omari, A. N. Mutere, Walter Jaoko, Christine Sekkade-Kigondu, Joan K. Kreiss, and Francis A. Plummer. 1991. "Long Distance Truck-Drivers, 1: Prevalence of Sexually Transmitted Diseases (STDs)." *East African Medical Journal* 68: 425–429.

Caldwell, John C., Pat Caldwell, and Pat Quiggin. 1989. "The Social Context of AIDS in Sub-Saharan Africa." *Population and Development Review* 15: 185–234.

Chua, Peter. 2001. *Condom Matters and Social Inequalities: Inquiries into Commodity Production, Exchange, and Advocacy Practices.* Unpublished dissertation, Department of Sociology, University of California, Santa Barbara.

Clumeck, Nathan, Michel Carael, D. Rouvroy, and D. Nzaramba. 1985. "Heterosexual Promiscuity among African Patients with AIDS." *New England Journal of Medicine* 313: 182.

Clumeck, Nathan, J. Sonnet, Henri Taelman, F. Mascart-Lemone, M. De Bruyere, P. Vandeperre, J. Dasnoy, L. Marcelis, M. Lamy, C. Jonas, et al. 1984. "Acquired Immunodeficiency Syndrome in African Patients." *New England Journal of Medicine* 310: 492–497.

Cohn, Victor, 1983. "Africa May Be the Origin of AIDS Disease." *The Washington Post,* November 27, A4.

Douglas, Mary, and Aaron Wildavsky. 1982. *Risk and Culture: An Essay on the Selection of Technical and Environmental Dangers.* Berkeley: University of California Press.

Enloe, Cynthia. 2001. *Bananas, Beaches, and Bases: Making Feminist Sense of International Politics.* Berkeley: University of California Press.

Family Health International. (FHI). 1992a. *AIDSTECH Final Report.* Vol. 1: *September 16, 1987 to September 15, 1992.* Durham, NC: Family Health International.

———. 1992b. *AIDSTECH Final Report.* Vol. 2: *Project Descriptions, September 16, 1987 to September 15, 1992.* Durham, NC: Family Health International.

———. 1996. *Assessment and Monitoring of Behavior Change Communication (BCC) Interventions.* Arlington, VA: Family Health International.

———. 1997a. *AIDS Control and Prevention Project, 1991–1997: Final Report.* Vol. 2. Durham, NC: Family Health International.

———. 1997b. *HIV Risk Behavioral Surveillance Surveys (BSS); Methodology and Issues in Monitoring HIV Risk Behaviors.* Bangkok, Thailand: Family Health International.

———. 1997c. *Making Prevention Work: Global Lessons from the AIDS Control and Prevention (AIDSCAP) Project, 1991–1997.* Arlington, VA: Family Health International.

Farmer, Paul. 2001. *Infections and Inequalities: The Modern Plagues.* Berkeley: University of California Press.

Foucault, Michel. [1978] 1990. *The History of Sexuality.* Vol. 1: *An Introduction.* New York: Vintage Books.

———. 1980. *The Foucault Reader.* Edited by Paul Rabinow. New York: Pantheon Books.

Fout, John C., ed. 1992. *Forbidden History: The State, Society, and the Regulation of Sexuality in Modern Europe.* Chicago: University of Chicago Press.

Giffin, Karen 1998. "Beyond Empowerment: Heterosexualities and the Prevention of AIDS." *Social Science and Medicine* 46(2): 151–156.

Gould, Peter R. 1993. *The Slow Plague: A Geography of the AIDS Pandemic.* Oxford: Blackwell Publishers.

Grover, Jan Zita. [1987] 1988. "AIDS: Keywords." In *AIDS: Cultural Analysis, Cultural Criticism,* ed. Douglas Crimp, 17–30. Cambridge, MA: The MIT Press.

Hall, Stuart. 1996. "The West and the Rest: Discourse and Power." In *Modernity: An Introduction to Modern Societies,* eds. Stuart Hall, David Held, D. Hubert, and K. Thompson, 184–228. Oxford: Blackwell Publishers.

Hanenberg, Robert, and Wiwat Rojanapithayakorn. 1998. "Changes in Prostitution and the AIDS Epidemic in Thailand." *AIDS Care* 10: 69–79.

Haney, Daniel Q. 1986. "Study Says Prostitutes, Customers May Be Key to AIDS in Africa." *Associated Press,* February 12.

Hartmann, Betsy. 1995. *Reproductive Rights and Wrong: The Global Politics of Population Control.* Rev. ed. Boston, MA: South End Press.

Havanon, Napaporn, Anthony Bennett, and John Knodel. 1993. "Sexual Networking in Provincial Thailand." *Studies in Family Planning* 24(1): 1–17.

Htoon, Myo Thet, Hla Htut Lwin, K. O. San, E. Zan, and Min Thwe. 1994. "HIV/AIDS in Myanmar." *AIDS* 8:S105–109.

Hunt, Charles W. 1989. "Migrant Labor and Sexually Transmitted Disease: AIDS in Africa." *Journal of Health and Social Behavior* 30(4): 353–373.

Labonte, Ronald. 1998. "Health Promotion and the Common Good: Towards a Politics of Practice." *Critical Public Health* 8(2): 107–123.

Leinbach, Thomas R., and Richard Ulack, eds. 2000. *Southeast Asia: Diversity and Development.* Upper Saddle River, NJ: Prentice-Hall.

Lewis, Gail, Sharon Gewirtz, and John Clarke. 2000. *Rethinking Social Policy.* London: Sage Publications.

Mann, Jonathan M., Nzila Nzilambi, Peter Piot, N. Bosenge, M. Kalala, Henry Francis, R. C. Colebunders, P. K. Azila, James W. Curran, and Thomas C. Quinn. 1988. "HIV Infection and Associated Risk Factors in Female Prostitutes in Kinshasa, Zaire." *AIDS* 2: 249–54.

Marcus, George E. 1998. *Ethnography through Thick and Thin.* Princeton, NJ: Princeton University Press.

Maticka-Tyndale, Eleanor, David Elkins, Melissa Haswell-Elkins, Darunee Rujkarakorn, Thicumporn Kuyyakanond, and Kathryn Stam. 1997. "Contexts and Patterns of Men's Commercial Sexual Partnerships in Northeastern Thailand: Implications for AIDS Prevention." *Social Science and Medicine* 44(2): 199–213.

Monitoring the AIDS Epidemic Network (MAP). 1997. *The Status and Trends of the HIV/AIDS/STD Epidemics in Asia and the Pacific: Provisional Report.* Manila, Philippines: Family Health International, Harvard School of Public Health, and the Joint United Nations Programme on HIV/AIDS.

Morris, Martina, Chai Podhisita, Maria J. Wawer, and Mark. S. Handcock. 1996. "Bridge Populations in the Spread of HIV/AIDS in Thailand." *AIDS* 10: 1265–271.

Morris, Martina, Anthony Pramualratana, Chia Podhisita, and Maria J. Wawer. 1995. "The Relational Determinants of Condom Use with Commercial Sex Partners in Thailand." *AIDS* 9: 507–515.

Orubuloye, I. O., Pat Caldwell, and John C. Caldwell. 1993. "The Role of High-Risk Occupations in the Spread of AIDS: Truck Drivers and Itinerant Market Women in Nigeria." *International Family Planning Perspectives* 19: 43–48.

Parker, Richard G., Regina M. Barbosa, and Peter Aggleton, eds. 2000. *Framing the Sexual Subject: The Politics of Gender, Sexuality, and Power.* Berkeley: University of California Press.

Patton, Cindy. 1997. "Queer Peregrinations." In *Acting on AIDS: Sex, Drugs, and Politics,* eds. Joshua Oppenheimer and Helena Reckitt, 235–253. London: Serpent's Tail.

Piot, Peter, Thomas C. Quinn, Henri Taelman, F. M. Feinsod, K. B. Minlangu, O. Wobin, N. Mbendi, P. Mazebo, K. Ndangi, W. Stevens, et al. 1984. "Acquired Immunodeficiency Syndrome in Heterosexual Population in Zaire." *Lancet* 2: 65–69.

Podhisita, Chai, Maria J. Wawer, Anthony Pramualratana, Uriwan Kanungsukkasem, and Robert McNamara. 1996. "Multiple Sexual Partners and Condom Use among Long-Distance Truck Drivers in Thailand." *AIDS Education and Prevention* 8: 490–498.

Said, Edward. [1978] 1990. *Orientalism.* London: Penguin.

Sawanpanyalert, Pathom, Kumnuan Ungchusak, Sombat Thanprasertsuk, and Pasakorn Akarasewi. 1994. "HIV-1 Seroconversion Rates among Female Commercial Sex Workers, Chiang Mai, Thailand: A Multi Cross-Sectional Study." *AIDS* 8: 825–829.

Schiller, Glick N., Stephan Crystal, and Denver Lewellen. 1994. "Risky Business: The Cultural Construction of AIDS Risk Groups." *Social Science and Medicine* 38(10): 1337–1346.

Singh, Yadhu N., K. Singh, R. Joshi, G. K. Rustagi, and A. N. Malaviya. 1993. "HIV Infection among Long-Distance Truck Drivers in Delhi, India." *Journal of Acquired Immune Deficiency Syndrome* 6: 323.

Sittitrai, Werasit, and Tim Brown. 1994. "The Emerging Epidemic of HIV Infection and AIDS in Asia and the Pacific." *AIDS* 8:S143–153.

Southwell, Brian. 2000. "Audience Construction and AIDS Education Efforts: Exploring Communication Assumptions of Public Health Interventions." *Critical Public Health* 10: 313–319.

Stern, Aaron, and Lawrence Crisman. 1998. *Maps of International Borders Between Mainland Southeast Asian Countries and Background Information Concerning Population Movements at these Borders.* Bangkok, Thailand: Asian Research Center for Migration.

Swaddiwudhipong, W., C. Chaovakiratipong, S. Siri, and P. Lerdlukanavonge. 1990. "Sociodemographic Characteristics and Incidence of Gonorrhea in Prostitutes Working near the Thai-Burmese Border." *Southeast Asian Journal of Tropical Medicine and Public Health* 21: 45–52.

Thuy, Nguyen Thi Thanh, Vo Tuyet Nhung, Nguyen Van Thuc, Troung Xuan Lien, and Ha Ba Khiem. 1998. "HIV Infection and Risk Factors among Female Sex Workers in Southern Vietnam." *AIDS* 12: 425–432.

Ungphakorn, Jon, and Werasit Sittitrai. 1994. "The Thai Response to the HIV/AIDS Epidemic." *AIDS* 8:S143–154.

United Nations Programme on HIV/AIDS, Joint. (UNAIDS). 1998. *Relationships of HIV and STD Declines in Thailand to Behavioural Change: A Synthesis of Existing Studies.* Geneva, Switzerland: Joint United Nations Programme on HIV/AIDS.

Van de Perre, Philippe, Dominique Rouvroy, Philippe Lepage, Jos Bogaerts, Philippe Kestelyn, Joseph Kayihigi, Anton C. Hekker, Jean-Paul Butzler, and Nathan Clumeck. 1984. "Acquired Immunodeficiency Syndrome in Rwanda." *Lancet* 2: 62–65.

Vandepitte J., R. Verwilghen, and P. Zachee. 1983. "AIDS and Cryptococepsis (Zaire, 1977)." *Lancet* 1: 925–926.

Wawer, Maria J., Chai Podhisita, Uraiwan Kanungsukkasem, Anthony Pramualratana, and Robert McNamara. 1996. "Origins and Working Conditions of Female Sex Workers in Urban Thailand: Consequences of Social Context for HIV Transmission." *Social Science and Medicine* 42(3): 453–462.

Weeks, Jeffrey. 1996. "The Body and Sexuality." In *Modernity: An Introduction to Modern Societies,* eds. Stuart Hall, David Held, D. Hubert, and K. Thompson, 364–394. Oxford: Blackwell Publishers.

Wilson, D, P. Chiroro, S. Lavelle, and C. Mutero. 1989. "Sex Worker, Client Sex Behaviour and Condom Use in Harare, Zimbabwe." *AIDS Care* 1: 269–80.

World Bank 1997. *Confronting AIDS: Public Priorities in the Global Epidemic.* Oxford: Oxford University Press.

Chapter 9

Genetically Modified Foods:
Shared Risk and Global Action

Francesca Bray

Genetically modified organisms (GMOs), or transgenics, are produced by transferring genes from one species to another. Whereas traditional plant and animal breeding involves the crossing of individuals with desirable traits within a single species, genetic engineering (GE) allows the grafting of genes from an Arctic halibut into a strawberry to confer frost resistance or the introduction of bacteria into corn to protect it from pests. Apart from GMOs designed for biomedical purposes, which I shall not discuss here, the main impact of genetic engineering on our everyday lives has been through the GM crops and other GMOs that enter our food system.

GM crops are new life-forms that promise great benefits: they may yield more than conventional varieties, resist disease or pests, require less water or pesticide, or incorporate extra vitamins. However, GMOs also entail complex risks that may not only affect our health and environment but also have social and political implications. Like nuclear power and DDT, GM crops and the foods made from them constitute what Beck (1999) calls a "manufactured uncertainty," a new technology that carries a range of complex risks and whose long-term global effects are impossible to predict.

Beck (1999) argues that we live increasingly in a world in which the control, predictability, and security characteristics of what he calls the "first modernity" can no longer be taken for granted. Like Douglas, Giddens, and other social theorists, Beck characterizes our current globalized world as a "risk society" where individuals as well as institutions are continually called upon to "decide about the undecidable" (Douglas and Wildavsky 1982; Giddens 1994; Beck 1999). We usually think of risk as a shadow of menace that affects individuals and groups

I would like to thank Nina Brown, Barbara Herr Harthorn, Jessica Jerome, Laury Oaks, and Sandy Robertson for their generous help with this chapter.

in negative terms, but Beck invites us to consider as well risk's liberatory potential. The contradictions that emerge in contests over definitions of risk help
sharpen a reflexive understanding and thus an effective critique of the modern
global world. Further, Beck perceives new, more generous possibilities where
people might *share risks* by linking their local issues to the global and their own
bodies to others' dangers. Beck sees new opportunities, in a period living beyond
its economic and ecological means, for "an escape from the 'bigger, more, better
creed'" (Beck 1999:10–11). Such risk-sharing offers the possibility of new coalitions and also the hope of a new global cosmopolitanism in which democratic action and solidarities would successfully transcend national boundaries.

The international debates and struggles over GM crops and foods neatly illustrate Beck's points. Beck notes that GMOs offer a classic example of a
manufactured uncertainty: industry insists there is no risk, while insurance
companies declare the new technology too risky to insure against (Beck
1999:106; Crook 2000). The biotech lobby (by which I mean the biotechnology
corporations producing commercial GMOs and their supporters in science,
business, and government) has tried to restrict the definitions of risk associated
with GM crops and foods to a few simple and quickly tested effects on health or
environment. In effect they have tried to normalize a scientific paradigm of risk
assessment that favors adoption of GMOs.

However, not only have environmental and consumer-safety groups engaged
the biotech lobby by contesting the scientific adequacy of their risk-testing paradigm, but a broad spectrum of opponents of GMOs around the world have in-
sisted on the need to take account of other significant dimensions of risk, not
susceptible to laboratory tests. Poor farmers immediately identified the threats
GMOs pose to their survival; other forms of risk identified by GMO opponents
include the dubiously democratic political procedures through which GMOs
are approved nationally and internationally and the heightened concentration
of corporate control over the global food system. Contest over defining the risk
of GM foods and crops has highlighted their role as emblems and agents of cor-
poratism and, as such, has placed opposition to GMOs at the heart of the current global anticorporate movement.

What unites Indian rice farmers with German shoppers is the shared convic-
tion that corporate GMOs are bad for the health at multiple levels, both physical and political. Using e-mail, the Web, and international rallies at Seattle and
its successors, anti-GMO activists have forged a coalition of consumer groups
and radical Greens, old-age pensioners and teenagers, Karnataka rice farmers,
Brazilian landless peasants, French sheep farmers, and Japanese housewives
whose forms of action include political protest, the destruction of GM crops, demands for long-term research, and a simple refusal to consume. By mid-2001,
we had witnessed several signal victories of the anti-GMO coalition, for instance, the temporary but dramatic collapse of biotech share prices, the elimi-
nation of GM foods from Western European supermarkets, bans on the release
of GMOs into the environment in Thailand and on the import of GM foods in

Sri Lanka, and the introduction of legislation requiring mandatory labeling in the European Union and Japan. Needless to say, each success of anti-GMO activists has been countered by the biotechnology industry, and the fortunes of war shift with dizzying rapidity as the day's field of battle moves from the World Trade Organization's offices to experimental fields in France, from mini-markets in Bangkok to the Indian parliament.[1]

The roller-coaster of biotech shares is just one example of how rapid and unpredictable the shifts have been: in early 1999, biotechnology was the darling of the market and investments were pouring into biotech companies, yet by July that same year, investment specialists were declaring that biotechnology had no future. By November 1999, the giant agro-biotech company, Monsanto, was about to be dissolved (Ramey 1999); however, by February 2001, biotech shares were soaring again and financial analysts were declaring that Monsanto had "made the transition from pariah to paragon" (Nicklaus 2001).

In the current neoliberal climate, most governments are tempted by genetic engineering and its promises of economic growth and progress. Biotech shares the glamorous ultramodern allure of the high-tech sector. Often governments are caught between consumer and small-farmer demands for tighter controls or bans on GM crops and foods and business-sector arguments that GMOs will generate wealth and give a competitive edge to their industrial and agricultural sectors. Meanwhile the transnational biotech industry has launched a huge, expensive PR campaign to convince people that GM crops will heal the environment, feed the hungry, and cure disease. Clearly the GMO war is nowhere near an end.

The biotech lobby has tried to discredit the opposition by insisting that "science" and "politics" are incompatible. The anti-GMO movement has countered by dramatically spotlighting the politics inherent in the science of biotechnology as practiced by corporations. This chapter argues that corporate and public-sector GMOs present different kinds and degrees of risk and concludes that the critique of corporate biotechnology and the shaping of risk-sharing alliances would be strengthened by a still sharper focus on the politics literally embodied in the artifacts we generically call GMOs.

THE POLITICS OF ARTIFACT

It is commonly said that technology is neutral in itself and its good or bad effects depend on the uses to which it is put. However, technological artifacts physically incorporate the values and goals of the social group that produces them. In other words, the social and political effects are—whether consciously or unconsciously—built into the design (Bray 1997:11). One crucial point often missing from the debate over GMOs is that different types of GMOs carry different kinds and degrees of risk. Even more significant than the biological characteristics of a particular GMO are the conditions of its production.

To clarify the risks, it is useful to distinguish between *public* and *corporate* *GMOs*. Public GMOs are developed in the public interest, usually in public research institutions, and not intended to be sold for profit (e.g., improved subsistence crops for peasant farmers). Corporate GMOs are developed by corporations for commercial use. In practice the boundaries are often blurred: corporations develop and patent information or techniques initiated in public laboratories; public projects negotiate free use of data generated by corporate research; corporations fund research in public laboratories; public institutions patent their products and purchase stock in biotech companies. But because public and corporate GMOs are engineered to fulfill distinct goals, the risks associated with each are significantly different.

As new life-forms, all GMOs present environmental and health risks that should be rigorously investigated. And as anyone familiar with the Green Revolution knows, new farming technologies intended to relieve poverty may actually increase the gap between rich and poor. But corporate GMOs present greater and more diverse risks than public GMOs, precisely because they are a *corporatist technology*. What do I mean by this term? Corporate GMOs are specifically designed as tools to increase corporate profits, extend corporate monopolies, and consolidate corporate control. The policies governing risk and responsibility that corporations have successfully imposed on the U.S. government and are urgently pressing for elsewhere embody the corporatist ideology that businesses have a legislated right to an *efficient* return (as large, as rapid, and as monopolistic as possible) on their investments and to the ownership of any knowledge they produce or even merely process, but they bear only limited liability for any adverse effects. The political and social risks associated with corporate GMOs are very high, and the environmental and health risks are likely to be much higher than for public GMOs because the drive for quick profits molds the science used to validate them.

Most arguments about GM crops and foods, whether against or in favor, proceed as if public and corporate GMOs were identical. This confusion of categories allows the biotech corporations to present their profit-generating transgenics as humanitarian products; it also encourages critics to dismiss all GMOs indiscriminately as tools of global capitalism. If we make the distinction between public and corporate GMOs, the mechanisms of the biotech lobby's propaganda machine are more clearly exposed, the articulations between different dimensions of risk are clarified, and a more open-minded weighing of the potential risks and benefits of this new technology becomes possible.

A CORPORATIST TECHNOLOGY

Perfecting a new GM crop can cost tens or even hundreds of millions of dollars. Although genetic engineering might offer significant scope for improving subsistence crops around the world—for example, breeding virus-resistant or drought-resistant varieties—few public labs can afford such research or obtain the many corporate patent clearances needed before they can distribute a new crop free to poor farmers. Not surprisingly, almost all GM crops currently released are produced by biotech corporations. As the corporations have accumulated intellectual property rights, it has become increasingly difficult for public research institutions to work on developing GMOs for noncommercial use.

The GM varieties produced by the biotech corporations are deliberately designed as a technology to increase corporate profits and control. The corporations that do the research and sell GM seeds also produce agrochemicals (fertilizers, herbicides, and pesticides). The interdependence of sales of seeds and chemicals makes the huge investments needed for GMO research worthwhile for conglomerates, eradicating small companies and raising the competitive stakes between the few remaining giants. After a series of mergers and buyouts, seven U.S. and European transnational corporations now dominate the industry, each with annual sales of over $2 billion. The biggest, the Swiss company Syngenta, was formed by the merger of Novartis and Zeneca in November 2000; then comes Monsanto, followed by Aventis, DuPont, Dow, Bayer, and BASF (PANUPS 2001).

In designing their GM crops, the goals for corporations are to increase overall sales, tie farmers into long-term cycles of dependency on their seeds and associated products, and maintain control over their "intellectual property." Monsanto has developed varieties of corn, cotton, and soy that are resistant to Roundup (glyphosate) herbicide. Because Roundup can be sprayed directly on the field without killing the crop, there is no need to weed mechanically. But Roundup-ready varieties will die if treated with any other herbicide, so Monsanto can count on selling its herbicide to farmers who adopt the seed; Roundup accounted for 67 percent of Monsanto's total sales in 2000. The logical next step in plant design is Genetic Use Restriction Technology (GURT), known to its enemies as traitor technology: an external chemical must be applied to switch the genetic traits of the plant on or off, so the farmer must buy extra products or the crop will fail.

One reason the biotech companies have not researched GMO improvements to subsistence crops such as cassava or barley is that it only makes economic sense for them to work on crops grown commercially on a vast scale around the world. In January 2001, Syngenta announced that it had mapped the genome of rice, and in late April the company launched its first base in the People's Republic of China (PRC), where rice is the principal crop. The Chinese government is very favorable to GM crops and recently passed a law that protects companies' rights to enforce genetic patents. Although the biotech lobby is concerned that Chinese consumers may not wish to eat GM foods, the official view is that "there is no room for GM critics in China." However, Syngenta is worried because the PRC is still a land of small farms. This is a serious obstacle to profit-making: transaction costs are high and scale-economies low, and small farmers are less likely to invest in more costly inputs (McGregor 2001).

It is to productivist farmers, growing commercial crops on a large scale and in highly competitive markets, that corporate-designed GM seed is primarily designed to appeal. *Productivism* is a term coined by critics to describe a system of production whose technical development is driven by the goal of continually increasing output to take advantage of economies of scale (Bové and Dufour 2000). Capitalist industrial agriculture is a prime example: competition lowers prices, driving farmers to invest in new technology, more inputs, and larger operations to survive. Farms must grow and specialize or die; as monoculture intensifies and spreads, so too does environmental contamination, vulnerability to pests and diseases and to market fluctuations, and the rate of bankruptcy and suicide among farmers (e.g. Kloppenburg 1988; Friedmann 1990; O'Hagan 2001).

The commercial farming sectors of North America and of parts of Europe, Australia, and South America have experienced relentless productivist expansion in recent decades. Working on a knife-edge between survival and bankruptcy, North American farmers were delighted at the prospect of maize varieties with inbuilt anti-borer pesticides or potatoes that, being blemish-free, were sure to meet the standards demanded by McDonald's (Pollan 1998). The first GM crop released for public consumption, the rot-resistant Flavr Savr tomato, was approved by the Food and Drug Administration (FDA) in 1994 (Bray, forthcoming). Since then, dozens of genetically modified field crops, fruits, and vegetables have been approved and released in the United States, as well as GM yeasts, pigs, poultry, and salmon. Roughly three-quarters of the total area of transgenic crops worldwide is in the United States; farmers growing cereals for export in Canada, Argentina, and Australia also make extensive use of GM seed (El Feki 2000:12).

The U.S. acreage under GM crops rose from 3 million acres in 1996 to 63 million acres in 1999; in 2001 approximately 24 percent of the maize acreage and 63 percent of the soy were GM varieties (Barboza 2000; El Feki 2000; Associated Press 2001). But American refrigerators have been invaded by the biotech industry without most Americans noticing; in the United States, GM varieties of crop or foodstuffs containing GMOs do not require special labeling. Although many Americans are still unaware of the fact, about two-thirds of the food items they routinely purchase in their supermarkets contain GM ingredients (Connor 2001).

Biotech companies patent their GM varieties and rigidly enforce these intellectual property rights, especially in cases where the successful cultivation of the GM variety does not depend on the purchase of other products from the same company. Companies such as Monsanto send out detectives, encourage neighbors to inform, and conduct DNA tests on fields to control the risk of "copyright infringement" by any farmer who might be tempted to replant the new variety from seed (Berlan and Lewontin 1998). Meanwhile farmers in the neighborhood face the serious risk of wind-borne pollen contamination. For organic farmers and beekeepers, contamination by GM pollen means losing their organic certification (Brown 2001a). But although farmers concerned about contamination stress that it is their property rights that need protection (Lambrecht 2001), Monsanto has brought suit against dozens of farmers in North America for copyright infringement. In the first case to come to trial, Percy Schmeiser, a Canadian farmer, was sued by Monsanto for a ruinous $105,000. Schmeiser argued that he had been unaware that the canola seed he replanted from his field had been contaminated by wind-borne GM pollen; the judge retorted that if he wasn't aware, he ought to have been and was therefore liable (Kaufman 2001b; Lambrecht 2001).

To short-circuit the problem of "seed piracy" completely, especially in Third World countries where control would be much more difficult, in the late 1990s Monsanto planned to incorporate into its GM varieties a chemical sequence that renders grain sterile at maturation so it cannot be used for seed, a technique patented in 1998 and immediately dubbed "Terminator technology" by GMO opponents. In traditional breeding, the functions of grain and seed are interchangeable: a kernel of wheat can be eaten, or it can be planted. Terminator technology ensures that grain cannot be used for seed. Seen from this perspective, the political risks of GMOs are clearly apparent. Third World farmers and crop scientists reacted with outrage. In 1999, after huge demonstrations by small farmers, the Indian government banned any use of Terminator technology (Griffiths 1999). "Terminator has finally become synonymous with corporate greed, and it was met with intense opposition all over the world," said the Research Director of the Canada-based Rural Advancement Foundation International (RAFI 1999) just before Monsanto's CEO undertook to withdraw the gene on October 6, 1999, in response to a public request by the president of the Rockefeller Foundation (Conway 2000). Though Monsanto suffered a setback, Terminator is too tempting a tool for profit generation to have been permanently removed from the biotech corporations' armory (RAFI 1999).

PACKAGING RISK

Before GM products can be planted or sold for food, they have to be officially approved and licensed by the government of the country concerned. It must therefore be demonstrated that the GMO presents either no risk or acceptable levels of risk. Even an officially approved product may fail, however, if consumers reject it. In the case of GM crops and foods, the biotech industry has had either to persuade farmers and consumers that the benefits of GMOs outweigh any possible risks or to conceal the fact that a crop or food is genetically modified.

The United States has always been the main center of biotech research, testing, marketing, and uptake. One reason is that the United States has the best labs and greatest number of biotech scientists. Another is that boundaries between science and capital investment are particularly permeable in the United States, providing big economic and intellectual incentives to adventurous scientists to join forces with venture capitalists. Biotech projects considered the domain of public science elsewhere are conducted as commercial enterprises in the United States.

Corporations producing GMOs have generally first submitted them for approval in the United States. One reason is that the U.S. administration has enthusiastically encouraged GMOs from the outset; regulation and testing standards are consequently more favorable than elsewhere. Another is that U.S. farmers grow huge quantities of bulk commercial crops, and U.S. farming is large scale, capital intensive, and highly competitive, so huge profits could be made quickly with approved GMOs. Finally, the United States exports large quantities of crops and foods. Once a GM crop has been approved in the United States, U.S. representatives can exert pressure in the name of free trade through organizations such as the World Trade Organization for the acceptance of American GM crops as imports, regardless of local regulations.

Corporatism and the Science of Risk Definition

The kinds of risk that modern governments are expected to investigate and regulate are in fact quite narrowly defined as risks to personal health or to the environment. Other dimensions of risk are not officially regarded as legitimate concerns, being dismissed as "political" and therefore "not scientific" (Heller 2001).

In the United States, three regulatory bodies, the Food and Drug Administration (FDA), the Environmental Protection Agency (EPA), and the U.S. Department of Agriculture (USDA), are responsible for controlling different aspects of GM crops and foods. Although proponents of GE imply that having three regulators must mean very strict standards, Pollan (1998) shows how easily one can be played against another. The many connections between research, corporate, and regulatory entities smooth the path for official support of corporate GMOs. As a result, the biotech industry has successfully imposed a scientific paradigm of risk-testing that favors rapid approval of GMOs. As we know from our emerging understanding of the environmental and health effects of nuclear power, pesticides, or BSE (mad cow disease), products and processes initially declared completely safe often prove to have complex long-term environmental and health effects. But the biotech industry has successfully convinced U.S. regulatory bodies that GM crops and foods can be tested adequately in a few experiments, on small samples, over just a few weeks or months—a practice scathingly criticized by some scientists (Marvier 2001).

The biotech industry has successfully persuaded U.S. regulatory bodies that allergies and cancer are the two categories of health risk for which GM foods should be tested and that short-term tests are sufficient for both. Biotech companies have been scrupulous in testing whether a GM product causes allergic reactions, perhaps because this is such a cheap way to gain the public's trust. Most recognized food allergies produce immediate, highly visible health effects that are easy to investigate and avoid in the course of designing of a GMO (e.g., Fulmer 2001; Kaufman 2001a).

Given all we now know about the long gestation period of cancer and of other immune system disorders, it is surprising how willing official authorities have been to accept the adequacy of short-term tests to investigate carcinogenic or other possible adverse health effects of GMOs. In 1995 Dr. Arpad Pusztai, a researcher for over 30 years at Rowett Research Institute in Scotland, was put in charge of a project funded at £1.6 million (about $2.5 million) by the British government to test genetically modified potatoes. This was the first (and last) independent testing of GM foods in the UK. Pusztai describes the initial attitude of the project workers as "very pro-GM"; then, however, the rats they were testing appeared to suffer depressed immune functions as a result of eating the GM potatoes. In 1998 Pusztai mentioned this on a BBC-TV current-affairs program, suggesting that current testing of GM foods might be inadequate. Within three days he was suspended, his team disbanded, and his research results confiscated, and all 20 scientists who had worked on the project were subjected by Rowett to a gag order. Pusztai's work was then publicly trashed as "bad science" by an anonymous panel convened by the Royal Society. It is true that his results, as subsequently published in *The Lancet*, were open to alternative interpretations. The incident does not, however, show the proponents of GMOs to be very open to genuine scientific debate (Clover and Irwin 1999; Freeman 2001; Walkom 2001).

Managing Public Opinion

In the United States, even before the first GM crops were approved in 1994, the biotech lobby began a media campaign to persuade farmers and consumers that GM crops and foods present no risks and that there are serious risks in refusing them. The campaign to convince U.S. farmers was relatively simple and very successful: GM crops would reduce the risks to their health and to their bank accounts. They were told that GM crops required the application of fewer dangerous chemicals and would guarantee higher yields of better quality. Farmers in the United States were quickly convinced. Although sometimes the adoption of GM crops led to higher use of dangerous chemicals (Cox 1998) or lower yields (Anderson 1999), only the crash of their export markets in 1999 jolted U.S. farmers into a new perception of the full range of financial risks that GMOs presented.

The campaign to convince the general public was somewhat more complex. At first the GM lobby feared people might worry about the "naturalness" or even the moral implications of what elsewhere are called transgenic foods. When genes from Arctic halibut are spliced into tomatoes, it could be that vegetarians would hesitate to eat them; if human genes are spliced into pigs, does it become cannibalistic to eat bacon? GM proponents point out both the naturalness of the artificial and the unnaturalness of nature. As one op-ed writer put it, "There's nothing natural about bread, or wine, or beagles. In fact there's nothing 'natural' about ourselves" (Cole 1999).

As it turns out, not many people in the United States seem to have been worried about the monsters that might result from tinkering with nature. To open the way for public acceptance of GM crops and foods, the biotech lobby astutely chose a rot-resistant tomato rather than a pesticide-oozing potato as the first GM food to be launched. When the FDA solicited public opinion on the genetic modifications used to produce the Flavr Savr tomato, it received only 43 responses (USDA 1994). But the biotech lobby was also able to count on the trust Americans place in their federal regulatory systems. A report published in July 1999 in *Science,* based on public-opinion surveys conducted in 1996 and 1997 in the United States and 17 European countries by researchers at the London School of Economics and the London Science Museum, found that 84 percent of U.S. respondents said they would trust a statement about the safety of biotechnology made by the FDA; 90 percent said they would trust statements made by the USDA. Europeans had almost no trust in the equivalent public bodies (4 percent) but had greater confidence in environmental (23 percent), farming (16 percent), and consumer (16 percent) organizations (Gaskell et al. 1999).

American scientists, politicians, and pundits tend to claim that European mistrust is well founded given the blatant official mismanagement of such public health threats as BSE and that public trust in the FDA and USDA is justified because the U.S. has watched the agencies responsible for managing such situations do so very effectively (McGloughlin 2000). Cynics might say this trust is based on illusion. The USDA, as well as being seriously understaffed and constrained in the types of investigations it is empowered to make, is unable, for example, to order a meatpacking company to withdraw contaminated meat from fast-food kitchens or supermarkets (see Schlosser 2001).

Furthermore, the American public was shielded from negative opinions about GM foods that might have aroused doubts or stimulated public debate. From the start, the biotech industry closely controlled the flow of information, generating almost all the available scientific data, lobbying legislators, setting up bodies such as the International Food Information Council to generate positive promotion, and hiring PR companies and individual journalists to mold public opinion (Rosset 2001).[2] Although some investigative journalists tried to document adverse effects, they quickly found themselves muzzled by employers fearing the application of new food antidefamation ("veggie libel") laws passed under pressure from agribusiness in several states (Hawk 1998; Anderson 1999; Schlosser 2001:266). For people in the United States who did not subscribe to environmental listservs or magazines, GM food did not stand out as a controversial technology that raised distinct issues. It was just another example of corporate research furthering science, technology, and progress.

Virtuous Consumption

As early as 1994, the International Food Information Council (IFIC) announced on its Web site that biotech research would soon give us potatoes that absorbed less fat when fried, GM plants with added vitamins, and GM foods that might even help reduce the risk of cancer. In other words, consuming the new GM foods would actually *reduce* health risks for those who consumed them (IFIC 1994). Facing a collapse of confidence in GM crops in late 1999, DuPont "released a series of TV commercials about the future, featuring the company's 'to do list,' which included research to 'find food that helps prevent breast cancer,'" a breakthrough that might induce greater acceptance among consumers, company executives said (Barboza 1999).

One exception to slowly developing second-generation GMOs is "golden rice," which should eventually provide enough beta-carotene to prevent vitamin-A deficiency disorders that commonly afflict those too poor to eat anything but rice. Golden rice represents a refinement of an argument that is repeatedly put forward by biotech supporters, namely, that GMOs are indispensable to feeding the world's growing population. If we do not avail ourselves of this opportunity, we risk condemning countless millions to malnutrition or starvation and the environment to complete despoliation. As the IFIC (1994) put it: "'Better Crops'—Global population will double to more than 10 billion people by 2030. Biotechnology will help push back starvation in the next century as traditional breeding has in this century." The IFIC Web site plays to American tastes and concerns, including the gratifying promise that U.S. know-how, industry, and generosity will once again help save the world from starvation and disease. In another, more recent example, Avery pushes a masterly set of buttons in his op-ed appeal to support genetic engineering:

If Europe's deception succeeds [in banning GM foods], genetic engineering will not be used to help the world's farmers meet a threefold increase in demand for food by 2050. As a direct result, the world's children would suffer more hunger and malnutrition while huge tracts of tropical forests—and many thousands of wildlife species—would be needlessly destroyed. People's needs would even be pitted directly against the food needs of cats, dogs and other companion animals. (1999)

Oppose genetic engineering and you will end up fighting your dog for kibble!

The specter of world starvation is one of the most potent and destructive weapons in the free-traders' armory. Avery and others offer the seductive argument that more corn in Iowa means less hunger in Ethiopia, but in fact, flooding local markets with cheap imported grain usually means ruin and starvation for small farmers. Farmers and governments in the South are well aware that in the hands of big corporations GMOs are a threat, not a promise. But to many Westerners, it seems clear that here is a technological solution that it would be sinful to refuse.

CONTESTING THE SCIENCE OF RISK

An alternative paradigm of risk assessment, increasingly prevalent in European institutions since the late 1990s, is the *precautionary principle*. This says that wherever long-term or complex effects are likely, all kinds of risk should be thoroughly explored before a process or product is declared safe and adopted.

American commentators have commonly blamed public resistance to GMOs in Europe and Japan on a series of health and food scandals—from blood tainted with HIV, through BSE (mad-cow disease) and dioxins in animal feed, to the recent foot-and-mouth epidemic—that have exposed the inefficacy of the European and Japanese regulatory bodies, inclined the public to mistrust their governments, and unreasonably prejudiced them against GMOs when science has definitely shown GMOs to be safe. GMO proponents are certainly correct that these scandals have entrenched an attitude of mistrust toward government and state "experts" (Gaskell et al. 1999). The biotech lobby argues that if only opponents would consider the matter rationally and scientifically, they would be convinced by the tests already carried out that "prove" the safety of GM foods. But the recent health and food scandals in Europe and Japan have fed into historical experiences since World War II in sharpening public perceptions of the long-term and unpredictable nature of biological or environmental risk. Post-Hiroshima, post-Chernobyl, in the age of AIDS and the exposure of the carcinogenic qualities of once-trusted materials such as asbestos, it seems unlikely that most members of the public in Europe or Japan would easily be persuaded that any short-term tests of GMO safety could be adequate (Taylor 1999).

Given how badly most European governments' images were tarnished in the wake of such scandals as the use of HIV-infected blood for transfusions in France, it is not surprising that most European governments too have now come round to public pressures in favor of adopting the precautionary principle (Boy 1999). This better-safe-than-sorry approach requires a very different science of testing from that used to gain approval for GMOs in the United States. For example, the use of growth hormones for beef, standard in the United States, has been banned in Europe since 1989 (Chauveau 1999). On the precautionary principle, the European Union (EU) is currently financing 17 research groups working on the potential harmful effects of hormones and antibiotics in meat. The resulting ban on U.S. beef imports almost led to a trade war between the United States and Europe in 1999 (Chauveau 1999). The EU also requires longer-term testing of GM crops and gives approval more sparingly. "Of 16 bioengineered varieties of canola, 14 are approved in Canada, but only 10 are sanctioned in Japan and three in the European Union" (Shadid 2001). As a paradigm of risk-definition, the precautionary principle conflicts directly with the preferences of free-traders and corporations (Chauveau 1999).

CONSUMER BACKLASH

Although governments and big farmers outside North America initially favored the adoption of GM varieties, public opinion quickly rallied against them, and the media across the political spectrum ensured that GM issues were brought dramatically and repeatedly to everyone's attention. Anti-GM activists skillfully intertwined the potential health risks to individual bodies with environmental and political risks at home and abroad, mobilizing a broad coalition whose forms of action included not only contesting the licensing of GM varieties and destroying experimental GM crops, but also the simple yet powerful refusal to consume GM products.

Although governments may be brought to heel by international regulations or by the threat of trade wars, consumers cannot be legally forced to buy products they do not want. Whatever the reason for the consumer's refusal to purchase a product, the seller has no redress but must try to find a more acceptable substitute or a more convincing label. The power of consumer choice, manifested through anti-GM boycotts in Europe and Japan, halved markets for mid-Western grain, toppled biotech share prices, and convinced both governments and the biotech industry that the opposition to GMOs was serious.

European consumers declared en masse that GM foods were risky. Some probably were most concerned about risks to their own or their family's health. Others were also using their refusal to consume to express anticorporate sentiments, rejection of a corrupt food system, critique of their government, environmental responsibility, and/or support for small farmers threatened by Terminator technology (e.g. Vidal 1999; Bové and Dufour 2000). As consumers, they demanded labeling, refused to buy foods containing GMOs, and threatened boycotts of companies. Local councils declared "GM-free zones," and school and hospital canteens banned GM ingredients. Food-manufacturing companies such as Unilever, initially an enthusiastic supporter of biotech, stopped producing foods that used GM ingredients. In May 1999, seven of the largest European supermarket chains announced they would distribute products "guaranteed GMO-free."

In Europe, every level of the food chain was affected by public opposition to transgenics. Most food brands or local specialties now have their own Web site and "Green phone line" for answering inquiries. Faced by a growing number of direct questions about GMOs in their cheeses, from individual retailers and consumers as well as from the giant supermarket chains, in 1999 the sheep farmers and cheese-makers of Roquefort decided to require their feed suppliers to guarantee the absence of any genetically modified product in the food. French sheep farmers changed from American soy-cake to soy-cake from the Brazilian province of Rio Grande del Sur, whose governor banned the planting of GM soy in spring 1999 (Laval 1999). Eventually even the politicians saw which way the wind was blowing, and in 1999 the European Community (EC) passed laws requiring food producers to label products containing GM ingredients (Blythman 1999).

In Japan as in Europe, public concern fueled public action. A 1997 government survey showed that over 80 percent of Japanese had "reservations" about GMO foods, and 92.5 percent favored mandatory labeling. Twenty million Japanese people belong to food cooperatives (Efron 1999); when the giant food conglomerate Kirin Brewery introduced a GMO tomato in 1996, the cooperatives immediately threatened a total boycott of its products. Kirin withdrew at once, and since then no Japanese companies have dared to propose selling GMOs, even though the Japanese government has invested billions of dollars in biotechnology (Efron 1999). As a result of public pressure, the Japanese government has proceeded with caution in approving GM varieties for cultivation or consumption and has imposed labeling of foods containing GM ingredients, though at a rather lenient level of 5 percent (Simon 2001).

It is not only in rich countries that consumers are exerting pressure against GMOs. Some Thai food manufacturers now regularly test their products in DNA laboratories to label them GM-free (Kultida 2001), and Thailand was the first Asian country to ban the release of GMOs into the environment. Sri Lanka announced a ban on GM foods starting in May 2001 (*Global News Wire* 2001).

Because of the U.S. refusal to label GMOs and the grain industry's habit of mixing GM and ordinary cereals, markets for all U.S. maize and soy (GM or not) crumbled starting in 1998. U.S. exports of maize to Spain and Portugal alone dropped from 70 million bushels in 1997 to 3 million bushels in 1998 (Palmer 1999). In summer 1999, grain futures plunged on the Chicago Stock Market. On December 14, 1999, a group of mid-Western farmers filed a class-action suit against Monsanto and other GM seed companies, claiming they had been defrauded by safety claims on GM seeds. They also accused the companies of illegally controlling the supply of seeds and of misleading them about public reactions against GMOs (*Los Angeles Times* 1999).

The U.S. grain-export sector is hoping to restore its markets by increasing sales of GM maize and soy as feed, but this may not work, either: Already major supermarkets in Europe have banned or are phasing out GM-fed products, including fish, poultry, and eggs as well as meat and dairy (Vidal 2001). Countries such as Brazil are rushing to fill the gap by offering GM-free grains, and in the face of a growing array of bans by importing nations and by the huge international food companies (even McDonald's USA has decided not to use GM potatoes for fear of a consumer backlash), "the danger to the United States's nearly $52 billion food export market has prompted even supporters of biotechnology ... to urge a reform in the way federal agencies regulate biotech and what seeds biotech companies market" (Shadid 2001).

FRANKENFOODS: BURSTING THE BOUNDARIES OF RISK

One reason GM crops and foods, quickly dubbed "Frankenfoods" by the British press, were so widely opposed by consumers outside the United States is that people were not willing to accept the narrow definitions of risk the biotech industry and its supporters had tried to impose. GMOs were seen not just as a form of food that was or was not safe for individual bodies or an environmental threat whose long-term risks were poorly understood, but as an emblem and agent of emerging global configurations of corporatist control.

When they first became aware of the mistrust brewing in Europe and Japan, the biotech companies and their proponents, including the Clinton administration's U.S. Trade Representative and many U.S. op-ed writers and media commentators, poured scorn on their opponents' scientific ignorance and their lamentable propensity to bring politics into what should be purely scientific debates. The biotech industry tried to turn the tide by launching campaigns to "educate" consumers abroad.

The main multinational biotech companies formed an association called EuropaBio, hiring as their adviser the U.S.-based company Burson Marsteller, whose previous clients included Exxon after the Exxon Valdez oil spill and Union Carbide after the explosion of their chemical plant in Bhopal. Burson Marsteller advised that "public issues of environmental and human health risks are communications killing fields for bioindustries in Europe … all the research evidence confirms that the perception of the profit motive fatally undermines industry's credibility on these questions" (Anderson 1999:91). But even Burson Marsteller did not apparently gauge the full implications of its own observations; its advice to EuropaBio on selling GMOs to the European public was to focus on "symbols eliciting hope, satisfaction, caring and self-esteem" (Anderson 1999). In the course of 1998, Monsanto spent millions on a campaign in France setting out the environmental friendliness, improved nutritional qualities, and rich, glowing flavors GM foods would offer. A series of witty and beautifully designed color advertisements were placed in newspapers and magazines and displayed on a Monsanto-France Web site, with a chat page that invited people to send in their comments on whether GM foods should be regulated. The comments posted in response stated that corporate capital could not be trusted and that companies would be unlikely to tell the truth about risks or to regulate responsibly if profits were at stake (Monsanto 1998).

POLITICAL RISKS AND CITIZENS' RIGHTS

Meanwhile, GM opponents around the world developed an alternative semiotics of greed, control, and destruction. Non-governmental organizations (NGOs) such as Greenpeace and Friends of the Earth countered Monsanto's positive symbolism for GMs with a terminology built around "the greed gene," "anti-farmer technology," and "the neutron bomb of agriculture." The rhetoric *and* the action against GMOs emerged from an unprecedented coalition of farmers and activists from around the world, and the language of protest is very specific about the corporate capitalist interests that have produced and promoted the new technology and its political risks.

From the perspective of small farmers in poor nations, the risks inherent in corporate GM crops are clear. GM crops are an anti-farmer technology that will act like a neutron bomb, destroying people but leaving property undamaged. Like the new varieties of the Green Revolution, corporate GM varieties require farmers to purchase seed whose success depends on expensive industrial inputs, many of which replace hand labor with chemicals, thus increasing costs for farmers and depriving wage laborers of jobs. They will thus favor richer farmers at the expense of the poor (Bray 1986).

Nor are many people in the nations of the South impressed by the promise that GMOs will provide a simple technological fix for world hunger. At present, world cereal surpluses stand at 118 percent of what is consumed in a year, and yet there are still 830 million hungry people, four-fifths of them dependent on farming for their living (El Feki 2000:14). Most GM crops are designed to help First World industrial farmers increase exports of cereals, feed, or oils. Cheap food imports tend to increase rural hunger by putting small farmers out of business (Bray 1999). Some genetic engineering is specifically intended to undercut Third World agricultural exports, as in the case of current research to develop GM substitutes for vanilla, coconut oil, and cocoa butter. It is therefore not surprising that poor nations have consistently opposed corporate GMOs. In 1998, African representatives to the Food and Agriculture Organization (FAO) of the United Nations voted *en bloc* to oppose approval of GMOs, complaining that the image of their poor was being exploited to benefit rich corporations (Anderson 1999).

Small farmers' associations in the United States and Europe have made common cause with their sister organizations in Latin America, Africa, and Asia, opposing corporate GMOs as one element in an increasingly destructive system of industrialized, productivist agriculture (Rosset 2001). An international farmers' movement against GMOs is sustained by global networks of information and exchange that connect farmers, environmentalists, and consumer groups. Canadian farmers visit India for advice on how to mount a campaign; farmers' organizations and NGOs circulate data by e-mail. In summer 1999, the Karnataka delegates (KRRS) of the so-called Intercontinental Caravan were hosted in France by the second-largest farmers' union, the *Confédération paysanne*, as they feasted and crop-trampled their way around France, bound for Cologne. There they joined peasants from Chiapas and landless Brazilians from the *Movimento Sem Terra* in a "global laugh parade" against the World Economic Summit. The KRRS, with a membership of ten million, had demonstrated against Monsanto and dismantled a factory owned by its sister company Cargill, helping to bring about the Indian government's ban on Terminator technology (Griffiths 1999).

Meanwhile in European nations, the 1990s saw an increasingly widespread distrust of industrial agriculture, with its close links to agribusiness and its corporatist logic of production. This kind of farming is now seen as polluting the local and global environment, destroying rural communities, being cruel to animals, and producing bland Mac-food as likely to poison as to nourish our bodies. In this broader political context, artisanal Roquefort cheese, organic carrots, fair-trade coffee, and GM-free supermarkets are not just frivolous foody fashions but symbols of commitment to a more just social future.

Quite apart from the health risks GMOs might pose, the lack of public debate concerning the introduction of GMOs has outraged their opponents. When the biotech lobby pressed for quick approval of GMOs in Europe, this was widely construed as a bullying corporatist attack on national sovereignty in the domain of health, safety, and environment. When governments approved secret experimental plots or bulldozed through approvals despite public opposition, protesters were quick to label this a *democratic deficit* (Taylor 1999). The rhetoric of citizenship features prominently among anti-GMO activists. Numerous complaints have been voiced in terms of "lack of government transparency," conferring a civic right to investigate and act (e.g., Amis de la Terre 1999, Meikle 2000).

Some radical institutional shifts have already come about, or are promised, under this pressure. They include the European Union's adoption of the precautionary principle, the EU's recognition in July 1999 that agriculture should be treated as multifunctional (i.e., protecting diversity, employment, the environment, and rural life), the proposal in 2001 by the Portuguese farm minister that farm support be decoupled from production (Norman 2001), the reforms proposed by the EU farm commissioner that the Common Agricultural Policy (CAP) should be reformed to support quality rather than quantity production, with substantial investment in environmental improvement and in sustainable rural development (Fischler 2001), and the planned publication of an EU Commission White Paper designed to "organise the use of expertise to improve the quality of policy-making and public debate ... [including] how issues of uncertainty and risk should be handled" (EU 2001).

Musing on the potential of shared risk in 1999, Ulrich Beck (1999:106) asked, "Are Britons' post-BSE food scares beyond the reach of government when faced with global corporate opponents? Are consumers and voters powerless in the face of global financial powers?" It seems that in Europe, at any rate, the anticorporate-GMO coalition and its sister movements for reform of farming have already contributed to a significant shift in mainstream political ideology.

GOLDEN RICE: WHY WE MUST DISTINGUISH PUBLIC FROM CORPORATE GMOs

In 2000, the invention of golden rice was announced. Golden rice contains daffodil genes to generate beta-carotene; its consumption might help reduce vitamin-A deficiency prevalent among poor people unable to afford a varied diet. It was developed ("invented") by Potrykus and Beyer at the Federal Institute for

Technology in Switzerland, with over $100 million in funding from the European Community Biotechnology Programme and the Rockefeller Foundation, and it is intended for free distribution to subsistence farmers (Potrykus 2001).

Golden rice is still very much at the prototype stage. According to scientists at the International Rice Research Institute (IRRI) in the Philippines, a public research institution working to develop varieties suitable for local conditions, it will be at least five years before golden rice is ready to go to field trials. Nor is the vitamin enhancement operational yet: in its present form, an individual would need to eat about 9 kg of cooked golden rice a day to get the recommended daily dose of vitamin A (Brown 2001b). Although golden rice's benefits are still promises rather than reality, the biotech industry has already invested $50 million in a publicity campaign. Though golden rice was developed in a public research institution with public money, the work was only affordable because various biotech corporations, including Syngenta and Monsanto, donated around 70 patents. Monsanto has given the patents unconditionally; Syngenta has retained rights over the commercial cultivation of golden rice (Fulmer 2001; Potrykus 2001; Shah 2001).

Around the world, many people now think of GMOs as synonymous with corporate greed, but in golden rice we are offered a GMO that will feed the poor and cure the blind. A recent full-page advertisement placed by the Council for Biotechnology Information in *The New Yorker* shows a girl of about five silhouetted against the plank wall of a hut, dressed in coarse striped cotton pajamas and feeding herself with chopsticks from a rice bowl as her mother offers a protective caress:

Biotechnology researchers call it "golden rice." For the color. For the opportunity ... Discoveries in biotechnology, from medicine to agriculture, are helping doctors treat our sick, farmers protect our crops—and could help mothers nourish our children, and keep them healthier. (*New Yorker* 2001)

Golden rice was a canny investment for the biotech industry. For the price of a few gene sequences and patents, they bought an opportunity to present themselves not just as technical wizards but also as disinterested benefactors of mankind. Those who oppose GM crops can then be vilified as indifferent to hunger and disease. In a dramatic claim about the risks of *not* accepting GM foods, Syngenta claimed that a single month of marketing delay for golden rice would leave 50,000 poor Asian children blind (Pollan 2001).

The president of the Rockefeller Foundation declared in exasperation in January 2001 that "the public-relations uses of golden rice have gone too far" (Pollan 2001). Although agreeing that genetically engineered rice may have a role to play in combating malnutrition, he stated, "We do not consider golden rice the solution to the vitamin-A deficiency problem" (Pollan 2001). Critics have rightly argued that technical fixes such as golden rice may simply distract attention or divert resources from the need to address the social and political roots of extreme poverty. Nevertheless, as at least a partial contribution toward addressing the problems of malnutrition, pests and diseases, or extremes of climate, golden rice-type research has important potential.

It seems that some environmentalist organizations, for instance Greenpeace, have decided to oppose all GM crops on principle and are not prepared to relax their opposition to testing even those crops designed by public scientists to serve the poor. Greenpeace's decision to condemn golden rice (reached after some dissent within the ranks) enraged Potrykus, who retorted that golden rice "will be given free of charge and limitations, via national institutions, to resource-poor farmers in developing countries for local use and trade. ... It also fulfills an urgent need, can be re-sown from its own harvest, does not reduce biodiversity, does not present any conceivable threat to the environment, and will be made available only if there is no risk to the consumer" (Potrykus 2001). Although no agricultural innovation can be guaranteed free of social risk or unintended consequences, Potrykus's statement indicates that he and his colleagues have taken the social and political lessons of the Green Revolution to heart and have deliberately tried to design a GM crop free of "greed" mechanisms as well as environmental risks.

Many public-sector scientists who do research on GM crops support them in principle, especially where they would be distributed free to subsistence farmers and designed to reduce their production risks (for example drought- or flood-resistant cereals, blight-resistant potatoes, or virus-resistant cassava). Though other plant scientists counter that old-fashioned cross-breeding is less environmentally risky and would be equally effective if adequately funded (Berlan and Lewontin 1998; Kloppenburg 1988), supporters of public-service genetic engineering argue that certain features simply cannot be achieved through cross-breeding—for example, in golden rice, the production of beta-carotene in the grain as well as in the leaves (Conway 2000; Potrykus 2001). Furthermore, as the IRRI plans for golden rice illustrate, public scientists tend to be much more cautious about the potential risks of GMOs than their corporate colleagues, preferring long-term testing—in other words, the precautionary approach (see Conway 2000; Pimentel 2000; Pollack 2001).

As long as we continue to conflate corporate and public-sector GMOs, however, we shall fail to give due consideration to the significant differences in risk between the two categories of artifact. On the one hand, this means we play into the hands of the biotech corporations; on the other, it will make it increasingly difficult, if not impossible, for public-sector scientists to pursue serious research into what could be very useful improvements in crop breeding.

Clearly it is in the interests of the biotech industry to present public and corporate genetic engineering as a single enterprise, implying that all GMOs are designed to be distributed free to the hungry and sick and that companies such as Monsanto are more interested in helping the poor than increasing their share prices. The Council for Biotechnology Information is an industry propaganda tool with a current 5-year operating budget of $250 million (Rosset 2001:23), but its name makes it sound like a public-interest organization disseminating objective information. In Scotland, a GM corporate consortium has sponsored 140,000 glossy brochures that "sing the praises of GM technology" for distribution to schools (Edwards 2001). Not only corporations play this game. The San Diego Center for Molecular Agriculture, "an alliance of scientists who work at public research institutions," has also produced a beautiful brochure listing the virtues of GM crops, containing no mention of profits nor even of the existence of biotech corporations, though it does take explicit swipes at organic farming and Greenpeace (SDCMA 2001).

Unfortunately, although the biotech lobby has painted GM crops uniformly golden, we in anti-GMO coalitions have usually painted them uniformly black. This rules out the possibility of productive collaboration between activists and public-sector scientists to explore the full potential of public GM crops. If anti-GMO coalitions were to differentiate between corporate and public GMOs, they could bring their considerable political muscle to bear to support public scientists in developing improved procedures and paradigms for testing the risks associated with transgenics and in pressing for the return of biological knowledge now covered by corporate patents to the public domain. And if we can discuss authoritatively the different implications of adopting public and corporate GMOs, it may help us win over some of the many people in the United States who are now becoming aware of the issues surrounding GMOs, largely through the biotech lobby's propaganda.

NOTES

1. In Bray (forthcoming) I provide a detailed account of the formation of the coalition and of the impact of its campaigns on the biotech industry up to September 2000.

2. The International Food Information Council is a nonprofit organization supported by the food, beverage, and agricultural industries.

REFERENCES

Amis de la Terre. 1999. *Manque de transparence des autorités françaises.* Available from www.amisdelaterre.org/campagnes/OGM.

Anderson, Luke. 1999. *Genetic Engineering, Food, and Our Environment.* White River Junction, VT: Chelsea Green.

Associated Press. 2001. "Farmers Will Plant More Genetically Altered Beans." *St. Louis Dispatch,* April 30, E8.

Avery, Dennis T. 1999. "Europe Engaged in a Phony War on Biotechnology." *Bridge News,* July 15, Opinion Section.

Barboza, David. 1999. "In Switch, Biotech Firms Join Food Fight." *New York Times,* November 12, A1.

————. 2000. "In the Heartland, Genetic Promises: If Farmers Sow Modified Crops, Big Companies Will Buy Them." *New York Times,* March 17, C1.

Beck, Ulrich. 1999. *World Risk Society.* Cambridge: Polity Press.

Berlan, Jean-Pierre and Richard C. Lewontin. 1998. "Racket sur le Vivant: La Menace du Complexe Génético-Industriel." *Le Monde Diplomatique,* December.

Blythman, Joanna. 1999. *How to Avoid GM Food: Hundreds of Brands, Products and Ingredients to Avoid.* London: Fourth Estate.

Bové, José, and François Dufour. 2000. *Le Monde n'est pas une Marchandise: Des Paysans contre la Malbouffe.* Paris: La Découverte.

Boy, Daniel. 1999. *Le Progrès en Procès.* Paris: Presses de la Renaissance.

Bray, Francesca. 1986. *The Rice Economies: Technology and Development in Asian Societies.* Oxford: Blackwell Publishers. Reprint, Berkeley and Los Angeles: University of California Press, 1994.

————. 1997. *Technology and Gender: Fabrics of Power in Late Imperial China.* Berkeley and Los Angeles: University of California Press.

————. 1999. "A Stable Landscape? Social and Cultural Sustainability in Asian Rice Systems." In *The Sustainability of Wet-Rice Agriculture,* ed. Noreen Dowling, 45–66. Manila: International Rice Research Institute.

————. Forthcoming. "How Wholesome Is That Soup? The Political Contents of the Refrigerator." In *Technology and Human Values on the Edge of the New Millennium,* ed. Roger T. Ames. Honolulu: University of Hawaii Press.

Brown, Paul. 2001a. "Outrage at New GM Crop Trials." *The Guardian,* February 7, 10.

————. 2001b. "GM Rice Promoters' Claims 'Have Gone Too Far.'" *The Guardian Weekly,* February 21, 5.

Chauveau, Loïc. 1999. "Les Mixtures du Dopage Animal." *L'Express,* June 10, 24–25.

Clover, Charles, and Aisling Irwin. 1999. "Heartfelt Fears of the Whistleblower Who Spilled the Beans over GM Foods." *The Daily Telegraph* (London), June 10, 10.

Cole, K. C. 1999. "Mind Over Matter: Genetically Altered Food Unnatural? Not Really." *Los Angeles Times,* October 21, B2.

Connor, Steve. 2001. "Biotechnology: Why Monsanto Thinks Its GM Wheat Is the Next Best Thing." *The Independent* (London), January 15.

Conway, Gordon. 2000. "Genetically Modified Crops: Risks and Promise." *Conservation Ecology* 4(1): 2 [online database]. Available from www.consecol.org/vol4/iss1/art2.

Cox, Carolyn. 1998. "Glyphosate." *Journal of Pesticide Reform* 18(3): 2.

Crook, Tony. 2000. "Length Matters: A Note on the GM Debate." *Anthropology Today* 16(1): 8–11.

Douglas, Mary, and Aron Wildavsky. 1982. *Risk and Culture.* Berkeley and Los Angeles: University of California Press.

Edwards, Rob. 2001. "Brochures Sponsored by GM Firms Such as Monsanto Are Adopted into School Curricula; Fury at Pro-GM School Magazines." *Sunday Herald* (Glasgow), April 15, 6.

Efron, Soni. 1999. "Japanese Choke on American Biofood." *Los Angeles Times,* March 14, A1.

El Feki, Shereen. 2000. "Agriculture and Technology." *The Economist* (special supplement), March 25: 16.

European Union. 2001. "Enhancing Democracy: A White Paper on Governance in the European Union." Available from http://europa.eu.int/comm/governance/index_en.htm.

Fischler, Franz. 2001. "A Three-Pronged Reform." *Financial Times,* May 8, 19.

Freeman, James. 2001. "Modifying the Argument." *Glasgow Herald,* March 31, 12.

Friedmann, Harriet. 1990. "Family Wheat Farms and Third World Diets: A Paradoxical Relationship between Unwaged and Waged Labor." In *Work without Wages: Domestic Labor and Self-Employment within Capitalism,* eds. Jane L. Collins and Martha Gimenez, 193–213. Albany, NY: SUNY Press.

Fulmer, Melinda. 2001. "Biotech Bears Fruit for Farmers, Not Consumers." *Los Angeles Times.* April 8, C1.

Gaskell, George, Martin W. Bauer, John Durant, and Nicholas C. Allum. 1999. "Worlds Apart? The Reception of Genetically Modified Foods in Europe and the U.S." *Science* 285: 384–387.

Giddens, Anthony. 1994. *Beyond Left and Right.* Cambridge: Polity Press.

Global News Wire. 2001. "India: Greens Seek Ban on GM Crops Import." News release, May 15.

Griffiths, Jay. 1999. "Noddy Is on Page 248." *London Review of Books* 25(12): 34–35.

Hawk, Ann. 1998. "Veggie Disparagement: Laws in 13 States Prompt Fears Activists—and Journalists—Will Be Stifled." *The Quill,* September.

Heller, Chaia. 2001. "From Risk to Globalization: Discursive Shifts in the French Debate About GMOs." *Medical Anthropology Quarterly* 15(1): 25–28.

IFIC (International Food Information Council). 1994. "Guidelines for Communicating Emerging Science on Nutrition, Food Safety, and Health." *Food Biotechnology, Health and Harvest for Our Times* [online magazine], September. Available from ificinfo.health.org/brochure/biobroch.htm.

Kaufman, Mark. 2001a. "Biotech Corn Is Test Case for Industry: Engineered Food's Future Hinges on Allergy Study." *Washington Post,* March 19, A1.

———. 2001b. "Farmer Liable after Biotech Pollen Blows Onto His Field." *International Herald Tribune,* March 31, 3.

Kloppenburg, J. R. 1988. *First the Seed: The Political Economy of Plant Biotechnology, 1492–2000.* New York: Cambridge University Press.

Kultida, Samabuddhi. 2001. "Food to Be Labelled to Show It's GM-free." *Bangkok Post,* April 22, 2.

Lambrecht, Bill. 2001. "Monsanto's Win in Court Sharpens Battle Lines in Biotech Fight; Farmer Says Patented Crop Fell or Blew into His Field." *St Louis Post-Dispatch,* April 1, A1.

Laval, Gilbert. 1999. "Le meneur anti-McDo reste en prison" [The Anti-McDonalds' Leader is Kept in Prison], *Libération,* August 21–22.

Los Angeles Times. 1999. "Biotech Foods: Second Thoughts." December 19, M4.

Marvier, Michelle. 2001. "Ecology of Transgenic Crops." *American Scientist* 89: 160–167.

McGloughlin, Martina. 2000. "Biotech Crops: Rely on the Science." *Washington Post,* June 14, A39.

McGregor, Richard. 2001. "Syngenta Discovers Education Is a Two Way Street in China." *Financial Times,* May 9, 34.

Meikle, James. 2000. "MPs Criticise Control on GM Crop Trials." *The Guardian,* August 4, 7.

Monsanto. 1998. Monsanto-France Web site. Available from www.monsanto.fr/discussion.

New Yorker. 2001. "CBI advertisement series," June 25.

Nicklaus, David. 2001. "After a rocky IPO, Monsanto Appears to Be Back on Track." *St. Louis Post-Dispatch,* February 17, Business Section, 1.

Norman, Peter. 2001. "Portugal Adds to Pressure for EU Farm Reform." *Financial Times*, May 23, World News Europe Section, 10.

O'Hagan, Andrew. 2001. "The End of British Farming." *London Review of Books* 23(6): 3–16.

Palmer, Doug. 1999. "US Laments European Stance on Biotech Foods." *Financial Express*, March 5.

PANUPS (Pesticide Action Network Updates Service Bulletin). 2001. "Top Seven Agrochemical Companies in 2000." May 23 (Based on figures from Agrow, *World Crop Protection News*, January 5, March 2, and April 13).

Pimentel, David. 2000. "Genetically Modified Crops and the Agroecosystem: Comments on 'Genetically Modified Crops: Risks and Promise' by Gordon Conway." *Conservation Ecology* 4(1): 10 [database online]. Available from www.consecol.org /vol4/iss1/art10.

Pollack, Andrew. 2001. "The Green Revolution Yields to the Bottom Line." *New York Times*, May 15, F1.

Pollan, Michael. 1998. "Playing God in the Garden." *New York Times Magazine*, October 25, 44.

———. 2001. "The Great Yellow Hype: Will the Latest Genetically Modified Food Save the World? Or Just the Biotech Industry?" *The New York Times*, March 4, sec. 6, p. 15.

Potrykus, Ingo. 2001. "Harvest of Hope or Fear." *The Guardian* (London), April 18, Society Section, 8.

RAFI (Rural Advancement Foundation International). 1999. "Terminator Terminated?" Press release, October 4.

Ramey, Timothy S. 1999. "Ag Biotech: Thanks But No Thanks?" *Financial Report for Deutsche Bank*, July 12.

Rosset, Peter M. 2001. "Toward a Political Economy of Opinion Formation on Genetically Modified Foods." *Medical Anthropology Quarterly* 15(1): 22–25.

SDCMA (San Diego Center for Molecular Agriculture). 2001. *Foods from Genetically Modified Crops*. San Diego, CA: San Diego Center for Molecular Agriculture.

Schlosser, Eric. 2001. *Fast Food Nation: The Dark Side of the All-American Meal*. New York: Houghton Mifflin.

Shadid, Anthony. 2001. "Biotechnology: Against the Altered Grain. Some North American Crops Grown from Bioengineered Seeds Face Bans in Certain Lucrative Export Markets." *Boston Globe*, May 2, C4.

Shah, Saeed. 2001. "Disquiet as Syngenta Maps Rice DNA." *The Independent* (London), January 27, Business Section, 19.

Simon, Stephanie. 2001. "Farmers Have Love-Hate Relationship with Biotech Food." *Los Angeles Times*, March 31, A13.

Taylor, Ian E. 1999. "Political Risk Culture: Not Just a Communication Failure." In *Risk Communication and Public Health*, eds. Peter Bennett and Kenneth Calman, 152–169. New York: Oxford University Press.

USDA (U.S. Dept. of Agriculture). 1994. "The New Tomato: An Inside View." *NBIAP News Report*, July.

Vidal, John. 1999. "Grim Reapers." *The Guardian*, August 17.

———. 2001. "Supermarket Giants Pave Way for 'GM-free' Britain." *The Guardian*, January 27, Home Section, 10.

Walkom, Thomas. 2001. "Biotechnology Researcher Pays the Price." *The Toronto Star*, February 13.

Chapter 10

Risk, Ethics, and Public Space: The Impact of BSE and Foot-and-Mouth Disease on Public Thinking

Jo Murphy-Lawless

AN EPIDEMIC OF A MILD VIRUS LEADS TO THE POSTPONEMENT OF A GENERAL ELECTION

We currently face a complex and contradictory range of positions about risk. On the one hand, there is a general presumption that the scientificity of the process of measuring what we term risk enables us to have confidence in the end results of schedules of risk. Thus, for example, when citizens are informed by national health authorities that our risk of contracting certain forms of cancer is significantly decreased by the daily consumption of fruit and vegetables, we can expect that an alteration in our eating patterns will prove genuinely beneficial. Science claims it can do this work of risk prediction and that this is a useful task in helping the larger nonscientific community to reach responsible decisions in dealing with ascertainable risks. We also ask science to take on that task, often with the remit to report back on its findings to the state, which can be said to represent our collective interests, for in many areas we need the state to act for us.

On the other hand, we often increasingly exercise agency, drawing on and utilizing our common-sense judgments about what constitutes a risk in our daily lives, because we sense that scientific rigor and reliability are not straightforward, not least due to the very social processes that produce scientific rationality.

A further complication about risk relates to where we—the citizens of democratic societies—stand in relation to the state. The definitions of risk and actions to reduce its occurrence have comprised an interventionist discourse used by regulatory bodies that have had authority from governments to oversee safety to ensure citizen protection in a seemingly objective manner. And yet what has been a compromise device of regulation and protection may now be in danger of breaking down completely.

This chapter explores the current uneasy relationships between risk, science, the state, and citizen protection with reference to the recent crises and food scares that have affected the agricultural industry in Britain, notably the epidemics of bovine spongiform encephalopathy (BSE) and foot-and-mouth disease (FMD). These crises raise questions about how damage has been done to the citizenry while this collective responsibility of the state toward us has been jeopardized in the interests of protecting agribusiness. A careful reading of government actions indicates that economic risks to the interlocking concerns of agribusiness have been placed ahead of health risks and status of life of individual citizens, raising along the way core ethical issues about how a practical science should function in tandem with government actions to further the welfare of all its citizens.

Unusually, FMD led to the postponement of a British general election in 2001. The election was widely expected for May 3, 2001, but had to be delayed until June 7 because the Blair government judged it too embarrassing to be seen seeking its certain return to office while the countryside was closed down by government-sanctioned restrictions to prevent the spread of the disease (see Hoggart 2001). The FMD epidemic, the most extensive ever recorded internationally, followed only a few short months after the publication of the lengthiest and most expensive government inquiry ever, *The BSE Inquiry, Vols. I-XVI* (Phillips, Bridgeman, and Ferguson-Smith 2000), on the scandal of BSE. BSE and FMD created huge problems within the single market of the European Union, where there is meant to be a flow of disease-free animals but where outbreaks of BSE and FMD are directly traceable to British agricultural practices.[1] The impact of these epidemics begins to cast doubt on the willingness of governments to protect the health and well-being of their citizenry in this era of expanding transnational agribusiness corporations and the agendas set by the World Trade Organization for the complete deregulation of trade.[2]

BSE or "mad cow disease" was identified very recently, in 1986 (Pennington 2000). It is a transmissible spongiform encephalopathy (TSE) that attacks the central nervous system of cows. This lethal pathogen becomes evident when a cow develops tremors and lack of coordination, becomes painfully thin, and displays erratic behavior. The first officially recorded case of a cow dying from the disease in Britain occurred in 1985. BSE is known to have killed 179,000 cows; 4.7 million cows were slaughtered and burned as a precaution against its spread. In 1995, the first known human victim of BSE in Britain died from human variant Creutzfeldt-Jakob disease (vCJD). Over a hundred British deaths from vCJD have since been recorded, all of them attributed to the BSE epidemic. The spread of the disease, first through cows and then to humans, has been traced by the Phillips Report to the use of meat remains and bonemeal, through the recycling of animal waste after slaughter through its conversion into animal feed. BSE is one of a number of TSEs, of which the most common is scrapie, known to affect sheep but never before known to jump from that species to any other. Prion protein, a form of membrane protein, becomes drastically altered in the brain, leading to the typical spongiform structure associated with BSE. This altered brain protein has appeared in all people who have died from vCJD. The reasons for the alteration are a source of huge controversy within the scientific community working on BSE (Pennington 2000). Two substantive theories are that sheep scrapie did finally jump species through the feeding of contaminated sheep remains to cows or that BSE is the result of a spontaneous genetic mutation of prion protein.

By contrast to the mysterious BSE pathogen, FMD is one of the oldest afflictions known to farming communities. It is a flu-like virus, the many strains of which produce lameness and loss of appetite in the animals that contract it: cows, deer, goats, pigs, and sheep. It can cause death in very young animals or those that are already ill. Otherwise, most animals recover within two to three weeks. They lose weight during that time but are otherwise unaffected. The virus is only rarely transferred from infected animals to humans and, if this does occur, the symptoms are again mild, flu-like symptoms (Woods 2001). Yet between February and the general election in June 2001, over three million farm animals were slaughtered in the UK because of FMD. Thus the countryside in the late springtime, usually a potent pastoral metaphor for British people, its hills and fields dotted with new lambs and calves grazing across the lush green, was eerily empty.

Similarly, the once equally potent metaphor of democracy has also come to be viewed as increasingly empty.

THE MULTIPLE DIMENSIONS OF CRISIS

The slaughter of infected animals and the culling of animals on farms contiguous to sites of infection meant that the public was once more seeing photographs and camera footage of pyres of burning animal bodies across the skyline, invoking the too recent memories of BSE. The concrete details of the slaughter policy slowly reached public focus. On the main BBC television news bulletin on Good Friday, the public began to be informed of how chaotic the culling was; the broadcast contained explicit verbal and visual descriptions of marksmen with their guns, aiming so poorly at herds of terrified animals and missing so badly that dying animals staggered wildly around the fields screaming, ewes and lambs smeared with blood (see Booker and North 2001:16–22; Chrisafis 2001; O'Hagan 2001:85–87).

Descriptions of modern abattoirs in the course of their daily work would be equally disturbing (Ahmed, Barnett, and Millar 2000). And of course, with the exception of dairy cows and wool-producing sheep, farmers raise animals almost entirely for slaughter, with approximately 500,000 animals killed each year in Britain for food. But there are uncomfortable disjunctures around the scale and purpose of the slaughter that now came to the countryside, often unannounced and spreading fear with it (Booker and North 2001; Mercer

2001). By Easter the epidemic was officially eight weeks old, with 1,344 confirmed cases, and 1.9 million animals slaughtered or awaiting slaughter.

Throughout this period, the media spoke of the FMD epidemic as a "crisis." There were widespread assertions that from one-quarter to one-third of all farmers would go out of business as a result of FMD. A discussion on the BBC's "World Tonight" program on April 12, 2001, centered on how many farmers would leave farming for good. Proponents of large-scale farming argued that this would lead to an increasingly "efficient" industry, but a spokesperson for the Soil Association (which oversees standards for organic farming in Britain) argued that what would develop from this crisis was not more intensive farming but a reform of the Common Agricultural Policy[3] and the firm establishment of an agriculture that would be less intensive and yield better quality food and a better way of working on the land.

Several sociologists have recently written about the notion of crisis in relation to the linked issues of governmentality, democracy, and social exclusion. Bauman argues that crises have the potential for "decisive change" (1999:141), but this change is difficult to achieve because agencies "capable or at least willing to carry the decision through" have vacated the space for action (1999:145). Yet Byrne argues that what appear to be "small disturbances or developments" can bring about transformation, one in which people can have agency over the way matters unfold from a situation of crisis (1998:41–42).

In relation to BSE and other food scares,[4] there is deep confusion about how to do any of this. There is confusion about the role of science in assessing disease, risk, and safety and concern about where and how political will arises to encourage the process of assessment and the subsequent policies to help us see our way through crisis.

One response has been to think in terms of the "precautionary principle," where science serves as a public health watchdog by applying this principle. In the absence of certain knowledge about a particular hazard "where all possible outcomes are known in advance ... and can be expressed as probabilities," science must work instead with degrees of uncertainty or even ignorance, acknowledging that many outcomes are unquantifiable (Harremoës et al. 2001). Writing in the wake of the Phillips Report, one commentator put emphasis on the precautionary principle, arguing that the "scientists and policy makers ... should accept that there is no shame in saying 'We don't know' when a threat is hard to assess by conventional 'probabilistic' risk assessment methods" (Bradley 2000). Thus when BSE was first confirmed, the announcement that beef was safe to eat should have been replaced by the statement that "we do not know" (Bradley 2000). Bradley does not comment on the nature of agribusiness in this era of free-market capitalism, where the scientific production of new technologies is embedded in the work of increasing consumption. She ignores the uncertain position of national governments seeking to retain and extend that work of consumption (Monbiot 2000). And without this link, Bradley (2000) cannot perceive how risk-creation in the name of modernity and progress is constantly transformed into a private burden for citizens who must deal with it as informed consumers. Instead she argues that to prevent similar catastrophes, we require better, tighter structures of regulation on the part of the state and better self-regulation on the part of agribusiness.

This formula of tighter regulation and self-regulation may sound vaguely comforting to the private citizen-consumer (except those families of citizen-consumers who have already been diagnosed with vCJD). But at a time when, in the words of cultural critic Thomas Frank, governments have fully "accommodated themselves to free market faiths" and the "democracy of the super-market" (2001:17), this formula constitutes a woefully inadequate political response.

BURNING PYRES AGAIN

February 19, 2001, marks the official beginning of another terrible nightmare in British farming. On that date, the British Ministry for Agriculture, Food, and Fisheries (MAFF) placed a five-mile exclusion zone around an abattoir near Brentwood in Essex, preventing the movement of all livestock. The MAFF press release on February 20 stated that veterinary investigations were underway into a case of vesicular disease in pigs and that, although no FMD was confirmed at that point, the Ministry had to treat the case with great caution. The MAFF announcement and subsequent confirmation by the Minister of State at MAFF to the House of Commons that FMD disease was present appeared not especially important unless one was involved directly with farming. Indeed, the hammer blow this outbreak represented had to be carefully explained. The necessity of spelling out the message stems from the fact that in 1998 agriculture contributed only 1 percent to the British annual GDP, a mere £6.9 billion, and represented only 5.3 percent of its export market (O'Hagan 2001:10). Tourism earns more money in Britain, an estimated annual £24 billion. Because the vast majority of the British population is completely removed from farming, they were unaware that the FMD virus is highly contagious and is transmissible by air as well as by spreading from animal to animal and being easily carried on car and lorry wheels, clothing, boots, hair, and so on.

MAFF officials began a complex epidemiological tracing of animal movements across Britain to try to establish the original source of the disease. MAFF halted the movement of all livestock for seven days and suspended all animals for export. Before the week ended, the initial reported infection had been traced to a farm in Northumberland where pigs had been shipped for fattening and then transported hundreds of miles south to the Essex abattoir, at which point they had infected other pigs at the abattoir. The government chief veterinarian stated that the virus had probably been present for four weeks in the Northumberland site and that it had also spread to a nearby cattle and sheep farm, probably by air, where it was confirmed on February 23.[5] Sheep from that farm had been sold at a market in Hexham, along with some 3,500 other animals from many other farms on February 13. Some of these infected sheep were sold to a Devon farm in the southwest of England and were then sent to a holding center near Carlisle, still in the north of England, before being shipped to Devon. Subsequent to their arrival, other sheep from the Devon farm were sent to a slaughterhouse in Wiltshire, carrying the virus there, and yet others were sold to farms in Herefordshire and Northampton. The Devon farm had also sold some of the sheep to Germany.

By February 27, the British public was confronted on the television and in the newspapers with maps of colored arrows to chart 12 confirmed outbreaks and suspected new outbreaks and told of the numbers of pigs (1,600), cattle (1,800), and sheep (3,500) that had already been slaughtered and then burned and buried to prevent spreading the virus. The spread of FMD was so rapid as to leave a meeting of European Union (EU) farm ministers in Brussels speaking of the "very serious threat" of "such a dangerous disease" (Castle and Karacs 2001).

Suspect pigswill, contaminated by illegally imported meat, was discussed as a possible source of the infection.[6] It was pointed out that in the year 2000 alone, 67 tons of illegal meat had been seized at the third largest London airport, Gatwick (Brown 2001a). According to the Institute of Animal Health, the UN's World Reference Center on FMD at Pirbright in England, outbreaks of the disease internationally have risen dramatically in recent years, with diseased food being fed to animals most often the cause; more than 60 countries had reported outbreaks in the past two years, and imports, legal and illegal, of infected material were implicated (Vidal 2001a).

Thus in as dramatic a manner as with BSE, the rapid spread of FMD highlighted the operations of intensive agriculture and its realities, where animals are fed infected material that circulates easily as part of international trade and are then transported hundreds and even thousands of miles to markets, holding centers, and other farms and finally to slaughter, whether in Britain or in other countries. The extent of this movement of animals, the numbers involved, and the distances they traveled seemed to surprise the very authorities who should have known about this pattern of an ever-longer chain of rationalized production, namely the Ministry of Agriculture (Vidal and Brown 2001a).

The strain of the virus, a pan-Asiatic strain known as Type O, was especially virulent; it was thought that ten times as many animals were already infected by the time the first case was identified as had been infected in the last FMD epidemic in 1967 (Connor 2001a; Vidal and Brown 2001a). Reactions to the crisis, as the slaughter teams closed in and farmers lost what was often their lifetime's work in building up their herds, were quoted in press reports such as this one: "The last few days have been the worst in my life. It's as if there has been a death in the family" (quoted in Donald and Green 2001). Families were closed off from one another and unable to leave their farms. Counseling lines were set up, and the Samaritans, a charitable support group to prevent suicide, launched an emergency campaign for farmers to help break the deepening isolation of sealed-off farms.

The iconic status of the British countryside as a site for nonrural people meant that not only farmers were affected. Countryside rights of way and public footpaths were closed, and tourism suffered. By March 11, it was estimated that while farmers were losing £10 million each week in lost exports of animals, tourism in the hill region of Cumbria alone was losing that figure (Mendick 2001b). With hotel and catering business down by 75 percent and workers being laid off as a result, calls for the countryside to be reopened became more frequent prior to the Easter holiday period.

Threats of civil disorder emerged. There were multiple protests about the effects of mass burning and burial of animal carcasses. People in Cumbria, Durham, and Devon marched about pollution of their water supplies from FMD burial sites and high levels of airborne dioxin pollutants (linked to cancer) that were released from the materials used for pyres (Hetherington and Vidal 2001). The government had to convene emergency meetings with scientific advisers on the risks of BSE contamination from cattle slaughtered, burned, and buried for FMD. Tests on many of these sites raised fears that the rogue prion proteins might have been present in cattle over 30 months of age who were slaughtered without being tested for the presence of BSE, and therefore that the special regulations for disposing of BSE-infected cattle, still thought to comprise 2 percent of herds in Britain, were not observed (Harris and Burke 2001).

The greatest levels of protest emerged over the mass slaughter policy of animals. Increasingly, Ministry officials had to resort to the courts to gain entry to contiguous farms where animals were not infected but where farmers were barricading entry against teams of veterinarians and slaughtermen. A spokesperson for Farmers for Action, representing smaller farmers, argued that the policy of mass slaughtering of uninfected animals would continue to be challenged despite threats to bring in police and the army to enforce it (Burke et al. 2001).

Media pictures of the impact of culling served to raise the emotional temperature in the largely untouched urban British population, with photographs of stranded baby animals. The case of the 12-day-old calf, named Phoenix by its owners, who refused leave to MAFF officials to come onto their farm for its slaughter, forced the government to back down and to announce an "easing" or a "refining" of the rules about contiguous slaughter of uninfected animals (Vidal 2001b). Yet despite claims by government scientists that there would be no new cases of FMD by the date of the general election in June, numbers continued to rise. The beginning of September saw the 2,000th case of FMD (Brown 2001b).

THE CONTEST BETWEEN FARMING AS LIVELIHOOD
AND THE NEEDS OF AGRIBUSINESS

By the middle of May, it was made clear that a third of "confirmed" cases of FMD later proved negative and that animals had been unnecessarily slaughtered. However, MAFF said it could not risk waiting for test results to return from laboratories (Chrisafis, Vasagar, and Brown 2001). The notions of risk, threat, and danger appeared in the official statements about FMD within the epidemic's first week, albeit with a different collective set of associations than those being reported by individual farmers who were facing the final ruination of their livelihoods. Thus, Bernard Vallat, the director general of the International Epizootic Office in Paris, stated, "If the virus spread to the continent, the entire EU would risk losing its status as free of foot-and-mouth disease. The reemergence of the disease in Britain presents a potential major threat to European exports" (quoted in Vidal and Brown 2001b).

On February 26, the government's chief veterinarian also spoke of FMD as dangerous because EU regulations would prevent animal exports to other EU countries until Britain was disease-free (Elliott and Webster 2001). One critic pointed out that "MAFF steadfastly refuses to countenance any relaxation of its zero tolerance policy. This contrasts sharply with the enormous tolerance it showed BSE, allowing hundreds of thousands of diseased animals into the food chain and permitting food controls—when introduced—to be poorly enforced and widely flouted" (Lean 2001). This journalist termed FMD not a dangerous disease but an "economic disease," and it became clear that perceived economic consequences for large-scale agriculture had led to the enforcement of the slaughter (Booker and North 2001; Woods 2001). Put simply, slaughter is justified by the fact that during the recovery time for animals, they cannot be moved on in the food chain and thus the economic losses for large-scale agribusiness are greater than the disruption of slaughtering, especially as the costs for slaughter and for compensation of the loss of the animals are borne by governments. Woods (2001) also argues that the mass-slaughter policy favored by many European governments, scientific advisers, and veterinarians is bound up not with the biological nature of the disease but with the kudos of having a country with disease-free status from FMD.

Arguments about slaughter and the role of vaccination as an alternative dominated the remainder of the epidemic. The government and its advisers continued to assert that the mass-slaughter policy, including contiguous culling of noninfected animals, was the only sure route to eradication.

Vaccination, including emergency vaccination within a ringed area around an infected farm, followed by a cull, is used in many other countries where FMD outbreaks occur. But objections to its use in Britain came from the National Farmers Union, the biggest farming lobbying group, and from food producers, both claiming that their exports would be permanently banned for being less than pure and safe (Vidal and Hetherington 2001). Ministry officials were eventually forced to observe that products from vaccinated meat and milk could be sold domestically with no threat whatsoever to humans consuming these products (*Guardian Weekly* 2001; Wilson and Watt 2001). Moreover, national BBC radio reported that between June 2000 and May 2001, 18,500 tons of meat were legally imported into Britain from Brazil, a country that vaccinates against endemic outbreaks of FMD. It had already emerged that in 1999 an EU report from the Scientific Committee on Animal Health and Animal Welfare stated that the risk of FMD in the EU remains extraordinarily high because of its endemic nature in much of the rest of the world.[7]

Despite mounting evidence about different approaches to handling FMD, the confusion about "pure" meat, food standards, and an export market continued. A lead editorial in *The London Independent* (2001a) stated that the government should continue to resist vaccination because it would end the meat export trade and devastate sales at home.

Yet the issue of who profits most from the way international food production is now structured also became part of the public agenda. For the poorest and most marginalized farmers, the government's mass-slaughter policy, following from that of the EU's Common Agricultural Policy (CAP), was truly an economic catastrophe. Under CAP, a system of sheep-headage grants had provided a survival strategy for these farmers, despite severe problems of overgrazing: it was no surprise that one-third of all cases of FMD occurred in Cumbria and Devon, which have some of the highest indices of poverty in the British Isles.[8]

The obvious query was how had these farmers become so marginalized despite the extensive system of subsidies in place for many decades. Farmers' income dropped by 60 percent between 1995 and 1999, hill farmers such as those in Cumbria earned an average of less than £8000 in 1998–99 (60 percent of which came from CAP subsidies), the value of pigs dropped by £99 million between 1998 and 1999, and for lambs the drop in value was estimated at £126 million (O'Hagan 2001). There was a "giant profit gap opening up" between the production costs, the selling price to food manufacturers and retail sellers, and the selling price to consumers (O'Hagan 2001:10–11). This gap was underlined in the middle of the epidemic by the profits announcement from Tesco, the giant British supermarket chain, of £1 billion profit from its £23 billion turnover, or a daily profit of £3 million for the year 2000–2001 (Finch 2001). O'Hagan (2001) documented what listeners to farming programs had been hearing for some time, that farmers were shooting livestock for which there was no market price in the late 1990s, especially pigs, and then not infrequently shooting themselves, such were the levels of their indebtedness. Suicide among small farmers was a social issue of increasing concern to groups such as the Royal College of Psychiatrists (O'Hagan 2001:11).

Luttwak (2001) describes a similar scenario in the United States, where the costs for small farmers involved in cattle-rearing have spiraled uncontrollably, with resulting bankruptcy and suicide. Luttwak traces this disastrous development to the increasing imposition of agribusiness methods, such as the use of commercially produced animal feed to stimulate unnaturally rapid growth and keeping cows pregnant as frequently as possible. He lists the heavy and hidden costs of this forced pattern of animal rearing, including constant monitoring of and treatment for consequent serious and recurring diseases. And whereas commercial animal foodstuffs and the associated pharmaceuticals make huge profits for the transnational corporations producing such products, the cheap meat that ensues for the consumer may also entail hidden costs, not least because it is "sick" meat.

The significance of cheap food began to be explored in Britain. "Both the BSE emergency and the current emergency point in one direction—that we need less meat, but of better quality," wrote *The London Independent on Sunday* (2001). Many analysts asked why successive governments had failed to confront the principal beneficiaries of the cheap food policy, namely the supermarkets and their long-distance economy of food production and distribution (Monbiot 2001; see also Fort 2001a; Humphrys 2001; O'Hagan 2001; Ramonet 2001). Government policies based on this dogma had paved the way for the FMD drama, which had spread with such speed because of the "pressures of this deregulated market economy" (Ramonet 2001), bringing about a dangerous reduction in safety throughout the food chain. The monopolistic practices of the supermarket chains and associated producers had created huge costs for society in general, as tax-paying citizens dealt with the aftermath of food scares (Browne 2000; Monbiot 2000; Budden 2001; Humphrys 2001; O'Hagan 2001). Berthelot (2001) argued that BSE, multiple other food scares, and the FMD epidemic had starkly highlighted the inadequacies of the current model of agriculture under CAP. Lean (2001) argued that MAFF did not care for either human health or animal health and welfare, that the emergency actions that had been its response to FMD showed its basic concern about "a threat to the profitability of agribusiness that has ruthlessly driven small farmers to the wall."

However, the argument that weaker, less efficient farmers should leave the industry while larger, more efficient farming operations remained was a frequent counter-discourse. Observations that farmers were workers as in any other industry, such as coal and steel, employed the language of deregulated free enterprise. If jobs vanished as they had in these other industries, this was how the free market operates. This language, however, as Frank (2001) argues, obscures the outcomes of deregulation and untrammeled free trade; the claim is that deregulation constitutes a kind of populist leveling, where those who remain in business do so through their competitive edge. Yet the reality of this "extreme capitalism" is a relentless "upward transfer of wealth" (Frank 2001:86). Farming is not an industry like coal or steel. As Bové and Dufour (2001:124) observe, the components of a farmer's job are, very immediately, economic, social, and environmental,[9] and whether these components are accepted as an integrated package or not defines the struggle with modern intensive agriculture. So a central issue arising out of the FMD epidemic was how to challenge this construction of farming, with its remit, in Budden's (2001) phrase, to manufacture a commodity for global trade at the cheapest price.

The BSE epidemic arose within this same overly intensive industry that became increasingly determined to extract profits. The Phillips Report states that the identification of BSE as a disease entity in 1986 was followed by 10 years of announcements by government scientific advisers and ministers assuring the public that there was either no risk at all or, at worst, a very remote risk to humans from the lethal BSE pathogen. The Report cites a "culture of secrecy" that took hold of civil service officials within MAFF who feared that raising the possibility of a risk factor would provoke public alarm and would create general food scares (Johnston 2000). In their formulation of endangerment, this was endangerment to the food industry and to some abstracted concept of public health but not risk or danger to the individual citizens whose everyday lives depend both on food from that industry and on guidance from the very government machinery that is meant to promote and protect public health. Thus Lord Phillips cited approach to the general public "whose object was sedation" because they feared an "irrational" response that would destroy the beef industry (Johnston 2000). The BSE epidemic led to worldwide bans on the importation of British cattle and British beef and a collapse in the domestic market, resulting in bankruptcy for many thousands of small farmers. As yet, there is no end in sight to the long-term impacts of the epidemic. The numbers of people who will develop vCJD are not known (Meek 2001).

The Phillips Report reached the obvious conclusion that the relationship between animal health and human health is intertwined and that a sound surveillance system for animals' diseases is therefore required as an essential safeguard. But that is what British people thought they had to begin with; that is why there was a Ministry for Agriculture, Food, and Fisheries with a legion of scientific programs and advisers to test and monitor animal and food safety and from which a stream of bulletins issued for a decade assuring the public that there were no concerns. The gap between government assurances and the reality is why there is now a crisis of confidence about food safety.

Much of the media attention at the time of the Phillips Report's publication concentrated on a breach of trust between citizens and their government and its scientific advisers. Yet the BSE crisis is not just about science getting it wrong or even about government departments working either foolishly, blindly, or covertly to ensure damage limitation with the country at large.

Both the Phillips Report and the media coverage return many times to the notion of risk. Trying to piece through this, *The London Independent* concluded that "where the risk of danger appears low, but the potential damage is on a catastrophic scale, the precautionary principle ought to guide public policy" (2000). This was a common theme in the commentaries on BSE, as we saw earlier. What failed to be discussed is the urgent need to initiate a wide-ranging debate about the socially embedded nature of the risks we create on the one hand and, on the other, the crippling incapacity of current political processes to comment effectively on the nature and source of those areas of risk. For example, this so-called precautionary principle will not be operative in a context where language about the advance of science contributing to the progress of humankind remains the dominant discourse. Science as an enterprise central to modernization is not only viewed as bringing more gains than losses, it is also seen as solver of all the problems and risks we create with it in the process of creating modernity itself. As Bauman (1993:200) argues, we accept what science says of itself and its enterprise, that it is promoting progress through its own critique of the "unwholesome nature of its past accomplishments;" we also accept its "indispensability" in cleaning up the "mess" it has previously made.

The reality is that there is no absolute safety from BSE in beef production. The reverberations from BSE continue, with reported cases in France, Ireland, and Germany up by 130, 58, and 88, respectively, in 1999–2000—due, we are told, to improved screening programs. But given the infectivity of even a tiny bit of BSE-infected material, how are we meant to respond to the lack of 100-percent effectiveness of any screening program? What do we now make of the problem of risk and safety? And how is a politics reflecting this complexity to be put in place?

LOCATING THE USES OF RISK

Risk has come to operate in multiple contexts since it was first used in the sixteenth century as a concept to aid the insurance industry in early modern capitalism. Ewald (1991:198–199) writes that risk was importantly "a neologism" of that burgeoning market activity that elaborated a particular kind of rational framework for the "treatment of certain acts capable of happening to a group of individuals" and to the "values or capital" they represented. The process of risk assessment earned healthy profits from the outset. Insurance depended vitally on a calculation of risk as a series of probabilities, for one never insures against real events but against the perception that any event can be a risk, with insurance itself scaling the probabilities of an occurrence over a given population. Ewald (1991) discusses a shift in thought in the nineteenth century, where industrial accidents are no longer defined as events that the individuals who sustained damage must prove in law as the fault of their employer, but as a risk. The cost of this risk is then to be borne by social insurance, redistributing the burden across the population of workers who pay for it.

Risk was progressively capitalized as an essential feature of an industrial economy. In this context, its use was effectively a compromise the state needed to strike between safety and profit. Thus, for example, a British government commission on child labor in the mid-nineteenth century ensured that mills would continue to run a 15-hour day while hours of work for children were limited to 9 hours only, permitting a shift system of child workers to keep up productivity at cheapest labor costs.

The citizenry came to feel that such regulatory bodies at least stated the facts of the situation, giving some voice to and representation about our daily realities. However, catastrophic events such as the BSE epidemic reveal how the value of this compromise device has broken down. Beck (1992) argues that the growing fragility of this arrangement has emerged as the foundations of industrial society, in terms of work, class, the family, and so on have shifted. In this late modern period, which Beck characterizes as the "risk society," the individual is expected to cope with anxiety and insecurity without the support of those traditional structures of industrial society.

There is a strong and correct sense now that people cannot any longer trust their government and its scientific advisers to safeguard them from future catastrophes (not that they ever could, but they claimed they could). Hence the Phillips Report was written up in one national newspaper editorial as not "truly" reflecting "public anger and outrage over the worst health and safety scandal of modern times" (*Daily Mail* 2000). This editorial concludes: "Why should anyone believe another word the politicians or government scientists say? After all that has happened, can there be the slightest confidence in official reassurances about the supposed safety of GM foods?"

Consumers are in "a state of bewilderment" about the "deeply flawed" system of agriculture and food production (Fort 2001b). That confusion is evident in a study undertaken for the Food Standards Agency, an advisory body the government launched in 2000 to oversee the public's health in relation to food. When respondents in the study group were asked about food safety and recent food scares such as BSE and salmonella, they revealed a broad skepticism about what are seen as intractable issues to do with regulating a food industry that may put profits ahead of safety (Cragg Ross Dawson Ltd. 2000). They expressed deep uncertainty about preventing more food scares and both concern and confusion about the effectiveness of regulatory bodies. Especially interesting was criticism of scientific experts who so often disagree with one another and the feeling that they thus failed to provide clear advice about food safety, based on evidence from which consumers could make an informed choice. Here we see an example of what Beck (1992) describes about the privatization of risk, of making it the responsibility of the individual as consumer to make choices and avoid dangers by using the tool of risk assessment. But if risk assessment is a tool of scientific rationality, its principal use, Bauman (1993) argues, is not to ask the underlying questions about why it exists but to continue to play the game of calculating the probabilities and size of disasters. "Risk information" is a form of "DIY survival kit," "dumping" the collective dangers produced by this technico-scientific machinery "into the privatized worlds of individual victims" (Bauman 1993:202).

Is the public to be reassured when the Food Standards Agency announces that there is no new evidence to query the limited ban on the consumption of sheep offal that has been put in place to protect consumers against the risk of BSE in lamb, while a former member of the principal government advisory

committee insists that the "precautionary principle" should be exercised because BSE has already jumped at least one species (Connor 2001b)? With the
tightly knit web of corporate sponsorship and links to government (Monbiot
2000), how can the public take as a serious policy commitment the recommendation from the Phillips Report that "in future when a new disease emerges
amongst animals which might have implications for human health ... the government should take precautions to prevent its spread" (Connor, Arthur, and
Woolf 2000)? This crisis of governance is as deep as the crisis of a science, which
acts as a "double-agent" (Bauman 1993:207), perpetuating a cycle of generating
new risks that it will then offer to solve on our behalf.

ISSUES OF GOVERNANCE AND THE CREATION OF NEW POLITICAL SPACES

The British government responded to the FMD crisis by setting up the traditional device of a commission of inquiry. However, there was no public inquiry
like the Phillips/BSE inquiry. The investigation of FMD comprised three separate closed inquiries. More significantly still, one of the inquiries on the future
of farming was chaired by the former head of the Meat and Livestock Commission (which was censured by the Phillips Report) and included as members
the chief executive of the Sainsbury's supermarket chain, the vice president of
Unilever, and the chairperson of Bird's Eye Wall's food producers. Additionally,
Lord Haskins, the head of Northern Foods, one of the largest food-processing
companies in Britain, was appointed as rural recovery coordinator. So the same
players who were entangled in the BSE debacle—government civil servants,
scientists, and corporate food producers—deliberated in closed sessions on the
FMD epidemic. The inquiries illustrate Bauman's argument that the state has
largely given up its previous capacity to supervise and directly administrate the
resources subject to its power in favor of its current position of making life as
comfortable and hospitable as possible for "cosmopolitan, stateless, and no-
madic capital-brokers to visit and stay" (1993:138–139). This sensitivity of government to corporate business as fickle employers is based on economic
contexts that national governments are reluctant to bring to the attention of
their electorates. As Gorz (1994), Bauman (1998, 1999), and others have
pointed out, the deregulated neoliberal discourse has led to a progressive free-
flow of capital and, with it, demands by transnational corporations for flexible
labor without the "once dense and numerous safety nets" (Bauman 1999:66)
that formed labor's protection in industrial society. It means governments can
exercise almost no control over the movement and relocation of labor.

The tensions between the state's working in this way and its citizenry are becoming more pronounced, even when their recognition is blunted by a sense of
political powerlessness. *The London Independent* (2001b) argued that public
suspicion "is unlikely to be allayed" as long as government policy on farming

and food production is being directed by the heads of two of the most powerful food producers in the country, Lord Haskins and Lord Sainsbury of the supermarket chain.

The outstanding issue coming out of the BSE and FMD epidemics is how to shift apparent public powerlessness and deep public suspicion into new political spaces. In Bauman's analysis, this is connected with working to retrieve or restore the "public/private" space of the *agora*, where the meaning of the "common good" and all its myriad differences can be debated and where "private worries" from everyday life become "public issues" (Bauman 1999). This currently "empty" space, which held the state's interest during industrial modernity when the state could imprint its stamp firmly on economic and cultural processes, has been abandoned in postmodern times, where instead there is a "separation and increasing gap between power and politics," with a consequent decline of trust in political institutions (Bauman 1999:97–98). The really "powerful and resourceful agents have escaped into hiding and operate beyond the reach of established means of political action" (Bauman 1999:97–98). These "agents" form an economic system with an "insatiable hunger" for "new and larger profits" that extend their expropriation and relations of inequality into new territories and new populations (Bauman 1993:214). At the same time, with the rapid fluctuation of both issues and the public's attention, when there is a question of what is to be done, the answer coming from near-bankrupt state institutions tends to be TINA (there is no alternative) because there appear no credible or willing agencies to carry out ideas, not that the ideas themselves are necessarily lacking (Bauman 1999:97–98).

Of course there is no profit for transnational corporate power to engage in the process of democratic negotiation, control, and collective action centered in the *agora*, but as the space is empty at present, it is there for the taking (Bauman 1999) and, along with it, the work on "the *revision* of profit definition" (Bauman 1993:216, original emphasis).

In relation to the issues discussed in this chapter, the origin and quality of the food each citizen needs every day, two tasks need to be undertaken in this reclaimed space.

The first task has to do with viewing differently the enterprises of science and technology and pushing on from the often unanchored notion of a precautionary principle (unanchored because it lacks sufficient agency or location in relation to the principal actors who must be confronted). The imperative to do everything we possibly can with and by science must be contested and, with it, there is a concomitant need to consider where science locates itself, now most frequently at sites of huge profit-taking.

In an essay on technology and responsibility that the philosopher Hans Jonas wrote in 1974, he made a distinction between traditional ethics and ethics for what he termed *homo faber*. Traditional ethics were typically anthropocentric and relationships with the nonhuman world were "ethically neutral": first, because the impact of humans did not impinge in such a way as to permanently injure the entire order of things and, second, because the pursuit of the nonhuman world was not the ultimate goal or concern of humankind. Our relationship with modern technology has fundamentally changed this ethical context, because as we have fostered with modern technology, we have changed the nature of human action. We have a newly created "causal agency" stemming from our actions that now has objects and consequences beyond previous ethical imagining. Jonas argued that the "recognition of ignorance becomes the obverse of the duty to know and the part of ethics that must govern the ever more necessary self-policing of our outsized might" (1974:10). This recognition of ignorance is not to be confused with Beck's concept of reflexivity in the risk society, wherein science can make all well that it first makes badly because it does not know its own power. In that sense, ignorance of our vast capabilities or of the reality that the train of cause and effect we now set in motion has a huge spatial and time-span spread can no longer provide "an alibi" (Jonas 1974:9–10). In this radically changed world, the reality that our "predictive knowledge" always "falls behind the technical knowledge" that encourages us to act comes to have huge importance as a basis for a changed ethics, an ethics that recognizes how these "new objects" and new domains of action have added greatly to where rules of conduct must apply (Jonas 1974:3, 10).

Applying Jonas's thinking to BSE permits us to see the simple equation that created the disease. Ruminants are said by biologists to be among "the most accomplished of all herbivores," if not the "most ecologically successful animals," because they accomplish that amazing task of efficiently digesting hard plant material, breaking down cellulose, and converting it to a usable source of energy (Tudge 2000:455–456). The hideous problem of BSE was created when the British farming industry sought profits from hitherto less profitable animal material. We ignored the rules of conduct when we overturned this primary ecological equation and in effect turned cows into cannibals by feeding the rendered parts of slaughtered cows back to live cattle.

We also created a new and terrible disease.

The *Review of the Origin of BSE*, from the government committee of scientific experts charged with analyzing the epidemic, concludes that this is the most probable hypothesis as to why the disease began in Britain. The report states that the risk of exposure to the pathogen that causes BSE was perhaps 30 times greater for young calves of only two weeks' age than it was for adult cows. Calves were already fed artificially (so that cows could be made pregnant again at once) rather than being permitted to suckle. When meat remains and bonemeal (MBM) pellets were first formulated in the 1970s as a cheaper alternative to powdered milk and soy supplements, sheep remains were used at the outset, creating the scenario for sheep scrapie or a scrapie-like agent to jump species through the very vulnerable immune systems of young calves. The committee judged that BSE was "one hitherto undescribed agent in sheep which possibly acquires new characteristics on recycling in cows" (Horn et al. 2001). Changes in the rendering process of sheep remains by dropping the temperature and dropping the quantity of some of the chemicals used "may have resulted in a ... clinically significant increase in the ... infectivity of this material" (Connor 2001c). And then as those infected calves went through food-chain production processes and also ended up in MBM, BSE was enabled to spread.

The Phillips inquiry had recommended that the government ensure future safety, and to this end, in the wake of the Horn Report, still dealing only with strong hypotheses and probabilities (which is frequently all science can do), the government issued a press release in September 2000 about the "theoretical" possibility that the BSE pathogen might be introduced into the sheep population (DEFRA 2001a). The government's Contingency Plan (DEFRA 2001b) to deal with this possibility if a worst-case scenario of BSE does emerge is to prevent transmission to humans through the slaughter of 40 million sheep per year until BSE is eradicated (DEFRA 2001b.).

This discouraging scenario leads us to the second matter we need to discuss in this space of the *agora:* how we make operational a relationship alluded to in the Phillips Report, where the common-sense observation is made that animal health and human health are closely intertwined. This is a nonanthropocentric ethical relationship, one in which we understand our responsibility to tend both to "human good" and to "the good of things extra-human" (Jonas 1974:10). There are some tentative beginnings for this "stewardship" (Jonas 1974:10).

The European Union actually included a protocol on animal welfare in the 1997 Treaty of Amsterdam, stating that member states must "pay full regard to the welfare requirements of animals" because there must be "improved protection and respect for the welfare of animals as sentient beings." This astonishing clause has been taken up by groups working for animal welfare reform that are calling for an end to the conditions of intensive farming. Campaign groups such as the Eurogroup for Animal Welfare (2001) and the Food Ethics Council are critically aware that making the EU protocol to the Amsterdam Treaty a reality will bring national governments and the EU into direct conflict with the World Trade Organization, because it will challenge WTO rules about unrestricted free trade that currently prevent the promotion of animal welfare.

Yet the Food Ethics Council (FEC) asks how we can work with farm animals and food production in more ethical ways (2000, 2001). It seeks to challenge what it terms "the high-tech scenario" in farming that has placed such a great burden of costs on animals, consumers and the state as food safety has been progressively ignored. Our future food system will depend, the FEC argues, on the outcome of the tension between these two opposing trends. Their Ethical Matrix suggests that respect for the welfare and the intrinsic nature of farm animals means we need "a notional contract with farm animals that requires us to repay the benefits we receive from them by ensuring as far as possible, that we care for them respectfully and compassionately" (Food Ethics Council 2000).

Strong programs of citizen action are also clearly required to open up and interrogate what currently present as the closed perspectives of government and corporate agribusiness. The FMD epidemic has produced some useful beginnings. Protests about culling, information on court injunctions, and investigations of breaches of welfare rules during the mass slaughter were all organized through e-mail bulletin boards and Internet sites. In Devon, one of the hardest hit areas, local authorities chose to hold an inquiry before any national action of this sort had been taken. The Devon Inquiry was pointedly a public inquiry to redress the trauma, voicelessness, and powerlessness so many citizens experienced. Its proceedings were carried via the Internet (Mercer 2001). Government officials refused to attend. The inquiry did request written answers from these officials and says of these answers: "Many statements in the DEFRA response invite further questions because they are vague, open-ended, or inaccurate" (Mercer 2001:1). By contrast, the Devon report, based on hard evidence, is a robust challenge to policy makers and civil servants.

These actions mark strong initial moves in opening up the *agora* to explore how food has become a complex source of risk and danger in modernity, as it has been captured for profit-taking and expanded scientific enterprise. The exercise of agency within a revitalized *agora* will require concise information, excellent channels for communicating this information so as to contribute to citizen understanding, and the identification of pressure points within the existing chaos of international commercial food production. At the conclusion of the FMD epidemic, it is thought that up to 10 million animals were slaughtered in unspeakable circumstances. The crisis epidemics of BSE and FMD have communicated vividly to all citizens the struggle over definitions of safety, ethics, costs, and efficiency in agriculture.

NOTES

1. BSE has been reported in countries across continental Europe and internationally. Limited outbreaks of FMD occurred on the island of Ireland, in France, and in the Netherlands. Precautionary culls of livestock also took place in Germany, Italy, and Spain.

2. Global agricultural trade is currently estimated at 300 billion dollars per year, with 10 United States-based corporations thought to account for over 60 percent of the international food-chain business, including seed, fertilizer and pesticide production, and food processing (Korten 1995; Vidal 2001c).

3. The Common Agricultural Policy (CAP), instituted in 1964 within the European Economic Community, was meant to ensure a stable supply of food production by using subsidies to improve farming productivity. It has led to substantial overproduction and stockpiled "food mountains." CAP was set up just as supermarkets were beginning to develop significantly in Europe. This was also the period of intensified research in the agrichemical industry that led to higher yields and factory farm methods. Taken together, these developments encouraged the trend away from family farms and toward large, rationalized farming operations. In Britain under CAP, the biggest farmers, the top

20 percent, absorb 80 percent of CAP subsidies. Calls for the reform of CAP have risen markedly in the wake of numerous recent food scares (Berthelot 2001).

4. On the extent of other recent food scares, see Fort (2001b) and Humphrys (2001).

5. It was argued that FMD had been present in Britain, probably in sheep, for many months before the outbreak was verified (see Booker and North 2001:5).

6. Substantive proof has not been produced that pigswill was the origin of the disease. But the virus survives well in bone marrow, and illegally imported meat on the bone from countries where the virus is endemic and untreated by vaccination was considered a likely route of infection (Mendick 2001a).

7. Escalating numbers of outbreaks internationally was attributed by the EU to "illegal smuggling of animals, increased traffic of refugees, tourism, weak veterinary and waste services and the globalization of trade" (Vidal 2001a). Cusimano (2000:45–46) has commented that a rising flood of legitimate goods is being shipped across state borders in an open global economy, where the technologies of mass containerization of goods make it impossible to check for contraband.

8. According to the Countryside Agency (2001), nearly a quarter of all people living in rural areas are living at or below the poverty line. Cumbria, the area worst affected by FMD, had the poorest households (Vidal 2001d).

9. As Budden (2001) observes, farming has to pay attention to the environment because it occupies more land than any other form of productive work.

REFERENCES

Ahmed, Khaled, Antony Barnett, and Stuart Millar. 2000. "Madness: How the British Government Betrayed the British People." *The Observer*, October 29, 19.

Bauman, Zygmunt. 1993. *Postmodern Ethics*. London: Blackwell.

———. 1998. *Work, Consumerism and the New Poor*. Milton Keynes, United Kingdom: Open University.

———. 1999. *In Search of Politics*. London: Polity Press.

Beck. Ulrich. 1992. *Risk Society: Towards a New Modernity*. London: Sage.

Berthelot, Jacques. 2001. "An Alternative Model for Agriculture." *Le Monde Diplomatique*. April 11. Available from www.en.monde-diplomatique.fr/2001/04/11agriculture.

Booker, Christopher, and Richard North. 2001. "Not the Foot and Mouth Report, a Special Investigation." *Private Eye*. Special Issue. November, 2–31.

Bové, José, and François Dufour. 2001. *The World Is Not for Sale: Farmers against Junk Food*. London: Verso.

Bradley, Anna. 2000. "Respecting Our Fears." *The Guardian*, October 27, 21.

Brown, Paul. 2001a. "Illegal Meat Trail Leads to Infected Countries." *The Guardian*, March 28, 4. Available from www.guardian.co.uk/footandmouth/story/0,7369 ,464312,00.html.

———. 2001b. "North of England Farm Virus No-Go Area." *The Guardian*, September 6, 11.

Browne, Anthony. 2000. "The Cost of Taking Nature Out of Farming." *The Observer*, October 29, 21.

Budden, Jo. 2001. "Cheap Food Is Exacting a Terrible Price." *The London Independent on Sunday*, March 4, 17.

Burke, Jason, Kamal Ahmed, Paul Harris, John Arlidge, Ed Helmore, and Kate Connolly. 2001. "Farmers 'Spread Infection': Army on Standby As Those against Cull Warn of Violence." *The Observer*, March 18, 9.

Byrne, David. 1998. *Complexity Theory and the Social Sciences*. London: Routledge.

Castle, Stephen, and Imre Karacs. 2001. "Belgians Revolt as Europe's Great Slaughter Starts." *The London Independent*, February 27, 6.

Chrisafis, Angelique. 2001. "Countryside Continues to Reel under Virus Outbreak." *The Guardian*, May 26, 11.

Chrisafis, Angelique, Jeevan Vasagar, and Paul Brown. 2001. "Third of All Foot and Mouth Cases Wrong: Many Infections Prove Negative, but Ministry Defends Slaughter." *The Guardian Weekly*, May 17–23, 9.

Connor, Steve. 2001a. "Sheep from New Cluster 'Had Virus a Month Ago.'" *The London Independent*, May 31, 13.

———. 2001b. "BSE: the End of a Mystery?" *The London Independent*, July 26, 8.

———. 2001c. "Food Watchdog Claims BSE Lamb Controls Are Adequate." *The London Independent*, August 29, 4.

Connor, Steven, Charles Arthur, and Marie Woolf. 2000. "The British Public Was Misled." *The London Independent*, October 27, 1.

Countryside Agency. 2001. "Cash into Communities—A Solution to Rural Exclusion." Press release, July 3.

Cragg Ross Dawson Ltd. 2000. *Qualitative Research to Explore Public Attitudes to Food Safety: Report for the Food Standards Agency*. London: Cragg Ross Dawson Ltd.

Cusimano, Maryann. 2000. *Beyond Sovereignty: Issues for a Global Agenda*. New York: Bedford/St. Martin's Press.

Daily Mail. 2000. "Mad Cows and a Question of Trust." Lead editorial, October 27, 21.

DEFRA (Department for Environment, Food and Rural Affairs, United Kingdom). 2001a. "Government Publishes Its Response to the BSE Inquiry Report." Press release, September 28.

———. 2001b. *Contingency Plan for the Emergence of Naturally Occurring BSE in Sheep in the UK National Flock*. London: DEFRA.

Donald, Kevin, and Nigel Green. 2001. "'It's Like a Death in the Family': The Farmers." *The London Independent on Sunday*, February 25, 6.

Elliott, Valerie, and Philip Webster. 2001. "Farmers Face Six Months of Fear." *The Times*, February 27, 1.

Eurogroup for Animal Welfare. 2000–2001. *Time for Change: The Future for Farm Animal Welfare in Europe*. Available from www.eurogroupanimalwelfare.org/.

Ewald, François. 1991. "Insurance and Risk." In *The Foucault Effect: Studies in Governmentality*, eds. Graham Burchell, Colin Gordon, and Peter Miller, 197–210. Hemel Hempstead, U.K.: Harvester Wheatsheaf.

Finch, Julia. 2001. "Tesco Sells Its Way to First £1bn Profit." *The Guardian*, April 11, 3.

Food Ethics Council. 2000. *Farming Animals for Food: Towards a Moral Menu*. Southwell, Nottinghamshire: Food Ethics Council.

———. 2001. *After FMD: Aiming for a Values-Driven Agriculture*. Nottingham: Food Ethics Council.

Fort, Matthew. 2001a. "Sacrifices on the Altar of Cheap Food." *The Observer*, March 4, 10.

————. 2001b. "Cheap Food Comes at Very High Price." *The Guardian Weekly*, March 1–7, 8.

Frank, Thomas. 2001. *One Market under God: Extreme Capitalism, Market Populism, and the End of Economic Democracy.* London: Secker and Warburg.

Gorz, André. 1994. *Capitalism, Socialism, Ecology.* London: Verso.

Guardian Weekly. 2001. "Government Gears Up for Vaccination: Foot and Mouth Policy Not Working Fast Enough." *The Guardian Weekly*, April 19–25, 8.

Harremoës, Poul, David Gee, Malcolm MacGarvin, Andy Stirling, Jane Keys, Brian Wynn, and Sofia Guedes Vas. 2001. *Late Lessons from Early Warnings: The Precautionary Principle from 1896–2000.* Environmental Issue Report no. 22, European Environment Agency. Luxembourg: Office for Official Publications of the European Communities.

Harris, Paul and Jason Burke. 2001. "BSE Crisis Talks over Risk from Cattle Cull." *The Observer*, May 20, 4.

Hetherington, Peter, and John Vidal. 2001. "Research Shows High Levels of Pollutants over Cumbria." *The Guardian*, April 28, 9.

Hoggart, Simon. 2001. "Deafening Silence As Countryside Dies a Slow Death." *The Guardian*, February 28, 2.

Horn, Gabriel, Martin Bobrow, Moira Bruce, Michel Goedert, Angela McLean, and John Webster. 2001. *Review of the Origins of BSE.* Available from www.defra.gov.uk/animalh/bse/bseorigin.pdf.

Humphrys, John. 2001. *The Great Food Gamble.* London: Hodder and Stoughton.

Johnston, Philip. 2000. "The Rolls-Royce System That Failed Whitehall." *The Daily Telegraph*, October 27, 4.

Jonas, Hans. 1974. *Philosophical Essays: From Ancient Creed to Technological Man.* Englewood Cliffs, NJ: Prentice-Hall.

Korten, David. 1995. *When Corporations Rule the World.* West Hartford, CT: Kumarian Press.

Lean, Geoffrey. 2001. "The Plague That Never Was." *The London Independent on Sunday*, March 4, 1.

London Independent. 2000. "Ministers Should Have Listened to the Scaremongers over BSE." October 27, 3.

————. 2001a. "Vaccination May Be the Only Solution for This Pestilence." *The London Independent*, August 29, 3.

————. 2001b. "It Is a Basic Right to Know If the Food We Eat Is Safe." *The London Independent*, August 10, 3.

London Independent on Sunday. 2001. "Too Much Meat Is the Problem." February 27, 23.

Luttwak, Edward. 2001. "Sane Cows, or BSE Isn't the Worst of It." *London Review of Books* 23(3) February 8: 26–27.

Meek, James. 2001. "Meat Trade 'Blocking CJD Investigations.'" *The Guardian*, September 7, 6. Available from www.guardian.co.uk/bse/article/0,2763,548044,00.html.

Mendick, Robert. 2001a. "45,000 Animals Slaughtered As Virus Spreads to Cornwall: The Causes." *The London Independent on Sunday*, March 4, 6.

————. 2001b. "Disaster for Tourism As Losses Far Outstrip Those of Meat Industry." *The London Independent on Sunday*, March 11, 6.

Mercer, Ian. 2001. *Crisis and Opportunity: Devon Foot and Mouth Inquiry 2001.* Devon, U.K.: Devon Books.

Monbiot, George. 2000. *Captive State: The Corporate Takeover of Britain.* London: Macmillan.

———. 2001. "Disease and Modernity." *The Guardian,* February 27. Available from www.guardian.co.uk/Archive/Article/0,4273,4143089,00.html.

O'Hagan, Andrew. 2001. *The End of British Farming.* London: Profile Books.

Pennington, Hugh. 2000. "The English Disease." *London Review of Books* 22(24) December 14: 3–6.

Phillips, Lord, June Bridgeman, and Malcolm Ferguson-Smith. 2000. *The BSE Inquiry: Volumes I-XVI.* London: Stationery Office.

Ramonet, Ignacio. 2001. "Britain: A Rolling Crisis." *Le Monde Diplomatique,* April. Available from mondediplo.com/2001/04/.

Tudge, Colin. 2000. *The Variety of Life: A Survey and a Celebration of all the Creatures That Have Ever Lived.* Oxford: Oxford University Press.

Vidal, John. 2001a. "Global Disease on the Rise: Finger Pointed at Illegal Trade." *The Guardian,* February 23, 4.

———. 2001b. "Confusion Rises over Cull Policy after Phoenix." *The Guardian,* April 27, 8. Available from www.guardian.co.uk/footandmouth/story/0,7369,479274,00.html.

———. 2001c. "Global Trade Forces Exodus from Land" *The Guardian,* February 28, 8.

———. 2001d. "Foot and Mouth Leaves Deep Scars on Rural Britain." *The Guardian,* August 30, 10.

Vidal, John, and Paul Brown. 2001a. "Chief Vet Hopes That Ban Will Slow Disease." *The Guardian,* March 2, 8.

———. 2001b. "Farmers' Hopes Go Up in Flames." *The Guardian Weekly,* March 1–7, 1.

Vidal, John, and Peter Hetherington. 2001. "Foot and Mouth Crisis: Food Lobby Forced PM into a U-turn on Plan for Vaccination." *The Guardian,* September 8, 7.

Wilson, Jamie, and Nicholas Watt. 2001. "Teams Get Ready to Vaccinate Cattle." *The Guardian,* April 16, 1.

Woods, Abigail. 2001. "Kill or Cure?" *The Guardian,* February 28, 8.

Index

About the Contributors

FRANCESCA BRAY is Professor of Anthropology at the University of California at Santa Barbara. Her publications include *The Rice Economies: Technology and Development in Asian Societies* (Blackwell, 1986; reprinted by University of California Press, 1994), and *Technology and Gender: Fabrics of Power in Late Imperial China* (University of California Press, 1997; winner of the Dexter Prize for the History of Technology, 1999). She is currently working on *The Tomato, the Telephone and the Toilet: The Politics of Everyday Technologies in California Today.*

PETER CHUA is Assistant Professor of Sociology at San José State University. He is working on a book titled *Condoms and Transparent Inequalities: Knowledge, Markets, and Social Change.* His research interests involve the interrelations of regional and global inequalities around race-ethnicity, gender, class, and sexuality.

KATHERINE B. DE VOOGD is Research Coordinator in the Division of Genetics and Metabolic Disorders, Department of Pediatrics, University of Texas Health Science Center at San Antonio. She has coauthored recent articles on abnormal Pap and cancer screening among Mexican-American women that have appeared in *Oncology Nursing Forum, JSRI Research Reports* (Michigan State University), and *Cancer Practice.*

BARBARA HERR HARTHORN is Assistant Research Anthropologist and Associate Director of the Institute for Social, Behavioral, and Economic Research (ISBER) and Co-Director of the Center for Global Studies (ISBER) at the University of California, Santa Barbara. Her research examines the social production of health inequality, farmworker and environmental health, immigrants and infectious disease, and gender and health in the Pacific. Her work has appeared in *Human Organization, Social Science and Medicine, Medical Anthropology Quarterly, Journal of Clinical Psychology, Medical Care,* and *Ethos.*

LINDA M. HUNT is Associate Professor in the Department of Anthropology and Julian Samora Research Center at Michigan State University. Her work examines ethnicity, medical ethics, culture of biomedicine, and health care policy, based on studies of Latinos. She is the lead author of recent research articles appearing in *Anthropology in Public Health: Bridging Differences in Culture and Society* (Oxford University Press, 1999), *Narrative and the Cultural Construction of Illness and Healing* (University of California Press, 2000), *Journal of Family Practice,* and *Medical Anthropology Quarterly.*

MARCIA C. INHORN is Associate Professor at the University of Michigan in the Departments of Health Behavior and Health Education (School of Public Health) and Anthropology and the Center for Middle Eastern and North African Studies. Her research has been devoted to infertility and new reproductive technologies in Egypt, and she is the author of three books on the subject: *Quest for Conception: Gender, Infertility, and Egyptian Medical Traditions* (University of Pennsylvania Press, 1994; winner of the Eileen Basker Prize of the Society for Medical Anthropology), *Infertility and Patriarchy: The Cultural Politics of Gender and Family Life in Egypt* (University of Pennsylvania Press, 1996), and *Babies in Global Test-tubes: Gender, Science, and Reproductive Technologies in Islamic Egypt* (Routledge Press, 2003).

JESSICA JEROME completed her Ph.D. in cultural anthropology at the University of Chicago. Her dissertation is titled *A Politics of Health: Medicine and Marginality in Northeastern Brazil* (2002). She is the author of the essay "How International Legal Agreements Speak about Biodiversity" (1998) and is currently researching the history of the Food and Drug Administration in the United States.

JO MURPHY-LAWLESS is an Irish sociologist and Research Associate in the Department of Social Policy at the University College Dublin. She is the author of *Reading Birth and Death: A History of Obstetric Thinking* (Cork University Press and Indiana University Press, 1998) and *Fighting Back: Women and the Impact of Drug Abuse on Families and Communities* (Liffey Press, 2002).

DOROTHY NELKIN is University Professor at New York University, teaching in the Department of Sociology and School of Law. She is the author of numerous books, including *Controversy: Politics of Technical Decisions* (Sage, 1979, 1984), *The DNA Mystique,* with M. Susan Lindee (Freeman, 1995), and *Selling Science* (Freeman, 1987, 1995).

MARK NICHTER is Professor of Anthropology at the University of Arizona and Coordinator of the graduate program in Medical Anthropology. He has conducted long-term fieldwork in South India and the United States, as well as shorter periods of research in the Philippines, Sri Lanka, and Thailand on issues related to the interface between anthropology and international health. The author of numerous articles and book chapters on medical anthropology, he is coeditor with Margaret Lock of *New Horizons in Medical Anthropology* (Routledge 2002), and coauthor with Mimi Nichter of *Anthropology and International Health: Asian Case Studies* (Gordon and Breach 1996).

LAURY OAKS is Associate Professor of Women's Studies and affiliated in the Departments of Anthropology and Sociology at the University of California, Santa Barbara. She is the author of *Smoking and Pregnancy: The Politics of Fetal Protection* (Rutgers University Press, 2001). Her articles on the social and cultural dynamics of reproductive politics in the United States, Ireland, and Japan have appeared in *Signs, Social Science and Medicine, Irish Journal of Feminist Studies,* and *Women's Studies International Forum.*

THERESA (TERRE) A. SATTERFIELD is Assistant Professor in the Faculty of Graduate Studies, Institute for Resources and the Environment and the Sustainable Development Research Institute, at the University of British Columbia. She is also a research scientist with Decision Research. Satterfield's research focuses on cultural interpretations of environmental disputes, risk and justice, and environment values. Her work has been published in *Society and Natural Resources, Land Economics, Risk Analysis, Journal of Anthropological Research, Journal of Social Issues, Human Ecology Review,* and *Ecological Economics.* Her book *The Anatomy of a Conflict: Identity, Knowledge, and Emotion,* on old-growth forests, was published in 2002 (University British Columbia Press), and *What's Nature Worth?* is forthcoming in spring 2003, coauthored with Scott Slovic.